D0805708

The Reflecting Team in Action

THE GUILFORD FAMILY THERAPY SERIES

Michael P. Nichols, *Series Editor*
Alan S. Gurman, *Founding Editor*

Recent Volumes

THE REFLECTING TEAM IN ACTION: COLLABORATIVE PRACTICE IN FAMILY THERAPY
Steven Friedman, Editor

REWRITING FAMILY SCRIPTS: IMPROVISATION AND SYSTEMS CHANGE
John Byng-Hall

INTERNAL FAMILY SYSTEMS THERAPY
Richard C. Schwartz

NORMAL FAMILY PROCESSES, Second Edition
Froma Walsh, Editor

CHANGING THE RULES: A CLIENT-DIRECTED APPROACH TO THERAPY
Barry L. Duncan, Andrew D. Solovey, and Gregory S. Rusk

TRANSGENERATIONAL FAMILY THERAPIES
Laura Giat Roberto

THE INTIMACY PARADOX: PERSONAL AUTHORITY IN THE FAMILY SYSTEM
Donald S. Williamson

HUSBANDS, WIVES, AND LOVERS: THE EMOTIONAL SYSTEM OF THE EXTRAMARITAL AFFAIR
David J. Moultrup

MEN IN THERAPY: THE CHALLENGE OF CHANGE
Richard L. Meth and Robert S. Pasick, with Barry Gordon, Jo Ann Allen, Larry B. Feldman, and Sylvia Gordon

FAMILY SYSTEMS IN MEDICINE
Christian N. Ramsey Jr., Editor

NEGOTIATING PARENT–ADOLESCENT CONFLICT: A BEHAVIORAL–FAMILY SYSTEMS APPROACH
Arthur L. Robin and Sharon L. Foster

The Reflecting Team in Action

COLLABORATIVE PRACTICE IN FAMILY THERAPY

Steven Friedman
EDITOR

Foreword by Lynn Hoffman

THE GUILFORD PRESS
New York London

A Division of Guilford Publications, Inc.
72 Spring Street, New York, NY 10012

Printed in the United States of America

This book is printed on acid-free paper.

Last digit is print number: 9 8 7 6 5 4 3 2 1

Library of Congress Cataloging-in-Publication Data

The reflecting team in action : collaborative practice in family therapy / Steven Friedman, editor ; foreword by Lynn Hoffman.
p. cm. — (Guilford family therapy series)
Includes bibliographical references and index.
ISBN 1-57230-003-5
1. Family psychotherapy. 2. Multiple psychotherapy. 3. Constructivism (Psychology) 4. Solution-focused therapy. 5. Group psychotherapy. I. Friedman, Steven, 1945– II. Series.
RC488.5.R43 1995 95-14307
616.89'156—dc20 CIP

To the individuals and families with whom
I have had the privilege to work . . .
to those with whom I've laughed . . .
to those with whom I've cried . . .
all have taught me so much.

Insight . . . refers to that depth
of understanding that comes by setting
experiences, yours and mine,
familiar and exotic, new and old,
side by side . . . [and] letting them speak
to one another.

—*Mary Catherine Bateson*

Contributors

Jukka Aaltonen, MD, PhD, Department of Psychology, University of Jyväskylä, Finland

Janet Adams-Westcott, PhD, Family and Children's Service, Tulsa, Oklahoma

Birgitta Alakare, MD, Western Lapland Health Care Organization, Tornio, Finland

Tom Andersen, MD, PhD, Section for Social Psychiatry, Institute of Community Medicine, University of Tromsø, Norway

"**Ben**," coresearcher, Diploma in Impurfection

Sally Brecher, MSW, Harvard Community Health Plan, Braintree, Massachusetts

Nollaig O'Reilly Byrne, MB, FRCP(C), Department of Child and Family Psychiatry, Mater Misericordiae Hospital, Dublin, Ireland

Victoria C. Dickerson, PhD, Bay Area Family Therapy Training Associates, Cupertino, California; Mental Research Institute, Palo Alto, California

Margaretha Edwardsson, Department of Child and Adolescent Psychiatry, Msc, Gällivare Hospital, Gällivare, Sweden

David Epston, MA, Family Therapy Centre, Auckland, New Zealand

Jennifer C. Freeman, MA, Graduate School of Professional Psychology, John F. Kennedy University, Orinda, California; private practice, Berkeley, California

Steven Friedman, PhD, Harvard Community Health Plan, Braintree, Massachusetts

James L. Griffith, MD, George Washington University Medical Center, Washington, DC

Melissa Elliott Griffith, MSN, George Washington University Medical Center, Washington, DC

Kauko Haarakangas, MA, Western Lapland Health Care Organization, Tornio, Finland

Deanna Isenbart, MS, Family and Children's Service, Tulsa, Oklahoma

Cheryl Jacques, MSW, The Beal Street Program, South Shore Educational Collaborative, Hingham, Massachusetts

Zeena M. Janowsky, MFCC, private practice, Santa Rosa, California

Jyrki Keränen, PhD, Western Lapland Health Care Organization, Tornio, Finland

Eva Kjellberg, MD, Department of Child and Adolescent Psychiatry, Gällivare Hospital, Gällivare, Sweden

William D. Lax, PhD, Department of Clinical Psychology, Antioch New England Graduate School, Keene, New Hampshire; Brattleboro Family Institute, Brattleboro, Vermont

Dean H. Lobovits, MA, Graduate School of Professional Psychology, John F. Kennedy University, Orinda, California; private practice, Berkeley, California

Stephen Madigan, PhD, Yaletown Family Therapy, Vancouver, British Columbia, Canada

Richard L. Maisel, PhD, California School of Professional Psychology, Alameda, California; Redwood Center Psychology Associates, Berkeley, California

Imelda Colgan McCarthy, PhD, MSocSc, Families and Systemic Therapies Programme, Department of Social Policy and Social Work, University College, Dublin, Ireland

Cynthia Mittelmeier, PhD, Harvard Community Health Plan, Braitree, Massachusetts

Timothy Nichols, MSW, The Beal Street Program, South Shore Educational Collaborative, Hingham, Massachusetts

Birgitta Johansson Niemelä, MSc, Department of Child and Adolescent Psychiatry, Gällivare Hospital, Gällivare, Sweden

Tomas Öberg, MSW, Department of Child and Adolescent Psychiatry, Gällivare Hospital, Gällivare, Sweden

Jaako Seikkula, PsD, Kerapudas Hospital, Tornio, Finland

Matthew D. Selekman, MSW, private practice and consultation services, Chicago, Illinois

Markku Sutela, MA, Western Lapland Health Care Organization, Tornio, Finland

Susan Swim, MA, Houston–Galveston Institute, Houston, Texas

Michael White,BASW, Dulwich Centre, Adelaide, South Australia

Jeffrey L. Zimmerman, PhD, Bay Area Family Therapy Associates, Cupertino, California; Mental Research Institute, Palo Alto, California

Foreword

The appearance of this collection feels to me like a lucky event—one of those times when the rain barrel for new contributions to the field is full to overflowing. Steven Friedman has gathered together a group of chapters describing what he calls *collaborative practice,* which derives from Norwegian psychiatrist Tom Andersen's reflecting team concept, the "collaborative language systems approach" of (the late) Harry Goolishian and Harlene Anderson in Texas, and the narrative approach of Michael White and David Epston in Australia and New Zealand. All these innovators—partly in response to the postmodern movement in the humanities and language arts—have cut loose from the problem-oriented tradition in family therapy and offered us a powerful new direction.

Let me indicate my own entry point on this evolving path. At the time that my book *Foundations of Family Therapy* (1981) was published, I was already becoming uncomfortably aware that the systems analogies used so widely by family therapists were in many ways limiting, if not downright wrong. In the decade that followed, it became clear that the major areas of study in the humanities would have to be rethought. But when my book came out, we family therapists had little inkling of the momentous shift that lay ahead. Postmodernism was a little understood French import, critical theory was a vague kind of Marxism, and hardly anybody had heard of social historian Michel Foucault. Narrative theory was just being taken up by cutting-edge psychoanalysts, and the very different frameworks of social construction theory and constructivism were being thoroughly confused. A few feminist family therapists, who were more literate than the rest of us, were ahead of the game; indeed, they attempted to warn us about what was coming.

When I finally did realize what postmodernism was trying to say, I began trying to catch up, and eventually pulled out what I thought were three particularly useful challenges to accepted ideas. The first is a philosophical challenge to the supremacy of scientific thinking. Ever since the Enlightenment, academic and practice fields in the humanities have sought to emulate the glorious successes of the natural sciences. Persuasive voices are now arguing that these fields cannot be understood using a language of what social constructionist Kenneth Gergen (1985) calls essentialism—a belief in the core essences of an outside reality. Where "modern" has come to be used as a term for a positivist, hard-facts outlook, "postmodern" is said to be social and interpretative. Critics of postmodernism complain of a dangerous ethical relativism, but defenders say that they are only substituting values for truth.

A second idea that the postmodern movement has challenged is the pervasive concern of social thinkers with internal systems of symbols or rules. When you look at the panorama of 20th-century social thought, you will easily see that all the major contenders in linguistics, literary criticism, sociology, anthropology, and psychology subscribe to a belief in structures thought to be tucked away within any human product or event. These structures have now been pulled out and branded as fairy tales. In fact, an entire "ism" was invented for this particular demolition derby: poststructuralism (Berman, 1988). According to this view, there is no set of symbols within (say) a novel or play that the accomplished critic can discern, any more than there is a dysfunctional structure within (say) a family that the skillful clinician can find.

The third challenge to accepted thinking is a new concept of social activism. This view has bypassed the old framework of a Marxist class struggle and focuses on a political critique at the level of social discourse. This stance derives from several sources. First is a German school of thought called critical theory, which advocates a type of emancipatory conversation that the social philosopher Juergen Habermas (Poster, 1989) has termed "ideal speech." Another source is the ancient field of hermeneutics, expanded from its original role of biblical exegesis to a more general art of interpretation. Finally, there is the radical work of Michel Foucault (Rabinow, 1984) who, in critiquing the invasive bureaucracies of the modern state, has given activists a powerful tool for resisting what has been called "the micro-fascism of everyday life."

These ideas supported my search for what I was calling a different voice, a term I had borrowed from the writings of psychologist Carol Gilligan. In her book *In a Different Voice* (1982), Gilligan had questioned the work done by Harvard researcher Lawrence Kohlberg on the stages of moral reasoning, because it was based on protocols only given to men. Her own research, using some of the same protocols and given to both men and women, suggested that women would bend the rules to protect relationships where men's choices were based on abstract principles of right and wrong. In offering the possibility of gendered value systems, Gilligan seemed to give me an answer to my dilemma. I began to see how I could opt out of the so-called masculine position, with its true–false imperatives, and find a style for therapy based on connection and partnership that would appeal not only to women but to like-minded men.

I had also written and talked about the wall of unfortunate inequities the profession of psychotherapy had built between therapists and their customers. Professional secrecy was one part of this wall, as was the barrier of technical training and what I called college words—the use of clinical in-language. I felt that Foucault was right in describing modern surveillance bureaucracies—the schools, the court system, hospitals—as a way vested interests enforce their power invisibly. But I still was hazy as to how one would dislodge this injustice. I didn't want just to criticize the institutions of family therapy but to find and put in place a set of practices that would of themselves create a change.

It was around this time that the Norwegian psychiatrist Tom Andersen electrified the field with a beautiful and dramatic format he called a reflecting team (1991). This method asked a team to share comments on the conversation between the therapist and family while the family watched and listened. The family would then comment on the team's ideas in turn. This innovation proved to be a great leveler, modifying the forbidding concealment that the use of the one-way screen had so long imposed. I also noticed that it changed the language of the professionals, which became simpler, more personal, and more appreciative. Feeling that this idea was heaven-sent in my search for ways to put a different voice into practice, I immediately adopted (more correctly, adapted) it.

Another helpful person during this stage of the journey was the late Harry Goolishian, an endlessly humane psychologist and family therapy pioneer who lived and worked in Galveston and Houston, Texas. Harry and his colleague, Harlene Anderson (Anderson & Goolishian, 1988), brought a stunning piece of learning into the family therapy field: the idea that the therapist should come from what they called a position of not knowing. This involved a method of talking with people that was so unprepossessing it shocked me. On the surface it seemed like an ordinary conversation, and indeed "conversation" was their description of what they did. I was particularly impressed by the fact that in their address and attitude I never felt that the "real" conversation they were holding was with colleagues, supervisors, or observers rather than with the people they were seeing. The philosophy behind their stance was tied in with hermeneutics and involved a definition of therapy as collaborative and based on postmodern linguistic theory.

A third break with systems concepts and the modernist methods of therapy that derived from them came with the extraordinary innovations of Michael White and David Epston in Australia and New Zealand. White and Epston's book *Narrative Means to Therapeutic Ends* broke upon the shores of family therapy in 1990, and the field has not been the same since. I think the immediate popularity of their approach rested in part on its use of the narrative metaphor, which fitted in with social constructionist ideas, and in part on its Foucauldian use of a liberation analogy for therapy. Seeing human predicaments in terms of "stories" held out hope for the possibility of transcending them, and seeing them as "stories of freedom" placed the practitioner and customer side by side.

All the approaches in this evolving postmodern tradition have dramatized a core shift from the unit-based thinking of older individual and family therapies. Instead of singling out an entity—the self or the system—the new practitioners treat the border between the two as if it were itself an entity—a loom, perhaps, on which rich tapestries are constantly being woven. There is a move here toward dealing with the concept of identity, which is always embedded in a social web. I would therefore call the work of therapists in this camp identity work. This is why they place such a huge emphasis on trying to construct a community that can positively influence its members' ideas about each other.

It is striking to note the degree to which all these innovators are defecting from the problem orientation that classic systems therapists are wed to, as well as from the language of change. Goolishian and Anderson are not interested in the problem as something to be fixed, but speak of it as "dissolving" in the context of a therapeutic conversation. Tom Andersen's reflecting team replaces interventions with poetic and affirming associations to the situation that comes in the door. White and Epston elicit what they call the problem-saturated story only to sideline it in favor of constructing a more optimistic one. All of these pioneers insist on holding up "a picture of the good," even if they have to create it themselves. Are they even therapists?

My answer is not in the old sense. I think they try to influence a novel area which I call the *community of perception*. This community is not the same as the bodies we think of as neighborhoods or towns, but consists of the shifting, face-to-face group of persons each of us travels in, like a school of fish, which maintains and shapes who we think we are. The conventional polarity between person and environment has dropped away, and we are now concerned with the type of communicational event that social psychologist John Shotter compares to a Ouija board (1993). There is no goal and no use in planning for one. Neither is there a leader. The outcome of the game is determined by the joint action of everybody's hands as they push the counter around the board.

One result of this shift is the appearance of a new kind of professional relationship, which psychiatrist Jeffrey Fortuna (1995), of the Windhorse Associates in Northampton, Mass., calls a therapeutic friendship. This ship allows far more parity between parties than does the traditional model. It includes a commitment to what White and Epston call transparency and I call forthcomingness. Ideas about process and the secrets of the craft are shared, as are many of the personal sides of life. Therapists will do humble, sociable things with and for their clients, like baking celebration cakes, going shopping together, or having cups of tea. Gestures of comfort or concern frowned upon by traditional approaches are also included. The sacred icon of the professional boundary is directly questioned by this ideal.

Let me end by mentioning one difference between White and Epston's work and that of the two other groups. The narrative approach is strongly therapist driven; in fact, it has an activist social frame. The universe of Tom Andersen, Harlene Anderson, and Harry Goolishian is far less intentional. It is characterized by a kind of purposeful planlessness (if there is such a thing), and this is where I place my "different voice" style too. Due to this divergence in philosophies of practice, the work of the latter group has a totally different feel to it from that of the narrative group.

Differences aside, I don't think anybody has yet considered what a radical departure this shift—from a focus on the unit to a focus on the exchange—represents. Shotter, in another effort to define the indefinable, has given us the phrase "knowing of the third kind." He means by this a knowing that is directed toward neither the internal world nor the outer one but is concerned with the space between the give and take of our most ordinary life. In this space, Shotter says, practical, political, and moral concerns are always present.

My colleague Mary Olson, also a writer, has said that one problem with social construction theory is that it has no theory of suffering. This may be why social activists complain about it, and why they complain about systems theories as well. The reason this collaborative practice seems so right to me is because I believe it allows us to acknowledge pain and still believe in transcendence, which is what the belief in a jointly created reality is all about. This is also why I feel this particular collection is so precious. Read it with care.

Lynn Hoffman
Brattleboro Family Institute, Vermont

REFERENCES

Andersen, T. (Ed.). (1991). *The reflecting team: Dialogues and dialogues about the dialogues.* New York: Norton.

Anderson, H., & Goolishian, H. (1988). Human systems as linguistic systems. *Family Process, 27,* 371–394.

Berman, A. (1988). *From the new criticism to deconstruction.* Urbana: University of Illinois Press.

Gergen, K. (1985). The social constructist movement in social psychology. *American Psychologist, 40,* 266–275.

Gilligan, C. (1982). *In a different voice.* Cambridge, MA: Harvard University Press.

Fortuna, J. (1995). The Windhorse program for recovery. In R. Warner (Ed.), *Alternatives to the hospital for acute psychiatric treatment.* Washington, DC: American Psychiatric Press.

Messer, S. B. (1988). *Hermeneutics and psychological theory.* Highland Park, NJ: Rutgers University Press.

Poster, M. (1989). *Critical theory and poststructuralism.* Ithaca, NY: Cornell University Press.

Rabinow, P. (1984). *The Foucault reader.* New York: Pantheon.

Shotter, J. (1993). *The cultural politics of everyday life.* Toronto: University of Toronto Press.

White, M., & Epston, D. (1990). *Narrative means to therapeutic ends.* New York: Norton.

✷

Acknowledgments

I wish to express special appreciation to the members of my family therapy team at the Braintree Center of Harvard Community Health Plan: Sally Brecher, Cynthia Mittelmeier, Ethan Kisch, and Madeline Dymsza. Working closely with this group of talented clinicians over several years has allowed me to take risks and grow both personally and professionally. Naami Seidman Turk, who joined the team as a postdoctoral fellow, made an exceptional contribution. Her intelligence and creativity served as a catalyst, broadening and enriching my clinical work. My colleagues in the mental health department at the Braintree Center of HCHP: Vicki Beggs, Rose Catalanotti, Stan Cole, Lauren Corbett, Ellen Frishman, Dan Gadish, Marge Lavin, Ted Powers, Jim Ritchie, Rob Schneider, and Ronnie Tilles, with whom I have worked over the past 10 years, have provided a context of stability, support, friendship and good humor in the sometimes turbulent world of managed health care. In addition, I want to acknowledge Margot Taylor Fanger, whose ideas have greatly influenced my own; Simon Budman, who has been a supportive colleague and teacher; and Michael Hoyt, who has been a consultant, advisor, and friend. I am also grateful to Harvey P. Katz, MD, Center Director at Harvard Community Health Plan in Braintree, for his support of this project.

I would like to give special thanks to the authors, whose dedication to their work is reflected in the outstanding quality of their contributions. I am also indebted to Seymour Weingarten, Editor-in-Chief at The Guilford Press, who encouraged me to pursue this book, and Anna Brackett and the production staff at Guilford, who put this volume together with great care. Finally, my deepest appreciation to my wife, Donna, who has been there for me over many years as consultant, friend, and general good listener and whose love provided the foundation that made this project possible.

Contents

II. The Reflecting Team: Hosting Collaborative Conversations

III. The Community as Audience: Reauthoring Stories

*

Opening Reflections

Steven Friedman

The field cannot well be seen from within the field.
—*Ralph Waldo Emerson*

I WAS THINKING back to 1978, when I was leading a training group at a child guidance clinic in Massachusetts. We were seeing a family on an alternate-week basis with the trainees observing from behind a one-way mirror. Two of my colleagues were serving as therapists and I was behind the mirror with this group of five or six trainees. One day the family came in reporting that there had been improvement in the child's behavior and that "things are better at home." We were all delighted with the changes. After speaking briefly with the two therapists who were meeting with the family, I suggested to the training group that we trade places with the family and allow them to overhear our observations and thoughts about the changes they had made over the few months we were involved with them. We spent about 10 to 15 minutes in conversation and then invited the family to return and comment on what they had heard. Family members seemed especially pleased with this opportunity to hear our thoughts and feel supported and encouraged in their successful efforts at home.

Many years passed and the experience was long forgotten when I read Tom Andersen's (1987) article on the use of the reflecting team and realized the powerful contribution that an audience can make to the therapeutic process as a medium for authenticating change, seeding ideas, and generating options. Over the past several years, my colleagues and I have been experimenting with the reflecting team format in our work in a managed health care setting. We have found the reflecting process to be time-effective in opening the client system to change.

Since Andersen's milestone article in 1987, the use of the reflecting team, and more recently a focus on the reflecting process itself, has dramatically altered the landscape of family therapy. In fact, these new ideas represent both the further evolution and, in some ways, dissolution of family therapy as we've known it. With conversational and narrative approaches, language and meaning, rather than the number of people in the room, become prominent and privileged. Refractions of meaning inherent in the conversational process emerge as opportunities to create new understandings and options for change.

The current interest in the use of teams and audiences seems linked to the earlier days of family therapy when emphasis was placed on the incorporation of extended family networks into the therapy process (e.g., Speck & Attneave, 1973). Multiple Impact Therapy (MacGregor et al., 1964), in which teams of therapists would join together for intensive interventions with families, or the multiple family group format developed by Laqueur (1976) are examples of other ways that historically therapists have "allow[ed] the outside world . . . to enter into the therapeutic relationship" (Laqueur, 1976, p. 409). In many ways the family therapy field is returning to its roots as a community endeavor. The idea of incorporating audiences or witnesses in the consultation process is a primary focus for this volume. The authors presenting their work here all utilize some form of audience as a means to open up the therapeutic conversation to new ideas.

The practice of psychotherapy in many ways mirrors the cultural milieu. The enormously popular self-help movement has offered people a public forum for dealing with individual problems. The Internet, or electronic superhighway, has created a "virtual" community, linking enormous numbers of people all over the world. One client told me that, during a recent difficult period in her life, she communicated about her sadness on the Internet and received hundreds of electronic letters of support and encouragement! Certainly in the United States the television talk show format has also made personal problems a public process.[1] Millions of people tune in every day to these talk shows that engage the audience both at home and in the TV studio in a dialogue about people's lives and relationships. In fact, Oprah Winfrey, one of most popular TV talk show hosts, just received a special career achievement award from the American Association of Marital and Family Therapy for educating the public about couple and family issues. Although we can see these kinds of programs as a purely voyeuristic pursuit, they do provide viewers with an opportunity to voice their point of view on the complexities and vagaries of people's lives. Communities of dialogue are created that offer a variety of views on a

[1] I thank Ben Furman for this idea. I find it interesting that this observation was made by someone living *outside* the United States.

multitude of personal and interpersonal situations. In the current volume, the contributors are also interested in how we can access community knowledges such that resources—professional and personal—can be brought forth to offer people options and choices on life's dilemmas.

This is a book about conversations between therapists and clients, conversations that make room for new ideas and new perspectives. Lest the reader be surprised, the contributors, while experts in the domain of conversation and language, are not especially deferential to the ideas of traditional psychotherapy. In fact, many of the ideas presented here are so discordant with traditional views about the therapy process that they represent a major "paradigm shift" in the field. The authors of the chapters to follow are not interested in the kind of conversations that assess and fix "problems"; they are not interested in psychodiagnostic labels and, in fact, find such labels pejorative and diminishing; they do not focus on the past unless these discussions can lead to change in the present, nor do they privilege one explanation over another.

The material presented in this book embraces a social constructionist view, that is, a belief that the conversational process with its meaning-generating potential provides the medium that creates our personal realities (Anderson & Goolishian, 1988). Problems are understood less as tangible structures and more as self-constructions or stories that have developed meaning over time in a person's life. Therapy becomes a forum for the reauthoring of stories and for the co-construction of new chapters that build on client strengths and successes. The narrative approach, pioneered in the groundbreaking work of Michael White and David Epston (1990), views the role of the therapist as bringing new stories of hope, resilience, and strength into the community ("going public") such that the newly defined narratives become embedded and extended into the social networks of which they are a part.

The chapters in this book continue in a tradition of moving away from hierarchical models and toward more collaborative, language-based approaches (e.g., Friedman, 1993; McNamee & Gergen, 1992). In the current volume, the contributors provide the reader with an opportunity to better understand the applicability of collaborative approaches to the domain of psychotherapy in all its complexities. New ideas and practices in family therapy are now emerging from all over the world, broadening and deepening both thinking and practice in the field. Representative of these trends, the contributors to this work come from eight different countries, bringing together a multiplicity of cultural perspectives, political ideas, and world views. The work represented here reflects a revision of the process of psychotherapy, one that privileges the dialogical process and provides opportunities, in our language-bound world, for new hope-generating narratives.

THE CHAPTERS TO FOLLOW

This book is divided into three sections. In the first section, the authors describe how to creatively structure the therapeutic conversation in ways that open space for multiple points of view and collaborative problem resolution. Featuring a diverse array of clinical and cultural contexts, the ideas and methods presented offer the reader a set of maps for generating respectful conversations that acknowledge and validate the voices of all participants, including people who have traditionally been "marginalized" or pathologized in society. Therapy becomes a dialogical process, a public and participatory forum allowing ideas to flow in recursive fashion. By allowing all voices to be heard, solutions emerge that affirm and respect the dignity of everyone involved.

Andersen (Chapter 1) takes the reader on a personal and historic journey, tracking the emergence and evolution of the reflecting processes. Believing that people are constantly in formation, he views the client as a coresearcher in a collaborative journey toward new possibilities. Andersen, in addition to outlining his clinical assumptions (or "prejudices"), details several valuable ways to apply the reflecting process in a variety of contexts. Kjellberg and her colleagues in Sweden (Chapter 2) describe the major shifts and dilemmas, as well as their own sense of liberation, in moving from a hierarchical, expert-dominated model to a more egalitarian, inclusive approach. Serving a rural community in which violence and child abuse are prevalent, the authors bring together the social service agencies and families in ways that allow all parties to be heard and treatment planning to be a more collaborative process. Seikkula and his colleagues in Finland (Chapter 3), working with people affected by "psychotic" behavior, describe the development and organization of a new, more open system of treatment that privileges dialogue and discussion over therapist-imposed treatment planning. Family members and hospital staff come together to create a "multivoiced discourse" leading to a reduction in psychotic episodes.

Griffith and Griffith (Chapter 4) share an impressive example of how the reflecting position serves to "rebalance power relationships" among professionals and patients in a medical setting and shifts the patient's "emotional posture" in ways that foster openness and reflectivity. Swim (Chapter 5), drawing on the innovative thinking of Harlene Anderson and the late Harry Goolishian, describes a novel application of the reflecting process to break down barriers and walls in a school context. Allowing the voices of all participants to be heard, including the students (who had histories of being labeled "emotionally disturbed"), creates a shift in which narratives of pessimism and pathology are transformed into narratives of hope and possibility. McCarthy and Byrne

(Chapter 6) show the usefulness of juxtaposing stories in helping people free themselves from constraining narratives. Drawing on the Irish heritage of story and myth, they weave together the dilemmas and process of the therapeutic team with the clinical material in ways that offer the reader a unique and valuable immersion in social constructionism. Their innovative team approach helps to "dis-spel" old myths that were holding the clients and themselves hostage to fear and isolation.

In the second section, the authors offer practical guidelines for incorporating the reflecting-team format in a variety of clinical situations. Drawing on both the narrative metaphor and solution-focused thinking, these authors suggest a wealth of concrete ideas and useful clinical examples on how to effectively organize the reflecting-team process. Ideas generated from team members and others invited into the clinical field support, intrigue, and activate the client/family in ways that facilitate change.

Lax (Chapter 7), drawing on ideas from hermeneutics and social constructionism, proposes a set of guidelines for reflections and places these "rules" in a context that values therapist transparency and the benefits of "misunderstanding" in therapeutic conversation. Janowsky, Dickerson, and Zimmerman (Chapter 8) creatively integrate the reflecting process within a narrative frame. Using a clinical example in which the client offers her own views on the therapy, these authors demonstrate the importance of soliciting client feedback on the therapeutic process. Friedman, Brecher, and Mittelmeier (Chapter 9) view the reflecting team as a "springboard for new ideas and options for action." The authors present several clinical vignettes from their work in a managed health care setting, illustrating the advantages of using teams in consultation with couples and families. Selekman (Chapter 10) describes the benefits of recruiting adolescents as peer consultants to the family in the therapy session. Using a solution-oriented framework, the author describes a number of ways to apply this innovative method in opening the family system to new ideas.

In the final section, the authors, using a variety of novel methods, extend the practice of therapy into the larger community. Audiences are recruited to promote the construction and circulation of preferred stories, liberating people from the constraints imposed by totalizing descriptions or the dominant influence of cultural ideologies. By separating the person from the problem, opportunities exist for people to construct and author revised narratives that lead to alternative perspectives and new possibilities. As people's struggles and successes are circulated in a community of caring—networks are created that embed these changes in contexts of hope and connection.

Lobovits, Maisel, and Freeman (Chapter 11) elegantly integrate theory and practice in presenting innovative ways for circulating preferred knowledges through the use of audiences. Special attention is also given to important ethical issues in therapy. Madigan and Epston (Chapter 12) further develop the idea of recruiting audiences for change in their discussion of Anti-Anorexia/Anti-Bulimia League. These "leagues" serve as resource banks or archives of preferred knowledges that can be circulated among participating "members." The authors demonstrate, with clinical examples, the effectiveness of these networks in freeing people from problem-saturated views of self. Epston, White, and a client coresearcher, "Ben" (Chapter 13), elaborate on ideas originally published in the *Dulwich Centre Newsletter*, suggesting that people can be consultants to themselves and others "in relation to solution knowledges that have enabled them to free their lives" from problems. Via a particularly humorous and engaging clinical interview, the therapist and client act as coresearchers, identifying and documenting alternative knowledges and circulating client ideas and achievements in ways that offer hope to others.

Nichols and Jacques (Chapter 14) creatively apply the narrative framework in a residential treatment center for adolescents. Recruiting members of the adolescent's community, a ritual of celebration ("rite of passage") is organized marking and authenticating the adolescent's accomplishments and progress. Adams-Westcott and Isenbart (Chapter 15) illustrate the usefulness of involving audiences of reflection in working with adults who were sexually abused as children. Using a group therapy format, and viewing the therapy process as a "journey," the authors offer examples of how an audience can effectively open space for new ideas and help authenticate an individual's evolving story. Finally, I offer some "closing reflections" that pull together the major threads that define the tapestry of ideas presented in the book.

★ ★ ★

A few years ago, having some free time while at a conference in Phoenix, Arizona, I decided to visit Taliesin West, a beautiful house set in the desert, designed by the architect Frank Lloyd Wright. Wright spent many winters here with his family and apprentices. This magnificent house seems to grow right out of the desert itself. Wright's work breaks free of the fixed rectangular world and opens space for light and imagination. Wright saw the design of a building as a personal process that required significant attention both to the site where the house would be located and to the inhabitants or local culture that would be using the space. In Wright's work, a house is "co-constructed" with the local landscape. The space indoors converges with the outside environment to create an integrated whole. The house takes on an organic fluidity matching the opportunities that adhere to its design.

The therapy process, from a social constructionist perspective, is very similar. The clinician and his/her team match the local culture by becoming immersed in the client's language and perceptions and collaboratively design ways to free the client from constraints and offer opportunities for choice and change. By so doing, the constraining or restraining structures (the walls) are shifted to make space for the generation of light as reflected in new meanings, understandings, and options for action. As Lynn Hoffman (1993) has said, "most of therapy consists of removing obstacles—the walls—and pointing out the hopeful factors—the windows. People will often find the doors on their own" (p. 155). My hope is that the material in this book will help open windows to new perspectives, allowing you to more easily find the doors on your own.

ACKNOWLEDGMENT

Thanks to Donna Haig Friedman, PhD, Naami Seidman Turk, PsyD, and Sally Brecher, MSW, for their thoughtful editorial assistance.

REFERENCES

Andersen, T. (1987). The reflecting team: Dialogue and meta-dialogue in clinical work. *Family Process, 26*, 415–428.

Anderson, H., & Goolishian, H. A. (1988). Human systems as linguistic systems: Preliminary and evolving ideas about the implications for clinical theory. *Family Process, 27*, 371–393.

Friedman, S. (Ed.). (1993). *The new language of change: Constructive collaboration in psychotherapy*. New York: Guilford Press.

Hoffman, L. (1993). *Exchanging voices: A collaborative approach to family therapy*. London: Karnac Books.

Laqueur, H. P. (1976). Multiple family therapy. In P. Guerin (Ed.), *Family therapy: Theory and practice* (pp. 405–416). New York: Gardner Press.

MacGregor, R., Ritchie, A. M., Serrano, A. C., Schuster, F. P., MacDanal, E. L., & Goolishian, H. A. (1964). *Multiple Impact Therapy with families*. New York: McGraw-Hill.

McNamee, S., & Gergen, K. J. (1992). *Therapy as social construction*. Newbury Park, CA: Sage.

Speck, R. V., & Attneave, C. L. (1973). *Family networks*. New York: Vintage.

White, M., & Epston, D. (1990). *Narrative means to therapeutic ends*. New York: Norton.

PART I

✵

THE REFLECTING PROCESS
Opening Dialogues

Uttering a word is like striking a note on the keyboard of the imagination.

—*Ludwig Wittgenstein*

The ethical imperative: Act always to increase the number of choices.

—*Heinz von Foerster*

Adaptation comes out of encounters with novelty that may seem chaotic. In trying to adapt, we may need to [behave] in ways we have barely glimpsed, seizing on fragmentary clues.

—*Mary Catherine Bateson*

CHAPTER 1

Reflecting Processes; Acts of Informing and Forming

YOU CAN BORROW MY EYES, BUT YOU MUST NOT TAKE THEM AWAY FROM ME!

Tom Andersen

> Concerning the psychology of the creative act itself, I have mentioned the following, interrelated aspects of it: the displacement of attention to something not previously noted, which was irrelevant in the old and is relevant in the new context; the discovery of hidden analogies as a result of the former; the bringing into consciousness of tacit axioms and habits of thought which were implied in the code and taken for granted; the uncovering of what has always been there.
>
> This leads to the paradox that the more original a discovery the more obvious it seems afterwards. The creative act is not an act of creation in the sense of the Old Testament. It does not create something out of nothing: it uncovers, selects, re-shuffles, combines, synthesizes already existing facts, ideas, faculties, skills. The more familiar the parts, the more striking the new whole.
>
> —*Arthur Koestler (1964, pp. 119–120)*

MY WAY OF TELLING about the origin and development of the reflecting processes has shifted over the years. At first I often referred to theories, as if these processes were born out of intellectuality. Now I do not think so. I think they rather were consequences of feelings. Although I was unaware of it when the reflecting process first appeared in March 1985, I now think it was a solution to my own feeling of discomfort as a therapist. Being a therapist is first of all being with others, and it is hard to be with others when they and I feel uncomfortable about that being together.

The rather personal start of this chapter might indicate its limited value for those who prefer objective descriptions. However, those who are attracted to the hermeneutic tradition and its assumptions about knowledge as context-bounded, time-bounded, and person-bounded will, I hope, find it of less limited value. I will first write a few words about the hermeneutic circle.

THE HERMENEUTIC CIRCLE

This concept has been discussed by two German philosophers, Martin Heidegger and Hans-Georg Gadamer (Wachthauser, 1986; Warnke, 1987). They said that what we come to understand is much determined by the life we already have lived. The life we already have lived has brought to us general assumptions of various kinds, that is, how human beings best can be understood.

Gadamer says that we are inevitably prejudiced when we meet with a person we are to understand; we have started to understand the person even before we meet him/her. Gadamer used the word "prejudice" and Heidegger used the word "preunderstanding" for this. Some people assume (have brought with them the preunderstanding) that what a person says and does is generated from an "inner core" of the person. Those who meet another with that preunderstanding will look for the signs in the other's behavior that reflect and indicate the dynamics of the assumed inner core.

An alternative preunderstanding to that of an inner core is that the center of a person is outside the person—in the conversations and the language the person takes part in. The other person will be best understood by concentrating on his/her conversations and language.

These are only two examples of several existing preunderstandings of human beings. When we try to understand another person (within the frames of our preunderstanding) we might see or hear something we have never seen and heard before. This new information might turn back upon and nuance or even change our preunderstanding. The preunderstanding's influence on the actual understanding and the actual understanding's turning back upon and influencing the preunderstanding have been called the hermeneutic circle.

Other Prejudices

The concept of preunderstanding applies not only to human beings but to all phenomena we are to understand (make meanings of), including the reflecting processes, the writing about reflecting processes, or the reader's reading about the reflecting processes.

My preunderstanding is that the reflecting processes are very different from my writings about them. These processes comprise much more than I am ever able to see or hear. The writing is therefore a simplified version and relates to what I (according to my prejudices) found useful to look at and listen to. What I heard and saw, when put into writing, is described in my metaphors and my language, and I can never take it for granted that the words of my writing create the same images and thoughts in the readers as they do in me.

What I will try to do in this chapter is to be in a language that is as close as possible to the everyday language of "ordinary" people. My prejudice is that readers will interpret within the frames of their prejudices, and such a chapter as this might offer a chance for readers to reflect upon their own work and their own preunderstandings.

A Nuance

The "aim" of this chapter is not only to describe the reflecting processes but also to describe the contexts in which they emerged and developed further. Because parts of those contexts are my own preunderstandings, I give space to elucidating how being part of various reflecting processes turned back upon, nuanced, and changed my prejudices and my being-in-the-world as therapist. The reflecting processes can be seen as hermeneutic circles.

NOTICING THE FEELINGS OF DISCOMFORT

This section discusses body and feelings and might be out of context for some. If it feels so, please leap to the preludes of the reflecting processes on page 16.

As a medical country doctor in the north of Norway, I learned about ordinary life and ordinary bodily complaints. Aches and pains and stiffness in the various parts of the body (neck, shoulders, lower back, etc.) were the most common complaints in general practice but "too ordinary" to be of interest in academia. The medical school I came from did not prepare us as doctors for how to deal with it, so we were left to our own wonderings. I was fortunate to meet with a Norwegian female physiotherapist, Gudrun Øvreberg, who introduced me to her teacher, Aadel Bülow-Hansen, another Norwegian female physiotherapist. They both let me see into a world I had not looked into before. Bülow-Hansen's work over the years taught her that breathing and movements are two crucial sides of life; our breathing influences our movements and our movements influence our breathing. There are two words in Norwegian for breathing: one the more physiological word, to breathe ("å puste"), and the other a more solemn, maybe even a sacred word, to spirit ("å ånde"). When a person passes away, Norwegians most often say he/she spirited out. We also say that we spirit the air when we are up in the freshness of the mountains or in places similar to that. Being-in-the-world is being-in-breathing. All our expressions and all our spoken words come with the exhaling phase of breathing; our laughing lets go of our happy feelings; our weeping elicits sad feelings; our barking voices convey angry feelings, and so on. And all the thoughts and feelings are brought to the fore during the exhaling part of breathing.

Our movements, sometimes nuanced and fine, sometimes rough and coarse, are part of the interplay between those muscles that stretch various parts of the body (e.g., the knee) and those that bend the parts. The stretchers in front of the knee and benders on the back side are opponents. When they both work, their work in common will balance the knee. We need them all, both stretchers and benders, to balance the various parts of the body when we walk, sit, get up, turn around, and so on.

Bülow-Hansen noticed that in difficult periods (e.g., when we are worried, angry, or sad and do *not* want to let others see), a person is brought out of balance in the sense that the benders increases their activity and the stretchers are constrained (by the benders) in their activity. The person as a whole tends to "creep together" and the body tends to be "closed." Readers have most probably seen those who cross their arms over the chest and lean forward, in an act of "closing" the body. In this closing act, the benders in front of the shoulders and upper arms, those in the back of the neck, those in the stomach, and those on the front of the hip take part.

Bülow-Hansen noticed that simultaneously with the stretchers being constrained the breathing was also constrained. She learned that if she was able to help a person stretch and open up the body something interesting happened. A spontaneous inhaling occurs when the body stretches, and with that inhaling there is a certain urge to continue the stretching, which stimulates more inhaling. This circle goes on until the chest is filled, and when the air passively leaves the lungs, some of the tension in all muscles (also in the benders) vanishes.

In this process of stretching and breathing and letting go of tension, the muscular balance of the body as a whole is changed. One can sometimes actually see the posture of the person changing.

Watching this work closely in order to write a book about it contributed to a certain knowledge "creeping under" my skin. While writing the book, between 1983 and 1986, I slowly began to understand that *how* Bülow-Hansen worked determined *what* she could reach. And *how* she worked was *in relation to the other.*

One of the ways for her to make the other person stretch a part of the body was to let one of her hands clench a tense muscle (e.g., the calf muscle) so that the clench produced pain. Pain is followed by a spontaneous stretch (of the knee), which is followed by inhaling. When her hand was too soft she could not see any response in the other's breathing. If her hand got a bit rougher, making more pain, she could *see* increased inhaling followed by a release of air during the exhaling part. If, however, her hand was too rough, causing too much pain or clenching too long, the other would inhale in a gasping manner and thereafter not let the air go but hold on it. Bülow-Hansen followed the process intensively by watching the other's breathing all the time. If her eyes saw that there was no increase of breathing, her hand worked harder, and if she saw that the breathing stopped because her hand was too rough, she let that clenching hand go immediately.

This taught me at least two things. First, it made Gregory Bateson's ideas about change visible. Bateson saw change as a difference that occurred over time. He also thought that a difference does not come by itself but with another difference; for example, if the temperature falls, one puts on one's jacket. In a few words, Bateson (1972) made the famous statement: "A difference makes a difference" (p. 453). Bateson's statement and Bülow-Hansen's work taught me that there are three differences of which only one makes a difference. What is too usual does not make a difference. What is too unusual also does not make a difference. What is appropriately unusual makes a difference. These nuances are widely applicable in many situations and under many circumstances, including conversations.

The other thing I learned from Bülow-Hansen was that she looked (and I assume she also heard and maybe even smelled) how the other responded to her hands *before* her hands continued to work. Applied to psychotherapy, it means that I have to wait and see how the other responds to what I say or do before I say or do the next thing. The next thing I say or do must be influenced by the other's response to what I just said. I have to go slowly enough to be able to see and hear how it is for the other to be in the conversation. If it is too unusual, the other feels uncomfortable and lets me know through one or many signs. There are many signs and I shall just briefly mention some examples that will remind readers of what they already know: talking less, looking down or away, conveying the feeling that it would be better to leave the conversation than to stay in it, and so on. We can *see* the other feeling uncomfortable.

We can also notice our own feelings of discomfort in moments when we push the other(s) into something too unusual for them. If we are aware, our bodies will tell us. For me this feeling appears behind the lower part of my breastbone. Some say they feel it in the stomach, some behind the eyes, some in the forehead, some in the lower back, and so forth.

TWO PRELUDES

The idea of being appropriately unusual to the others brought a more calm atmosphere to the therapeutic conversations in which I took part. That idea was one of two preludes to the first reflecting team in March 1985, and I believe it influenced the next prelude, namely a new way of giving interventions.

Our team initially worked using the Milan approach; in 1984, however, a shift occurred in the way we intervened with the families. We started to say, "In addition to what you saw, we saw this," and "In addition to what you tried to do you might try this [what we suggested]."

This was to underline that both what the families and what we had considered were of value. Previously we had a clear tendency to try find *the* correct interventions, and if the families disagreed with our interventions a dispute easily broke out: Either they or we were right. This shift from an earlier either–or stance to the new both–and stance made everything more "democratic."

In hindsight it seems that these two preludes were significant preparation to let the idea of open talks (reflecting) happen. The idea about such open talks had emerged already in 1981, and I mentioned it to Aina Skorpen, with whom I worked at that time. However, our fears that we might talk in a hurtful way about the families in front of them restrained us from trying. When we finally began to use this mode we were surprised at how easy it was to talk without using nasty or hurtful words. Later it became evident that how we talk depends on the context in which we talk. If we choose to speak about the families without them present, we easily speak "professionally," in a detached manner. If we choose to speak about them in their presence, we naturally use everyday language and speak in a friendly manner.

REFLECTING TEAM

The idea of open talk lay dormant for four years before we began to use it in March 1985 (the team members were Magnus Hald, Eivind Eckhoff, Trygve Nissen, and myself). The young therapist talked with a mother, father, and daughter about their sad family life. The mother, who had difficulties seeing a positive future, had been to the mental hospital several times (sometimes because she had tried to kill herself). The therapist was drawn into their hopelessness and could not find questions to elucidate an alternative future. The team members, who followed the talk from behind a one-way screen, called the therapist to our room and gave him our optimistic questions. He brought them back to the family, only to be drawn back to pessimism immediately.

We tried the same tactic three times, with the same pessimistic consequences. Then, after a short discussion behind the screen, we launched the idea to the family and the therapist that we might talk while they listened to us. Our fears made us hope they would not accept the offer, but they did.

In those rooms in which we worked there happened to be loudspeakers and microphones. Therefore, we turned on the light in our room and they dimmed it in their room. We turned on the microphone in our room and they turned off theirs; we turned off our loudspeakers and they turned on theirs. And there we sat in the lit room: visible and unprotected. (We finally realized how the families with whom we previously met might have experienced these arrangements: frightening and exciting at the same time.)

At first we stumbled over our words; we wondered whether there were possibilities that the family, for various reasons, had not yet seen? Our speculations became more and more lively as we envisioned an optimistic future. When we turned back sound and light, the family was totally changed: They talked eagerly about what they might do in the future. They even laughed. My immediate thought was that this is very different and this gives me a good feeling.

It did not take long before we stopped the switching of sound and light. We instead swapped rooms. The therapist and the family talked in one room with the team listening to that talk from the room behind the one-way screen. Then there was a shift when the team walked over to the "talking room" as the therapist and the family walked to the "listening room." When the team was through with their talking, the rooms were swapped again, and the family commented on the team's talk from the "talking room." The therapist is always together with the family, always separated from the rest of the team.

TWO DESCRIPTIONS

It took some time before it was possible to describe our process. At first we described it with the word "heterarchy." Many have not heard that word before, but everybody has heard the opposite word: "hierarchy."

Hierarchy governs from the top and down, and heterarchy governs through the other.

Therefore, the feeling of relief in March 1985 was most probably related to leaving the hierarchical relationships of therapy and entering the heterarchical ones. More common words for a heterarchical relationship might be a "democratic relationship," an "even relationship," or a relationship with equally important contributors.

Sometime later, another description came to mind, namely, that the reflecting team process comprises shifts between talking and listening. Talking to other(s) can be described as "outer talk," and while we listen to others talk we talk with ourselves in "inner talk." If we let a particular issue be passed from outer talks to inner talks back to outer talks, and so on, we might say that the issue is passed through the perspectives of various inner and outer talks. Bateson was very concerned with the significance of multiple perspectives: One might understand the same issue differently in the various perspectives, and when these different ways to understand are put together (as in this reflecting process), they might create new ideas about the issue in focus (Bateson, 1980).

DIFFERENT REFLECTING PROCESSES

Once we grasp the idea that the shifting between inner and outer talks is an important element, we might set up these processes in many ways in many different contexts. Here are some examples:

1. There could be a team in the next room behind a one-way screen, or we might use only one room with the team listening and talking from a corner.
2. A therapist without a team could have one colleague present to talk with during "reflecting" intervals.
3. If the therapist is alone without a team, he/she could speak with one member of the family (person X) while the others in the family listen. Then the therapist talks with these others while person X listens to that talk, and later turns to person X for comments and eventually further talk. In this case the family and the therapist become a reflecting team.
4. If the therapist is alone with one client, they might talk about an issue from the perspective of one who is not present (e.g., a mother). For example, the client is asked to talk about what she thought her mother would think (inner talk) and say (outer talk) about this or that. When the mother's thoughts have been

presented, the client might be asked, "What are your thoughts about your mother's thoughts?"

5. If a workshop or conference consultation goes on in a large room with an audience listening to it, the whole audience might serve as a reflecting team.

The applied forms are infinite and I assume that the limiting element is our own inventiveness. These processes might also be applied in several contexts besides therapy. Here are some examples:

1. In supervision, the supervisee might talk with the supervisor while other supervisees listen to that talk. Then the other supervisees and the supervisor talk while the supervisee listens, whereafter the supervisee and supervisor talk.
2. Staff meetings could be organized so that one half of the staff talks about a certain issue while the second half listen, whereafter the second half talk while the first half listen, and thereafter back to the first half, and so on.
3. Management leaders might come together to discuss certain issues. The group could be divided into smaller groups. One group could start talking about one particular issue while the other groups listen. Thereafter the discussion is passed over to the next group, which talks for a while before the discussion is passed over to the next group, and so forth.
4. In qualitative research the researcher might talk with another, for example, about his "data" and his attempts to search for something in his data, either a specific category or something unknown or not yet "discovered." Others who listen to that talk can then talk about what they were thinking when they heard about the researcher's search and about the not yet known, before the researcher gives his/her comment on what he heard.

SOME GUIDELINES

I would be the first to warn about a particular practice of a reflecting process. The less planned the process the greater the possibility of letting the situation determine its form. It is important that those who take part in the process can say and do what feels natural and comfortable.

When I am the person who speaks with the family, I never take it for granted that there shall be a reflecting team's talk even when a team sits by ready to give it. I always ask the family: "There have been some people listening to our talk. Would you like to listen to what they have been thinking or what will be the best for you? We could stop our talk here, or we can continue without the team's talk. What would be the best?"

If the team's reflections (speculations) are requested I usually say to the family: "When the team talks you might find it interesting to listen to them. However, it might happen that your thoughts go other places. If so, just let it happen since you do not have to listen to the team. Or maybe you would rather rest and not listen or think so much. Or maybe you would like to do something else. Do what you feel comfortable with."

I would never tell another team member how he/she should be as part of a reflecting team's talk. However, I have three guidelines for myself. The first is to talk (speculate) from something I saw or heard in the family's talk with the therapist. I usually start by referring to what I heard or saw: "When the mother said that she still thinks much about her father who just died, I could see her husband discreetly nodding in agreement, and I could see the children listening carefully to their mother even though they did not look at her." Then I try to talk in a questioning manner; for example, "I wonder if talking or thinking of him is easy for all of them or if it still is painful for some? If it is still difficult for some to talk about him, what could they do so that those who want to talk about him have that possibility and those who are not yet ready for it do not need to take part in those talks?"

Statements, opinions, or meanings are avoided. Meanings can very easily be heard by the family members as something they should consider or even do, and if the team's meaning is different from their own, they might easily feel it as "better" and their own second best. If that happens some families might even feel criticized.

If I am on a team when one of the other team members comes up with a strong meaning (e.g., "I absolutely think the father should do this or that"), I might ask that person: "What did you see or hear in the talk [the family had with the therapist] that made you come up with that opinion?" That allows the possibility of discussing what was heard or seen. If that which was seen and heard was discussed, other opinions might be launched in addition to the first one. If the other sticks to his/her opinion, we might discuss how that opinion fit in the various family members' perspectives: "What do you think the father himself thinks of that opinion? What would the mother think of it? The father's brother?" These few exchanges might remind everybody about what they already know, namely, (1) if one saw or heard something else one might come up with another opinion, and (2) an opinion shifts its meaning according to the context (perspective) it is part of.

The second guideline is that I feel free to comment on all I hear but not on all I see. If a person in the family tries to cover something, for example, the mother clenches her teeth in order not to let the others see how sad she is, or the father tries to hide his angry feelings, which might be seen in his clenching fists, I never comment on that. I often remind myself about the talk between Zeus and Hermes, when Hermes took the post as a messenger god (to pass further the messages): Hermes promised Zeus not to lie, but he did not promise to tell the whole truth. Zeus understood. Mothers, fathers, and others should have the right to *not talk about* all they think and feel.

I use my third guideline when both the family talk and the team talk occur in the same room. I usually say to the team (with the family listening), particularly when there are members on the team who have never been in such open talks before: "I shall not instruct you or myself, but I have collected some experiences over time that I would like to share. When you are to talk I would recommend that you talk with each other and not include the family in your talk. If you include them in your talk, either by talking with them or by looking at them, then you force them to listen to you, and they cannot let their mind go other places if that is what they prefer [and I think: If that is impossible it is impossible, so let it happen]."

FOUR QUESTIONS

Four questions emerged from these processes. One is raised only to myself in my inner dialogue, two always in the open, and one sometimes in the open and sometimes only to myself.

The first one is constantly repeated to myself: "Is what is going on now appropriately unusual or is it too unusual?" If there are signs that tell me that it is too unusual, I have to change, either by talking about something else or by talking in another manner.

The second and third questions are tied together and they are usually asked in the beginning of a session and seem particularly important in the first meeting. The second question is about the history of coming here today. Who had the idea? How did the various others respond to the idea? Were all in favor of it, or were some reserved? The idea is for me to learn which of those who are present would like to talk and to learn whether any of those present would not like to talk. That helps me to be sure that I talk with those who want to talk and do not talk with those who do not want to talk. The third question is simply to ask all present how they would like to use the meeting. Everybody is invited to give an answer. Those who were reserved about coming to the meeting often have no answer, but those who wanted to come usually have one. This question is the most open I have found thus far. It allows for very

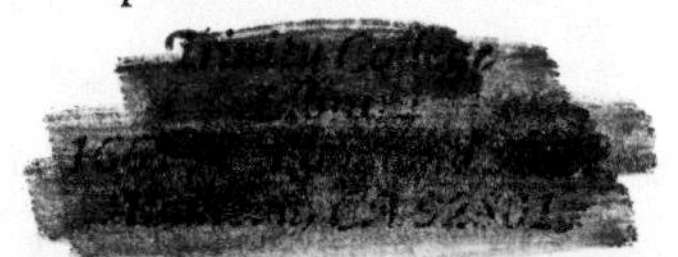

different answers: "I want to discuss my life philosophy," or, "I understand that I cannot proceed without making a point, and I would like to discuss how that might happen," or, "I am so tired and so exhausted that I want to just sit here and rest without thinking or talking."

It is most important in responding to the answer to the question ("How would you like to use this meeting?") that I talk about what they would like to talk about, and that I do not talk about what they would not like to talk about.

I might ask the fourth question if I feel that a new issue that is raised creates a certain tension. We must not take it for granted that everybody can talk about everything every way at any time. Therefore, this question, either raised in the open or only to myself, might be of value: "Who might/can/ought to talk with whom about which issue in which way at which point in time?" It might be that the original group is better divided into smaller talking units. This is to ensure that those who want to talk about the issue will have a chance to do so and that those who at the moment are not prepared for it are excused from that talk.

THE PROBLEM-CREATED SYSTEM

Harold Goolishian and Harlene Anderson launched the concept of the problem-created system (Anderson & Goolishian, 1988; Anderson, Goolishian, & Winderman, 1988). They saw that a person with a problem often attracts attention from many other persons. These others might be family members, friends, neighbors, colleagues, official persons, and even therapists.

These others create a whole system of meanings about how the problem can be understood and how it can be solved. If these meanings are appropriately different, the talks between those who hold the meanings may create new and even more useful meanings. If the meanings are too different, the talks between those who hold the meanings will easily close down.

Goolishian and Anderson say that the big problem arises when the conversations stop. When a therapist enters such a scene, already full of meanings, he/she should be careful about bringing more meanings. It is safer to ask questions and be interested in the meanings that are already there. If the therapist connects in a friendly way with the persons in the meaning system, these persons will more easily put their meanings into conversation. Maybe such conversations might loosen up and even change the various meanings so that the stalled conversations can start again.

GOING TO THE MEANING SYSTEM

When a local therapist wants my assistance, I go to the therapist and work together with him/her and the client(s) in the therapist's office. The therapist and I can be a reflecting team during the meeting. The therapist and the clients determine whether I shall continue working with them, but very often one meeting is enough for them to continue the work without me.

FOLLOWING THE OTHERS

Those family members who want to speak talk as long as necessary. It feels intuitively right that clients should be given the time they need in order to tell me what they want me to know. That means that I, as the listener, must be cautious not to interrupt. It is interesting to follow the monologues of the various clients, as the undisturbed monologue seems to comprise shifts between inner and outer conversations. The inner talks occur when the client stops talking (to the other) and makes a "pause." This is, however, not a really pause; the client just "withdraws" or "moves to an other place" or "meets someone else." We can see that when his/her eyes move away and look somewhere else. I imagine that the client searches through all the "pauses," or stops and "rests" at something somewhere (i.e., searches for meaning[s]). Then, after the pause, the eyes turn back to the other(s) present and the outer talk can continue.

The talk therefore comprises something that can be *seen* in addition to what is said and can be heard. These shifts between outer and inner talks are most meaningful if there are other(s) there to see and hear. Peggy Penn and Marilyn Frankfurt (1994) call the other(s)' contribution "witnessing." (See also Lev Vygotsky's [1988] discussion of so-called ego-centric talks.)

To Hear Is Also to See

Not only the pauses can be seen but also the "openings" that we, the professionals, might take as the points of departure for our questions. I used to think that the questions more or less were intuitively chosen. Now I do not think so; the person who listens, besides listening to all the spoken, also *sees* how this is uttered. There are the small shifts in the way to utter that might make one think: "What I just heard, which was followed with what I saw, seems to be meaningful for her. It might be worthwhile to talk more about that."

These small shifts can be so many: a look in the eyes; the head drops;

a cough; moving on the chair; the hands folded on the neck; one hand searching for something in the other hand without finding it; and so on.

These moves seem to occur when the person, while saying some words, hears the words as particularly meaningful; that is, the person's own word(s) move him/her. And the verb "to move" has in all languages two meanings: a physical and an emotional aspect.

New Questions

I often notice that the person who is given the opportunity to talk undisturbed quite often stops and starts over again, as if the first attempt was not good enough. The client searches for the best way to express him/herself; the best words to tell what he/she wants to tell, the best rhythm, the best tempo, and so on. The expressions that come (of which the words are a part) and the simultaneous activity (the way the words are expressed) have attracted my interest. Therefore, it has been natural to discuss not only the utterances themselves but also the way they are uttered. One of the questions that has emerged is: "I noticed that you said this or that. If you were to search for something more in that word, what might you find?" For example, one woman said that independence was the big word in her family. Not only did she repeat the word "independence," but she said it with such a look on her face that it was natural to let it be a starting point for the next question: "If you were to look into that word, what might you see?" She: "I don't like that word very much." "What is it you don't like when you look into the word?" Crying, and with her hands covering her face, she said "For me to talk about loneliness is so hard . . . yes it means staying alone. . . ."

Another example is of a young father who had left his wife and 7-year-old son. Some time after this happened he said that both he and his son often felt sad. When he said "sad," there was an audible and visible sigh, and he was asked, "When your son is sad, is his sadness totally filled with sadness or are there other feelings in his sadness?" The father, who said there was also anger in his son's sadness, was asked, "If your son's anger could speak, what would the words be?" He said, "Why did you leave me? You said I was the most important person for you. Why did you leave me?"

To give another example, a man spoke about the relationship between him and his wife in such a way that in the middle of fear and uncertainty, war (or anger) broke out. He was asked, "Is the fear in the anger or is the anger in the fear?" He sat long, bewildered, and thoughtful before he could answer. This question remained with him all the time for three months.

A fourth example is a question that was related to a man who in fierce anger and without words hit another with his fist. The question was: "If the fist, as it moved toward the person it was to hit, could speak, what might the words be?" There were several answers: "I feel stupid." "I am not listened to." "Nobody understood that I was hurt."

A finally, a woman spoke about peace and when asked said that "peace" was a very big word for her. She was then asked what she would see and hear if she walked into the word. She said that she walked into a landscape where she heard the final part of Gustav Mahler's second symphony. She was asked whether she was with someone or alone. When she mentioned whom she would have liked to be with she began to cry.

A commonality in these questions is that one searches for what is *inside* the expression; *in* the word; *in* the feelings; *in the movements, and so on. One does not* ask for what is behind or under or over but what is *in* the expressed. And that requires that the listener see and hear what is expressed.

These questions, which the clients surprisingly often like, are actually very sensitive in that focusing on such words is sensitive. I do not take it for granted that anyone can talk about these words right away because the emotions *in* them might be very strong. Therefore, I find it safer to introduce a few "outside" questions before "looking-into-the-words" questions. For example, the lady who talked about independence was first asked, "How was that word 'independent' expressed [in your family], was it in the open or was it implicit?" She said it was in the open. Then a second question: "Was it such that you should be independent or was it independence in general?" She said that she should be independent. As she replied to both of the questions she stayed with the word; she did not avoid speaking about it. Her ability to stay with the word told me that she was ready for the next question: "What do you see if you look into the word?"

An important prerequisite to being able to both hear and see carefully and precisely is for the listener (e.g., the therapist) to *avoid* thinking that the person who speaks means something else than what he/she says. There is nothing more in the utterance than the utterance; there is nothing more said than what is said; there is nothing more shown than what is shown. Nothing more.

Other, even simpler questions also have value, namely, after an introduction: "I noticed you said this or that . . ." and thereafter: "Can you say more what you were thinking when you said that?" or, "What flew through your mind when you said this or that?" or even more simply, "Can you say more?" Other possibilities are: "If you were to choose a word that is very similar [this or that word] what might it be?" or, "If you should choose the opposite word what would that be?" All are questions that can elicit nuances so that we might see and hear more than we previously could see and hear. However, these questions do *not* escape the overriding question: "Is this an appropriate unusual question or is it too unusual?" And the answer to *that* question is found, as I hope the reader has grasped, in the small signs the other person expresses to let the therapist know whether it feels uncomfortable or not.

If we accept the idea about the appropriately unusual, how can we increase our sensitivity to the other? A simple procedure might be useful.

THE CLIENTS AS CORESEARCHERS ON THE THERAPISTS' CONTRIBUTIONS TO THE THERAPEUTIC TALKS

During the last three years, in collaboration with a team in Harstad, North Norway, and a team in Stockholm, Sweden[1] I have tried to find a way to increase therapists' sensitivity for their own contribution to therapy (Andersen, 1993).

The procedure is that therapists, a while after therapy has ended (e.g., one year), ask the clients to return to discuss how it was to be part of the therapeutic meetings. In addition to the clients and the therapists, a visiting professional is present. The meeting starts with the therapists underlining that they wanted the discussion. The therapists, or the visiting professional, refer to reports about evaluation of various treatments that indicate that the collaboration that develops between clients and therapists contributes much to the therapeutic outcome, either making it better or making it worse (Lambert, 1989; Lambert, Shapiro, & Bergin, 1986). That makes it reasonable to research the therapeutic sessions together with the clients.

The visiting colleague thereafter talks with the therapists about what they want to focus on and clarify during the meeting, while the clients listen to this talk. In the next step the visitor invites the clients to comment on the talk they just heard (between the therapists and the visitor) and also asks them whether there is something from the therapeutic sessions they want to discuss.

The visitor then talks again with the therapists about what the therapists thought when they heard the talk between the clients and the visitor. The reader will probably notice that this is a variation of the reflecting processes.

There is something the visiting professional should bear in mind, namely, that his/her task is to talk about *the process* of the therapeutic talks and *not the contents* of these talks. If the issues of the therapeutic talks are touched on, that should only be to clarify the process.

[1]The members of the team in Harstad were Leif Hugo Hansen, Ingeborg Hansen, Torill Ida Aandahl, and Torgeir Finsås; and in Stockholm, Annica Forsmank, Marianne Borgengren, and Bo Montan.

If the clients want to talk more about the issues they once talked about in therapy, the visitor should recognize that as a wish to resume therapy and leave that to the therapists. In other words, the visitor should withdraw.

In dealing with the process of therapy the visitor should feel free to raise any questions. However, it seems most interesting for the therapists to talk about those parts of the therapy in which impasses occurred, where there were tense and uncomfortable periods, or when the therapists were uncertain and in doubt or, in hindsight, where the therapists felt they failed.

The clients' comments on such issues might be very valuable. The visiting colleague may be guided by the idea that the therapists now have the opportunity to hear what might have been *too unusual* for the clients, what might have come at an improper point in time, what might have been talked about in a improper context, and so on, and thereby to become more aware of they should *not* do again in future work.

Those therapists who have taken part in this "evaluating process" have made some interesting comments:

> "The process is as unique as the therapeutic process, but only those questions are relevant that all present can talk about. Standard questions that belong to standard evaluations would be felt as artificial, and I would not have been part of that."
>
> "The experience, *the feeling,* to sit there and hear how difficult it was for a client to be part of a way of talking that she had not had any impact on, has led me to understand how important it is for the client(s) and me to find a way of talking together we both appreciate, before we start the 'real' talk."
>
> "After being part of this I feel more and more convinced that the clients are the best supervisors. This is an alternative to professional supervision. Actually, hereafter I want both."
>
> "This experience has taught me to be inside the therapeutic relationships and *also* for me to 'move' out of it and look at it all, inclusive myself, from outside."
>
> "It was very special to be in this particular kind of triangle; in the sense that I felt we came so close to each other. When I was listening and felt so close to the clients I thought: maybe we should dare to talk more openly what we feel in those moments when we [the therapists] fight with them."
>
> "I was so surprised how much they remembered from the [therapeutic] talks. I had forgotten most of it."
>
> "It was a unique experience to feel so close and be on a basis of equality."

The clients have not been asked how they felt about this process, but some have spontaneously said that they appreciated learning what the therapists thought about the therapy they once had together. For some, namely, those who left therapy with the feeling that both they and the therapy had failed, experienced this aftertalk as a repairing process that brought them dignity. The process seemed to serve them well.

The Circle Is Closed

The reflecting processes appears to be a useful practice that is relatively easy to apply and can be used in many different circumstances. It is also a practice that studies itself. Clients and therapists are not only collaborators but also coresearchers. In many ways I believe this is a good evolution.

REVISED ASSUMPTIONS (PREUNDERSTANDING)

Maybe it is *not* a waste of time to discuss whether the reflecting processes represent an alternative way to reach knowledge, and maybe it even brings forth alternative knowledge? Maybe the reflecting processes can be regarded as an alternative, in correspondence with much else in the so-called postmodern period?

Being part of various reflecting processes has definitely contributed to my revisiting certain of my own basic assumptions, and has stimulated me to read about what others have written about these assumptions.

The postmodern era is for some a concept of time, namely, the period after "the modernism," which many say begins with Descartes. For others, postmodernism represents reactions to modernism, not at least *the way* knowledge is developed and *the assumptions* on which this way of knowing is based. It is a reaction not only to what kind of knowledge is said to be relevant but also to how this knowledge, and the process by which it emerges, influences us and forms our lives. Several books focus on these issues (see Polkinghorne, 1983, 1988; Gergen, 1991, 1994; Kvale, 1992; Shotter, 1993).

In the following discussion, I will point to a few, but central, "modern" *assumptions.*

1. True (objective, correct) knowledge about human beings can be reached (which means that this knowledge is generalizable and applicable for all human beings in all contexts at all points in time).

2. Human beings function from a basic "inner core" (which one can reach true knowledge about).
3. Language is a tool to express what one thinks (which stems from "the inner core").
4. The language, which must be unambiguous and literal, is in the service of information.

Inspired by the progress of engineering techniques and the progress in the physical sciences, we have been tempted to understand human beings in the same way as we understand those parts of nature that stand still; objective assessments of external signs (utterances and behavior) can mirror and explain the "underlying" (the inner core).

There is a need for experts who know how one can reach true knowledge (the methods), and also possess the knowledge that tells whether what one reached was true or not (know the norms). Collegia are established to protect and make more perfect the methods and the norms.

Quite naturally a hierarchy is developed: experts and nonexperts. This is what I see as a sign of the modern period.

Within the frames of the hierarchical someone became a helper and someone helped; someone a governor and someone governed; someone an observer and someone observed; someone a controller and someone controlled; and so on.

The divisions of people mentioned here separate people not only in terms of their functions but also in relation to privileges. It has been common to claim that the culture of knowledge mentioned above (modernism) was developed in a period of Western culture where economic and material conditions favored persons being independent and self-reliant, and independence and self-reliance became prerequisites for the economic and material life of constant expansion (Samson, 1981).

I consider a hierarchical culture dangerous because the unevenly distributed privileges so easily create bitterness among the underprivileged, and that bitterness easily creates a desire for revenge. And if the bitterness and the desire for revenge are oppressed, that might lead to more bitterness and maybe even violence.

Alternative Assumptions

I will first mention *other assumptions* about human beings and humans being-in-the-world.

1. One alternative to the stable and generalizable explanations of human life (e.g., the diagnosis of character disorders) is that a human

being is constantly shifting and adapts to the various contexts, which in turn (as everybody knows) shift all the time. A person might therefore be understood contextually at a given point in time. Such understanding of human beings is compatible with the concept of multiple realities: The same person can be understood in many ways—not only the person shifts (talks and acts differently) with shifting circumstances in different periods but also the others who try to understand. Those who try to understand do so from what they see and hear. If the person who understands were to listen to something else (than what he/she listened to and heard) and see something else (than what he/she looked for and saw), his/her understanding would, of course, be different.

2. An alternative assumption to the idea that a person is governed from an inner core is that the person is not in the center but the center of the person is outside him/her, in the collectivity with others. The inner core does not form the individual or the collectivity, but the collectivity forms the individual and the inner core; if this inner core exists at all (Shotter, 1993). Significant in the collectivity are the conversations that are there, and significant with the conversations are the language the participants of the conversations are *in*.

3. An alternative assumption of language is that besides being *informing,* language is *also forming.* Many have been inspired by what Wittgenstein said, namely, that the language we are *in* gives the possibilities, on the one hand, and the limitations, on the other, for what we come to understand (Grayling, 1988). Language will be part of forming what we come to think and understand. John Shotter, inspired by Bakhtin and Volosvinov, takes this even further and says that the utterances we perform not only form what we come to think but actually form the person as a whole, including the physiological makeup. Inspired by Bülow-Hansen's work and my collaboration with Gudrun Øvreberg I have reached the same conclusions (Andersen, 1993).

Language must be understood as an activity, not only the words that are uttered. "Utterance" is a bigger and more open word than "word." Utterances comprise all that activity that occurs when the spoken word is uttered, and that activity comprises not at least the physical movements and the breathing, the interplay between creating a muscular tension and letting it go. It is in the interplay between letting the tension come and letting the tension go that the forming occurs. What is formed (uttered) may be various things: The sculpture becomes the sculptor's utterance; the crescendo the musician's; the widely open, searching eyes with the closed, stiff mouth the refugee's; the disease the patient's; and so on. The expressed becomes impression for the person and others (e.g., the painting, the text, the music, the house, the dance, the stone wall, and the patient's record). The impression is, in short, related to what was expressed (uttered), or one might say a result of what was uttered (the product).

Products are given much attention in our culture and are quickly evaluated, for example, as good or bad, useful or useless, expensive or cheap. *How* it was uttered (to become a product) (i.e., the method or the skill) may also be given attention, even though not as much as the product.

A third aspect of the whole is that the person who expresses herself, by expressing herself as she does forms her life and her self(selves). Because every person is constantly in some kind of activity (i.e., constantly expressing oneself), every person constantly is in the process of being formed—transforming, reforming, or conforming oneself. Shotter (1993) says that an essential part of forming oneself is "positioning oneself" in relation to those who are in the surrounding (i.e., those who see and hear the person's utterances).

Not all I might say and do is acceptable for society. The other who is present, having a notion of what society accepts, will in his/her response to how he/she sees and hears me inform me whether I am within or outside those limits.

It will be in the eyes of the other(s) that we might find an answer to the question about what is or is not acceptable for society. And it is my own response to the other's response that contributes to the forming of me as a responsible person. These limits, reflected in the face of the other, to which I am supposed to respond are tied to the tradition and the culture of society and its surrounding nature.

In the hierarchical culture, the products are of primary interest, the methods (skills) of secondary interest. To what extent is there an interest for the individual's being-in-the-world when the skills are applied and the products shaped? I doubt there is much interest.

An alternative to this might be interesting: First, let a society refuse those products that are *not* acceptable. Then let people, in their forming of various acceptable products (which were not to be ranked according to sales value or standard), search simultaneous formings of their "own selves"; selves they feel comfortable with and are responsible in relation to.

4. An alternative assumption of words as they are heard, spoken, and written on paper is that the words only refer to some other words. It is the French philosopher Jacques Derrida who makes this assumption (Samson, 1989). Words have meanings in their similarities and differences to other words. The word "dark" will, for example, create a meaning as we simultaneously think of gray or white. Derrida writes that words refer to other words and not to the objects "out there." The particular impression of, "picture" of, or ideas about that which is "out there," and

which we talk about, are formed by the words we choose for our descriptions.

The Vienna circle in the 1920s, which represented the physical sciences and was much concerned with applying an unambiguous language, thought metaphorical language should be avoided (Polkinghorne, 1983). This opinion has been challenged by many during the last three or four decades by stating that we cannot *not* talk metaphorically (Johnson, 1987; Lakoff & Johnson, 1980). All words (metaphors) are all ambiguous and refer to other words (other metaphors). All words might therefore be nuanced and, after being nuanced, be further nuanced.

At this point I will refer to "the new questions" that I mentioned in this chapter, and which seem to have a certain value in the therapeutic work. For example, "I noticed that you at some time said this or that word. Is that a small or a big word?" If the answer is that the word is big, we might ask: "If the word is so big that you can walk into it, what would you see and hear?" Many interesting "stories" might emerge as a result of such questions.

Talking Habits and Moving Habits

Wittgenstein said that we are *in* the language. I understand him to mean that the language is not inside us but we are *in* the language. Correspondingly, I see that we are *in* movements, *in* conversations, *in* collectivities. A collectivity exists *in* a culture, and a culture is *in* a nature.

Martin Heidegger's word "being-in-the-world" might be nuanced to life is being-in-movements, being-in-language, being-in-conversations, being-in-collectivities, being-in-culture, being-in-nature.

The person's habits, which exist within these various frames, give possibilities to and limitations for what can be expressed.

A significant matter is to which extent a conversation, a collectivity, or a culture provides new possibilities for new talking and moving habits.

Outer and Inner Dialogues

Throughout his whole (but short) professional life, Lev Vygotsky was preoccupied with the relationships between inner and outer dialogues (Vygotsky, 1988). He thought that a small child at first, in the interplay with adults, learned to imitate their sounds and thereby gained an "outer" language, which means a language that did not yet have personal meanings for the child. However, in the period from approximately three to seven years of age the child develops an "egocentric" language, as the child talks with him/herself during play. Vygotsky noticed that the presence of a listening adult increased the tendency for the child to talk to him/herself. The adult did not participate in the talk but was present and listened.

Vygotsky regarded this outloud speaking of the child as a precursor to the inner (not audible) talks where the words have personal meaning. I tend to think that we receive ideas we did not have before from the outer talks, and that our inner talks (with ourselves) sort out which of the new ideas we want to include in our talking habits.

Bakhtin points to the significance of the responses our utterances evoke in those who listen to and see them (the utterances). We might both expand our habits of uttering and have them corrected by the responses from the other(s). Simply spoken, one *cannot* see one's own face when the face utters something (and the living face is such a crucial part of the utterances). Bakhtin thinks that the closest we can come is to see our face reflected in the eyes of the other. And the same will be for the other. One "lends one's eyes to the other."

Three types of *inner talks* must be mentioned. The first is those we have in our dreams; they are richly composed of rapidly changing "scenes" where most of what happens (everything?) is experienced simultaneously. The second is those we have in daily life when we talk inaudibly with ourselves; those are more coherent than dream talks but sometimes disruptive. The third is those with ourselves when we write: The writing forces us to form longer and more coherent sequences. Writing, for example, about our own work, might therefore give a significant and alternative perspective compared to that which emerges when talking to another. Be reminded of what I wrote earlier about multiple perspectives, with which Gregory Bateson was preoccupied, and differences (between the various perspectives) that make differences (in the particular perspectives).

If the Language Forms, It Forms the Person Who Speaks

One might enter the observer's language and become distant and cold, the language of the participant and be near and warm, the language of the technician and become standing still and lonely, or the language of religion and become distant and violent.

Whatever question one asks is chosen from many possible questions, and whatever answer is one of many possible answers. Every question raised and every answer given can therefore be regarded as limiting the possible (a process of simplification).

The metaphors one selects to construct one's questions and answers will be likely limiting in the same way as the scientist's method is limiting in his/her search for knowledge.

A saying such as "Many senile people suffer from depression" will create a certain understanding by the person who hears these words. A simple reformulation, "Many who seem to be senile are lonely," most probably creates another understanding, maybe even an understanding that provides ideas about how to relate to the senile person. A further reformulation is, "Many elderly people who find it difficult to take part in conversations appear lonely." These three formulations indicate that the language (the utterances) might be part of forming both "the helper" and "the helpless," in making them either more incompetent or more competent.

When the Language Creates Deficiency

Gergen (1990a, 1990b) seems to be the first to have mentioned "deficiency language" (e.g., the language of pathology). This language, first developed by professionals, has become everyday language for everybody. Goolishian organized the second Galveston conference in San Antonio, Texas—with the title "The Dis-Diseasing of Mental Health"—together with Harlene Anderson in November 1991, shortly before he died. In the announcement of the conference one can read:

> The central theme of this conference will be the exploration of the Wittgensteinian concept that the limits of the reality that can be known are determined by the language available to us to describe it. This theme will permit us to dialogue around the implications of the "deficiency language" of the mental health field and the effect these words have on our theoretical, clinical and research work. This theme will also address the pragmatic distinction to be made between the concepts of constructivism and social constructionism.
>
> It is our impression that over the last century of the mental health movement we have contributed thousands words to the vocabulary of the world. Unfortunately, most of these contributed and constructed words reflect some central sense of deficiency. It seems that in many ways the deficiency language has created a psychological and theoretical reality that can be metaphorically described as a black hole. This is a socially constructed black hole out of which there is very limited escape for meaningful clinical and research activity.

Alternative Descriptions

What might happen if we, the professionals, started to mention and describe what we do in a different manner?

It is quite usual to say that during a conversation, one is listening and one is talking. What would happen with our conversation if we were to choose other metaphors and, for example, say that the person who listens is touched by what the other expresses (utters)?

The person who becomes touched will, the next time, be moved. However, the person will not be passively moved. The person will actively take part in the sense that he/she will be active in the moving of him/herself. One way to clarify what the moved person wants is for that person to search through the language to find how to understand the situation and what to do. The next would be to express that meaning. The expression, in turn, will be a touching of the other(s).

Touchings might take many forms: stroke, press, push, grab, hold, hit, and so on. If we were to "look into" the touches we give others when we utter something, which of the words above (or other words) would we see?

I imagine that there is a wide spectrum of possibilities, and maybe only the endpoints should be avoided? On the one end to avoid *not* touching (overlook and ignore) and on the other end to avoid clenching fiercely or pushing away? Which other word might be found in the words: overlook, ignore, clench fiercely, and push away? Maybe our responsibility should make us constantly search for what shall limit us from the endpoints?

The corresponding endpoints for the listener might be to avoid *not* being touched and moved on the one end and on the other end to escape being held and being pushed away?

The more I write (and think) about this the more it all becomes a matter of a collective responsibility.

Assumptions Have to Be Chosen

In this chapter the word "assumption" has been used purposely several times. Much of what we consider good or bad, right or wrong, or essential or nonessential is based on our assumptions of being so. Assumptions of these kinds cannot stem from something observed and assessed. They are rather results of our speculations, or if we dare to use a bigger word, of what we reach through our "philosophizing." *Webster's Dictionary* defines philosophy as "a search for a general understanding of values and reality by chiefly speculative rather than observational means." Much in "therapy" and "research" and in everyday life concerns knowledge based on assumptions we have already made. The choice of underlying assumptions (preunderstanding) is what I call philosophical choices. Koestler (1964) calls these the ego, the collectivity, the language, the conversations, the emotions, the desires, the talking, the listening, the expressed, the created, the formed. The new, or what might contribute to the new, comes from combining what we already know in new ways.

It is in this respect that the assumptions become significant, as does the choice of assumptions. Which of the bits are essential and which of the bits should be put together with other bits in which way? In the end, these questions comprise choices about which assumptions we find most useful.

What might help in this search is to participate in various conversations as we work with the following question: "Is that with which I am occupied the most essential or is there something else that is more essential?"

Words at the End

It would be interesting to speculate on how the body participates in creating meaning. Johnson (1987) discusses how the body is thought to perceive (sense) shift in the surroundings before the thought has grasped it. He thinks that the sensing is connected to something learned in the very early part of life; the body senses the difference, for example, between out and in; between up and down; between being against a force and being with a force. The earliest experiences of sensing become habits and basis for the metaphors we later develop (learn from others) in language, through which we become "ourselves."

It is also tempting to speculate on how our understanding of the other becomes an expectation that he/she lives up to (Jones, 1986). The other's eyes, in this sense, do not passively mirror (reflect) me. It therefore might be useful to consider which other's eyes one is to borrow, so that one does not borrow them from whomever.

REFERENCES

Andersen, T. (1991). *The reflecting team: Dialogues and dialogues about the dialogues.* New York: Norton.

Andersen, T. (1993). See and hear, and be seen and heard. In S. Friedman (Ed.), *The new language of change: Constructive collaboration in psychotherapy.* New York: Guilford Press.

Anderson, H., & Goolishian, H. (1988). Human systems as linguistic systems: Preliminary and evoking ideas about the implications for clinical theory. *Family Process, 27*(1), 371–394.

Anderson, H., Goolishian, H., & Winderman, L. (1986). Problem created system: Toward transformation in family therapy. *Journal of Strategic and Systemic Therapies, 5*(4), 1–11.

Bateson, G. (1972). *Steps to an ecology of mind.* New York: Ballantine Books.

Bateson, G. (1980). *Mind and nature. A necessary unity.* New York: Bantam Books.

Gergen, K. J. (1990a). Therapeutic professions and the diffusions of deficit. *Journal of Mind and Behavior, 11*(3), 353–368.

Gergen, K. J. (1990b). Therapeutic professions and the diffusions of deficit. *Journal of Mind and Behavior, 11*(4), 107–122.

Gergen, K. J. (1991). *The saturated self.* New York: Basic Books.

Gergen, K. J. (1994). *Toward transformation in social knowledge.* London: Sage.

Grayling, A. C. (1988). *Wittgenstein.* New York: Oxford University Press.

Johnson, M. (1987). *The body in the mind.* Chicago: University of Chicago Press.

Jones, E. E. (1986). Interpreting interpersonal behavior: The effects of expectancies. *Science, 234,* 41–46.

Koestler, A. (1964). *The act of creation.* London: Pan Books.

Kvale, S. (Ed.). (1992). *Psychology and postmodernism.* London: Sage.

Lakoff, G., & Johnson, M. (1980). *Metaphors we live by.* Chicago: Chicago University Press.

Lambert, M. J. (1989). The individual therapist's contribution to psychotherapy process and outcome. *Clinical Psychology Review, 9,* 469–485.

Lambert, M. J., Shapiro, D. A., & Bergin, A. E. (1986). The effectiveness of psychotherapy. In S. Garfield & A. Bergin (Eds.), *Handbook of psychotherapy and behavior change.* New York: Wiley.

Penn, P., & Frankfurt, M. (1994). Creating a participant text: Writing, multiple voices, narrative multiplicity. *Family Process 33*(3), 217–233.

Polkinghorne, D. (1983). *Methodology for the human sciences.* Albany: State University of New York Press.

Polkinghorne, D. (1988). *Narrative knowing and the human sciences.* Albany: State University of New York Press.

Samson, E. E. (1981). Cognitive psychology as ideology. *American Psychologist, 36,* 730–743.

Samson, E. E. (1989). The deconstruction of the self. In J. Shotter & K. J. Gergen (Eds.), *Texts of identity.* London: Sage.

Shotter, J. (1993). *The politic of everyday understanding.* Buckingham, England: Open University Press.

Vygotsky, L. (1988). *Thought and language.* Cambridge, MA: MIT Press.

Wachthauser, B. R. (1986). History and language in understanding. In B. R. Wachthauser (Ed.), *Hermeneutics and modern philosophy.* Albany: State University of New York Press.

Warnke, G. (1987). *Gadamer: Hermeneutics, tradition and reason.* Stanford: Stanford University Press.

CHAPTER 2

Using the Reflecting Process with Families Stuck in Violence and Child Abuse

Eva Kjellberg
Margaretha Edwardsson
Birgitta Johansson Niemelä
Tomas Öberg

THIS CHAPTER IS ABOUT how we, a team in an ordinary outpatient psychiatric clinic for children and adolescents, met the challenge of treating clients from a culture different from our own, for whom our old theory and practice did not provide us with the necessary tools. Indeed, when our customary methods were applied as a basis for clinical work, they even proved to be harmful in some of the most difficult situations. Our theory and practice, based on experience in middle-class urban society, got us stuck, and thus we turned to the clients themselves for guidance as to what kind of help they wanted, and how it should be provided to them. In this way we found it possible to build new understanding as well as to develop a new practice that was better suited to our reality.

CULTURAL CONTEXT

Gällivare, where we work and live, is a community situated above the polar circle in the northernmost part of Sweden, Lapland. The area is large and covers about one eighth of the total Swedish land area. Alpine mountains, widespread subarctic heath land, and large swamps constitute the landscape. The climate is hard; the land is covered by snow and ice eight months of the year. In midwinter the sun does not rise above the horizon and during the short summer it never sets. The population is small. About 60,000 persons live here, most in the two communities Gällivare and Kiruna, which grew up around two iron ore mines 100 years ago. The area was originally populated by the nomadic Lapp people, making their living out of herding reindeer, hunting, and fishing, and also Finnish settlers.

In order to transport the iron ore, a railway was built through the wasteland to the open sea at the coast of Norway. Also at this time the large waterfalls in the alpine streams were exploited to produce electricity. All these huge industrial projects demanded laborers who came from the southern parts of Sweden and the adjacent northern parts of Finland and Norway. So, people from many countries with different traditions and totally different languages met and now live together, thus forming a new culture of Lapland.

The area is rich and poor: rich in natural resources as iron ore, waterpower energy, and wood, which have constituted the solid base for economic welfare of the whole country. For a long time the miners were proud of their professional skills and were the best paid laborers in the country. With economic recession this has changed. The unemployment rate is high and many have been forced to leave the area, especially the young people. The hard climate makes earning a living a challenging enterprise. The Lapp people have had to fight for their existence as modern society has intruded upon the grazing land of the reindeer, thus threatening the basis of their culture. Because of these rapid changes there has been a long period of frustration in developing alternative ways to survive in the face of modern technology.

Statistics indicate that alcohol consumption is highest in the country per capita; youth in the area have a criminal record twice the average; and violent crime is more common than in other parts of Sweden. Suicide rates are higher than average in the Swedish population and many persons are diagnosed with schizophrenia. Medical statistics also show high figures for accidents and violent death.

It is also true that a high proportion of citizens here are concerned with and take an active part in politics; unions are the strongest and most independent in the country. Families are often large, with close contact between generations. Dependence on relatives, neighbors, and work mates is a natural part of life. An orthodox religious movement, the Laestadianism, has many members with strong affiliation to special values shared in that community. The area is also known as paradise for adventurers and others fascinated by a simple lifestyle in a wild landscape of extraordinary beauty. The inhabitants are friendly and generous to newcomers. Three languages, Swedish, Lapp, and Finnish are spoken. In the south, Laplanders are thought to be silent, reliable, and direct.

CLINICAL CONTEXT

Until 20 years ago, psychiatry in this district was known only in terms of the mental asylum situated 200 miles to the south, where the mentally ill were brought. These people were thought of as "living dead" as they often had to stay there forever, cut off from communication with their families and communities. Thus there is a long history of fear and mistrust toward psychiatry in the community, leading to a tradition of taking care of "craziness" and solving difficult problems within the family. The families kept their secrets and hid their problematic members rather than let society hide them in a locked asylum.

In the 1970s a modern hospital was built in Gällivare with a psychiatric clinic and 10 years ago the outpatient clinic for child and adolescent psychiatry was started. Our team has eight members: four psychologists, three social workers, and one psychiatrist. In addition to our shared work in the central community, we work in pairs of two in each of the other three communities on a regular basis. We are responsible for all care in the four communities of our area. The work includes diagnostic evaluations and treatment of the usual broad spectrum of disorders such as anorectic disturbances, autistic and other neuropsychiatric disorders, suicidal behavior, school refusal, psychosis, aggressive acting out, posttraumatic stress, and so on. We are also obliged to do evaluations at the request of social authorities and courts when children are involved in situations in which legal authorities must act. Another task involves acting as consultants to social workers, school health personnel, and other colleagues in the medical system.

THE NECESSARY CHALLENGE

The team members all live in the community and have everyday contact with our clients, who are our hairdressers, supermarket cashiers, teachers, or friends to our children. We encounter them in our professional lives as various coworkers. This means that we must offer help in a way that does not endanger mutual respect.

For many years we were uncomfortable with the knowledge that many children and adolescents in our communities were living under tough psychosocial circumstances and showing obvious symptoms of disturbed behavior. We seldom succeeded in our efforts to be helpful. When social authorities were alarmed they often tried to persuade the families to seek our help because the families almost never came to us voluntarily. It was obvious that we needed a model for cooperation that enabled us to work together in order to fulfill our different obligations.

Having few professionals working in a very large area forced us to a systemic approach. We had to trust others in the clients network to be capable of handling difficult dilemmas, sometimes with help from us. So the main thing was to be available and predictable as to what assistance they could get from us. We also had to be careful not to take over any task other professionals or families could handle themselves, thus making them less capable. Thus they could use our expertise in a way that they found most useful. Being available means not having waiting lists. We must be prepared to meet those who want to see us as soon as possible.

The hardest dilemma for us was how to be a resource for the social authorities—controllers with power to seriously interfere in the clients' private lives—and also a resource for the clients subject to this authority. In order to be helpful to the children at risk, we think of these tasks as being of equal importance. Often these questions are dealt with by splitting the assignment between different psychiatric teams with airtight walls in between. One agency is asked to investigate how things really are—What is the capability of the parents? Are they violent? Are they unable to care for the children? Was the child abused? Are the symptoms to be understood as an aftereffect of trauma? How strong is the bond between parent and child?—and to recommend direct action and identify treatment needs for different members of the family. Then another agency is asked to do the therapy because an evaluation of this kind is thought of as being so detrimental that it destroys the necessary trust and faith to form a therapeutic alliance.

In the beginning we would have preferred to work under this structure. However, because we were "the experts," both the clients and the social authorities, (i.e., courts and other professionals seeing children) had to come to us. And we had no other colleagues but ourselves to ask for help. We had to find a way to do "both–and."

Another dilemma we faced was that because we lived and worked in the health care system of a small community, we shared the collective beliefs and "knew" the histories and fates of many families for generations. From a viewpoint of social heredity, this knowledge could easily lead us to think that the story would continue to repeat itself, which is not helpful if the goal is to break the pattern. To free ourselves from this assumption we had to find a form that permitted us to elicit an understanding built on present reality, not one deduced from the past.

TOWARD A NEW PRACTICE

In the mid- and late 1980s we were overwhelmed by the emerging knowledge of the number of sexually abused children in our community as well as in other parts of the world. We found ourselves confused and angry with the perpetrators and determined to rescue the children. To counteract our own strong feelings and confusion we tried to build strict cooperative models between ourselves and various authorities on how to handle these cases (i.e., who was to be responsible for what, who should talk to whom, in what order, etc.). The goal was for justice to be done: the offender sentenced by the court, the mother back in charge and protective of the children, and the children getting individual psychotherapy to overcome the harm done to them so that they would be able to live a normal life as grownups. It was very well intended but not so easy to achieve. Reality proved to be more complicated than "good and bad," "crime and punishment," and "rescue of victims." The stronger we pushed and tried to do the "right" things the stronger the resistance from those we tried to cure. More often than not family members vigorously fought our attempts to be helpful. We always had some reluctance to deal with the task of evaluating clients forced to come to us by authorities and were unsure whether our contribution was really more help than harm in the long run as it often led to split positions and "lost" families. There were many arguments with the authorities in which we tried to free our part of the work as much as possible from control issues in order to be able to do "therapeutic work." In this way, neither the clients nor the social authorities got help.

A light in the tunnel was lit when we learned about the Irish team of Nollaig O'Reilly Byrne, Imelda McCarthy, and Philip Kearney (1988). They developed the idea of a free space, a fifth dominion, for conversation in which the incestuous family system and their "helpers" all took part. The Irish team was interested in the shifting and strong loyalties between all concerned that seemed to maintain stability in the system. They did not see their roles as involving an evaluation of right and wrong or who is telling the truth, thus enabling them to have "freeing talks." We found their ideas very helpful in dealing with our own seemingly hopeless and complex situation. We then met Tom Andersen and his colleagues from Tromsö, Norway, who were working with reflective processes. All our team members took part in their two-year educational program. This training in systemic work and reflective conversation helped us to do the investigational work. Guiding us has been Tom Andersen's constant reminder to ask ourselves and our clients: "For whom is this conversation useful. Who wants to talk about what, when, where, and in what way." Moreover, we try hard to be attentive and listen and talk in a way that makes the different people present feel comfortable to communicate.

USING DEMARKATION AS PREMISE FOR REFLECTION

When social authorities refer a client family to us, they are alarmed about the welfare of a child and have started their own investigation, according to the law. They ask for our expert knowledge in a psychological/psychiatric evaluation. Nowadays we always ask the referring person to be present at the first meeting of the family and the team. Before this meeting we receive a written list of the questions they want answered and the issues they want to be addressed. This is shown to the client and is thus known to all before the meeting starts.

During that first meeting one of us interviews the different people present. Other team members are in the room in a reflective position. When we have discussed the premise for our meeting we make sure to ask those most uncomfortable or afraid how they will feel safe to express themselves. We also discuss how their dilemmas can best be communicated to those concerned. First we talk with the social worker, because he/she as referring agent has requested this meeting and thus is the one who owns the problem. We ask referring agents what their worries are about this child and what they want our contribution to be. The family and the other team members listen and are then asked to comment. We then try to find out whether the different family members in any way agree with the social worker and in what ways they don't agree. Most often we can find some areas of agreement. We then ask the social workers to be specific as to what will happen if the family chooses not to cooperate. They might say that they are so alarmed by the child's situation that they must have an evaluation and if the parents refuse the child will be removed from their custody. Or, they might say we could bypass some issues but we must evaluate whether the teenager is, for example, suicidal. We then ask family members whether they themselves are worried about something that has not yet been brought up which they think we might be able to help them to elucidate. We try to be as clear as possible to find out which problem belongs to whom. There may also be a problem that belongs to us as "psychiatric experts." For instance, during the interview we might become aware of certain issues and propose them as worthy of more discussion. We ask the family whether they want other persons to be brought in (e.g., relatives, teachers, friends, or a lawyer). We also try to make the settings as comfortable as possible, meeting at the clinic or perhaps in their home. We make a timetable and also stipulate that we will not discuss the case with the referring person unless the parents are informed or present.

So the talking and listening goes back and forth. The meeting is finished when we are all in agreement on what issues we shall work on, how, and in whose interest; what parts the family is forced to agree to; and which parts are mutually agreed on. We have found it to be of vital importance that everyone present sticks to his/her problem and that we don't try to push family members into accepting the social worker's problem as their own if they don't want it. It is also very important that the clients very clearly know what they can say no to and what they cannot say no to.

This is the stable frame we have found necessary for everybody to be as safe as possible to be able to talk and share relevant information with us. We always act to inform the family of what we think and do. We also ask for their opinions and consider how we can meet their different wishes. In so doing we invite them as coworkers even in situations that are framed by societal power and control.

During the whole conversation the other team members take a "listening position" in order to give the system some supportive reflections. This talking process provides the opportunity for different topics to be brought up. In this way family members are invited to take part in the reflecting process between the interviewer and the person in the listening position.

When an evaluation of the child is requested we assess the child's emotional status and cognitive functioning using ordinary methods and tools. We talk to the parents with and without the children and other relevant persons connected to the family. We talk with the parents about what we think when we meet their children and discuss how this can be understood in relation to the issues to be elucidated.

We make sure to get the parents' own understanding of the present situation, and, if asked, we evaluate together their capability to meet with the needs of their child and what support might be useful to them. These pieces of information are listened to and reflected upon, giving the participants a more nuanced understanding. This often liberates parents to find new ways to act even during difficult life crises, including societal control. Many times the original problem seems to dissolve during the evaluation period. Even if the problems themselves are not dissolved, the social workers often report they have a better working alliance with the family after our meetings. The evaluation period is completed with our delivery of a written document. At this point our contract is fulfilled.

Sometimes the parents come back to us for further discussions, or the child might need extra help from us concerning some dilemma. In this case a new contract is formed. This phase is characterized by voluntary participation and wishes for working on special aspects of problematic issues now defined by the family members themselves. Or the family might choose to go to another context more suitable to deal with their problem. In the last years our main efforts have been to move from a cooperating approach to one that is more collaborative.

CLINICAL ILLUSTRATIONS

Case One

A mother and her two children, a girl age seven and a boy age five, were referred to us by a social agency. The request was for psychiatric treatment for the mother and her children. She had been battered badly by her husband in front of their two children. The father's assaults on his wife had been going on for several years, especially when she was pregnant and when she expressed her needs for independence.

Treatment started with mother and children in a traditional way. The focus was on the trauma and the symptoms of the mother and her children. During the treatment period of approximately one year, two main themes crystallized: protection and information.

First, the mother and her children were in need of protection from the father in their everyday life. For a long time after the trauma they were extremely afraid of him. For a period they considered going underground and remaining anonymous. At this time the father was sentenced by the court and placed in a locked facility at the regional mental hospital several miles away.

Second, the mother needed information about her husband's attitudes toward what he had done and his intentions for the future. She could not get this kind of information from the staff at the hospital because they had not managed to establish any contact with her husband. In other words, she felt stuck between the lack of protection and the lack of information. The mother solved this problem by maintaining communication with the father through everyday telephone calls. She made it possible for the father to call her without his knowing their present address. She thought this was necessary to prevent him from finding them and being able to continue his violent behavior. More and more we became a support to the mother in her efforts to get necessary information to orient herself and the children to the future. We were in a reflective position in regard to the ongoing communication between the mother and the father while the children maintained a listening position (Andersen, 1991). In the beginning these telephone calls were extremely stressful for the mother because the man was threatening and aggressive toward her. She still continued this communication, and after some months the father stopped his destructive behavior and turned to a more responsible and respectful attitude toward the mother. He began to ask about the children, which he had not done after the trauma. When we finished treatment, the primary symptoms of the mother and her children had faded away and were no longer defined as problems.

A New Request

Two years later we received a new request from the same social agency. This time the father raised the question of his rights to meet his son and daughter. To us the assignment was to evaluate the father's parenting ability.

In comparison to our previous work with the mother and her two children, when she herself defined the aim and the extent of the treatment, we were now obliged to present enough information to the social authority for them to decide whether or not the father could meet his children. This request raised a dilemma. How could we take a position without supporting the father's need to meet his children against their wishes (they were still afraid to meet him) or preventing the father's approach to his children?

When these questions were sent to us, the father, after almost three years in a locked facility, was about to leave the hospital. He was taking psychotropic medication and had been diagnosed as "Schizophrenic with paranoid features." We were aware of the fact that the outcome of our evaluation could never guarantee that the father would not continue his battering behavior. It made us even more unsure how to handle this assignment.

We decided to incorporate the reflective processes in our work with this family (Andersen, 1991). The way the mother had solved her dilemma when she felt stuck between the needs of protection and information also became a great help to us. We started this project by meeting with all participant authorities and family members. (The father came separately.) The main idea was to create a context that provided a mutual and continuous communication without the participants feeling stressed.

Here are some of the voices from the family members.

MOTHER: I understand that he has the right to see his children, but they are still afraid to meet him. Myself, I will under no circumstances meet him since he almost killed me.

DAUGHTER: I do not want to meet him, not yet, not after what he did to my mother.

[The son did not say anything. He just looked at his mother's face, scared.]

MOTHER: He [the son] has told me that he is afraid of his father. Afraid that his father is going to hurt him because he tried to protect me that night when his father almost killed me with the knife.

[We met the father separately.]

FATHER: I want to meet my children now, I have not hurt them. I do not understand why they are afraid of me.

How We Worked

We videotaped the interviews and asked the father whether we could let the mother and the children see his videotape together with us, and vice versa. They all agreed to this experiment. The social authority agreed too but wanted a continuous report of the work. We continued this "ongoing conversation" (Anderson & Goolishian, 1988) with no other purpose than the mother had when she tried to solve her contradictory needs for protection and information. While the mother did not want the father to see her on the videotape, the children demanded that she stay close to them during the meetings. The children wanted to watch their father but not to meet him. They wanted him to watch them. The father wanted to meet his children as soon as possible. We arranged these conversations in a special way. The way we positioned ourselves during the sessions is described in Figure 2.1.

The interviewer talked to the children in front of the camera after the children (and the mother) had watched the videotape of the father and the interviewer. The mother and the reflective person listened to this conversation. Twice during the conversation, the interviewer turned toward the reflective person and talked to her about the talking that had taken place, while the children and the mother served as listeners.

In the next session with the father, the interviewer talked to him in front of the camera, after they had watched the videotape with the children and the interviewer. A few times the interviewer turned toward the reflective person and then talked about the talking that had taken place, with the father as listener, and so on.

Here is an excerpt from a videotaped session that was shown to the father.

MOTHER: (*to the children*) Tell them about your telephone calls with your father.

INTERVIEWER: What does your father say?

DAUGHTER: He asks about the school. . . .

INTERVIEWER: And more?

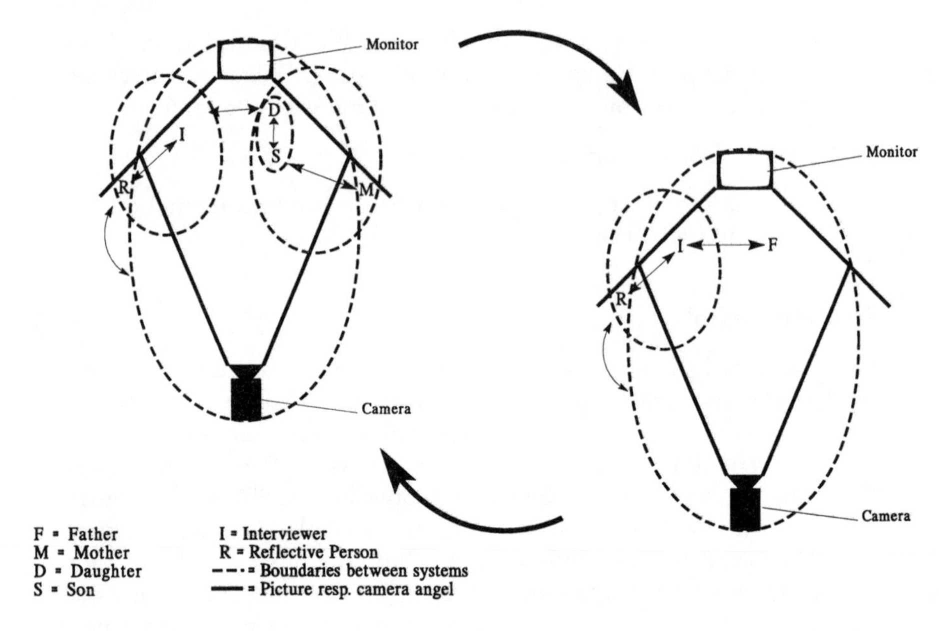

FIGURE 2.1. The arrangement of participants in interview sessions with the children (left) and father (right).

DAUGHTER: He wants to see us. . . . Once he said that I should say that I want to see him. . . .

SON: Me, too. . . .

INTERVIEWER: What about it?

MOTHER: My son became so scared and said: "Mother do I have to? Mother I am afraid."

DAUGHTER: I told him that it is my decision whether I want to see him or not . . . and after that he asked, "Does the fear never stop? . . . What could I say? . . . I don't know."

INTERVIEWER: Do you feel more or less afraid of him than before?

DAUGHTER: A little bit less.

[During this session the children talked in detail about the trauma. At the end of the session the interviewer turned toward the reflective person.]

INTERVIEWER: What are your thoughts?

REFLECTIVE PERSON: The children remember details. . . . Mother tells them to remember . . . they express both anger and fright about what their father has done.

[The next session was with the father after he had seen the videotape.]

INTERVIEWER: What are your thoughts about what you have heard and seen?

FATHER: My wife is still afraid of me, and so are the children.

In the beginning we met with the mother and the children and with the father once a month. Nowadays they are satisfied with about four meetings a year. After about one year we changed the arrangement for these conversations from communication via video to communication via one-way mirror.

Feedback from the Family Members

Here is some feedback from the family members about the ongoing conversation they have participated in for two years.

MOTHER: The children have begun to watch him . . . he doesn't look as ghastly as they imagined. . . . They have carried this for a long time now, but when they saw him through the window they said he didn't look dangerous. . . . Then I thought, this has been good for us. . . . They looked so calm after that, and then they wanted to paint pictures for him. . . . Despite that it has been hard . . . it has been good to take it slowly. . . . He [the father] seems to understand it, that it has to take time.

INTERVIEWER: (*to the son*) Was there anything you liked of what we have done?

SON: The possibility to watch father behind that window . . .

INTERVIEWER: How come you continued despite that you were afraid?

SON: Mother was beside me.

INTERVIEWER: (*to the daughter*) What did you like the most?

DAUGHTER: To watch him! . . . He didn't seem as stupid after having watched him.

INTERVIEWER: (*to the mother*) For how long should this work continue?

MOTHER: The children guide us.

[We interviewed the father separately.]

INTERVIEWER: What is your opinion about our meetings?

FATHER: I don't know . . . some progress . . . but slowly.

INTERVIEWER: Whom does this form fit?

FATHER: It is good for the children. I can see that they are less afraid of me nowadays, that is good.

At present the children have met their father a couple of times in the same room. They have a lot to talk about after all these years.

Discussion

This case describes a process that has passed through several steps. The development of this form of work has been guided by the opportunities presented in every new meeting.

The "fuel" for this ongoing conversation has been the flexibility of participation. Everyone had the opportunity to take a both–and position to the conversations—a listening and a talking position. Providing space for an ongoing conversation has been an aim in itself. In the words of Anderson and Goolishian (1988), "It is the therapist's role to take part in the system's process of creating language and meaning and to keep the dialogue going toward dis-solving the problem and the dissolving of the system itself" (p. 372).

Case Two

Anna, a 35-year-old woman who lived in a small village in the Lapp countryside, had been known to the social agency since she was rather young. As a teenager she gave birth to a girl who was adopted by a family in the south of Sweden. Later on she had five more children, all girls, ranging in age from 2 to 15 years old. She drank so much alcohol that she was incapable of taking care of her children. The eldest girl had been placed in the home of Anna's parents. The rest of her children were placed, in pairs of two, in two different foster homes. One of the girls had been moved from home to home until the latest foster parents decided to take care of her and her youngest sibling.

Some years ago Anna told the social agency of her suspicion that two of her children had been sexually abused by their stepfather. Anna and these two girls were referred to us for evaluation. Although there were some odd findings in their playing and drawings, they didn't admit to any abuse. Later on their stepfather was sentenced by the court for sexually abusing some other girls and he was sent to prison for two and a half years.

During the evaluation process we were very worried about Anna's capacity to take care of her children. Soon after, all the girls were placed in foster care. After some time, one foster family realized that the girl in their home was very insecure and was constantly thinking of and worrying about her mother. She also expressed suicidal thoughts. Once at the day-care center she had climbed up a tree and threatened to jump, telling the personnel that she had no reason to live. The girl came to our clinic with her foster mother and we met for some time in therapy. Anna told us that it was okay, but she expressed negative feelings about this contact with her daughter. Anna wouldn't define any problems. The girl couldn't cope with this situation and we found it impossible to continue in the same manner.

We and the social workers decided to try something different. All the persons concerned with the children's well-being saw that these girls needed to have a healthier contact with their mother, and we all feared that they would be at risk as grownups.

The "case" of Anna and her daughters was considered very difficult, which was reflected in the large number of professionals involved. We were curious about the consequences of bringing together those involved and generating a conversation adapted to the "family's" needs instead of being formed by the "experts." Our wish was to create a context in which all the participants could freely express their feelings, thoughts, hopes, and fears.

The social workers liked the idea. As a result, we decided to invite Anna, her four daughters, and their foster parents to a common meeting with us and the social workers.

The First Session: Demands on the Mother

At the first session everybody showed up. Anna also brought her new fiancé with her. She wanted him to stay outside the room, a decision that the social workers supported because of a rumor that he was being sentenced by the court as a child sexual abuser. Anna expressed both aggressive and sad feelings toward the social workers and the foster parents.

During the session Anna took a break to connect with her boyfriend. After a while she came back and we continued. Anna and her children were all confused concerning why they were not allowed to live together. One of the results of this session was that all the participants agreed to write down their thoughts about what had to change for Anna to be able to take care of her children and then to send their writings to the social workers.

One of the daughters wrote:

> "I don't want to be used by the social agency to determine whether my mother is healthy or not."
> "I want my mother to stop drinking beer."
> "I think my mother falls in love with strange men."

Another daughter wrote:

"How come my mother has the power to stop me from doing fun things like going on holiday with my friends?"
"Can my mother get a telephone from the social agency so that I can phone her easily?"
"Can I visit my mother at her home together with somebody from the social agency?"

The foster parents also took time to think about what children need from their caretakers. In her writing, Anna showed that she really cared for her daughters, and she had several suggestions about how she could take part in their daily activities. At this session we decided that we would meet again to develop a program for Anna.

The Second Session: The Children's Voices and Thoughts about Absent Fathers

Before this session the social workers made a list of the most important things the participants had written down. The list was transformed into a program for Anna, which included her own wishes. By the time of the second session Anna already had started and followed the program for one week. We discussed the plan. The children were very interested, and they had clear ideas about what they thought would be fair demands on a good mother. They also pointed out how important it was to have contact with their fathers. We discussed the different fathers and where they were at the moment. We looked for different ways to contact them. One girl's father lives in India and she suggested how she might meet him and that she at least would like to talk with him on the telephone. The siblings were very quiet at first, listening to the talk of the grownups, but after a while they joined the discussions and were able to tell Anna what they expected from a caring mother.

The plan made by the social workers was read out loud. The children commented spontaneously as follows:

"A real good mother must be healthy before she can take care of her children."
"She must be nice"
"She must be able to help children who are caught in barbed wire, or who got lost in the woods."
"She must care for them so they won't be caught in a fire and burn."

When the children talked about what they thought were the most important things for a mother to do, Anna nodded her head in agreement. At the end of the session Anna talked about her own father. He had rejected Anna and will not let her visit him until she has sorted her life out. We tried to find different ways to make Anna's father more interested in our work and take part in it. The social workers and the grandmother decided that they would try to meet the grandfather in his home in an attempt to engage him in the process. The second session ended with a discussion on how to proceed if Anna did not succeed with the program. The group agreed to continuing evaluation.

The second session gave us a new insight about the importance for the children to meet with their mother and their foster parents and with the social authorities. They dared to say things they had been thinking about and they extended the context by bringing their different fathers into the conversation.

The Third Session: Failure or Lack of Flexibility

Anna did not succeed in sticking to the program. She started to drink again and she sent a message that she wouldn't be attending the meeting.

This time the session took place in an atmosphere of disappointment. Many accusations between the different foster families surfaced. The fact that Anna did not succeed disappointed the foster parents and they expressed it by getting angry and accusing the others of being too soft about Anna's drinking problem. A discussion took place about whether it was right for the children to be part of this big group. This discussion didn't lead us any further in the process and we started to think about what had stopped the ongoing conversation that we wanted to achieve. Maybe the group members should have made the plans together instead of letting the social workers do this job. If Anna had been a part of that process she might not have failed.

A New Session

After summer vacations we met once again with the larger group and with Anna and her family. She had now entered a home for addicts.

The meeting was started by one of the foster mothers:

FOSTER MOTHER: I don't like these big meetings when we all sit together. I thought we decided last time that those big meetings should stop. I think the children won't talk and feel free to talk when there are so many people here that they don't know. They are afraid of talking about the things that bother them with so many people in the room. I want these meetings to stop but I still want each foster family to have the opportunity to get help from the clinic and for myself, that is exactly what I want. (*small pause*) It's so difficult sometimes at these meetings when you say something to somebody that slips off of your tongue. Well, at least for me, I have great problems trying to repair it afterwards. You say something to somebody else that hurts and then you regret the things you said.

THERAPIST: Okay. that's how you feel. What about the rest of you. How do you feel about this?

ANNA: I think these meetings have been very good. It's my chance to see all my children together. But I agree with you. (*nodding her head toward the foster mother*) It's hard for me sitting with a lot of people. . . . I don't know. . . . I know I'm not good at expressing myself, I don't know how to say this but I think it's good to meet everyone at the same time and yet it would be easier if I could see each foster family and those of my children that they are taking care of at different times. I want you to be present, of course. (*pointing at the therapists*)

THERAPIST: I wonder about you Ruth. For you as a social worker, have these meetings been positive in any way?

RUTH: I'm very anxious that these sessions continue. I have an almost impossible job acting both as the police, guarding you Anna, and at the same time helping you and your children. I have to follow the law that says that I must keep my eyes on Anna so that maybe at some point in the future she can take care of her children and I must also make sure, that the children are safe and will grow up in a positive way. Before we started these group meetings I was mostly confused by all my tasks and very split up between them. For me these meetings are important and a big help to give and get information about what's happening.

THERAPIST: What about you Carl? You have been working as a social worker with these people before. How do you feel about this?

CARL: I, myself, prefer small group meetings but I can see the advantages with this bigger group. I don't know, but perhaps we could do both. We could have the big group and then split up and also have smaller groups so that the children can talk to their mother and feel more free to do so.

SECOND THERAPIST: I have been sitting here listening to your conversation and I hear you talk about two different settings. It seems to me that we are talking about two different levels of need. This big group is good for the children in the sense that they can meet and talk to each other. And it is an opportunity for everyone to get information about what happens around Anna and her girls. You can also give information to the others. But it seems important to split up into smaller groups if we want the girls to feel secure and talk about things that they want to take up with Anna and us.

ANNA: Yes, that's what I want. I want to talk to my eldest daughter and my mother because I . . . I'm worrying about my contact with her. She avoids me . . . maybe it's her age . . . I don't know.

After this conversation about the advantages and disadvantages of meeting as a large group we agreed that the both–and solution was the most acceptable. We thought that there were two different needs in the group: Information needed to be mutual between the social workers and the rest of us on the one hand and, on the other hand, between the foster families and Anna. Another need was to continue the dialogue among Anna and her girls and the foster parents as an ongoing process. The foster families expressed that their foster children showed symptoms and problems they needed to talk about with both Anna and us at the clinic. As a result of this meeting, we split up the big group and one of the foster parents met with Anna, one of her daughters, and the team from the clinic.

Discussion

In this case our aim was to form settings that allowed all persons concerned to meet in a way that made it possible for everyone both to listen to and to express their own meanings to be reflected upon by the others present. The original problem, the threat by one of Anna's daughters to commit suicide, disappeared. However, other problems surfaced.

One daughter's biological father asked for custody of her. Both Anna and the social worker both had serious doubts about the father's ability to take care of his daughter. In our discussions of how to handle the problem, we chose to meet the parents involved together with the social agency.

Another issue for the social agency was the ability of Anna and her fiancé to take good care of their new baby. We intend to continue to invite all concerned into this system, guided by the needs of the participants.

Case Three

Mary, a woman in her early 40s, mother of three children, had her first contact with our clinic in 1990 during an evaluation dealing with a question of child sexual abuse. Mary raised this suspicion herself. Her forceful way of questioning her ex-husband's ability to take care of their son Peter after the separation, which at times became abusive to the son, finally made the social agency ask for a complete evaluation of parental ability and of the boy's psychological health. The agency also wanted to know what kind of support the parents and child needed.

We made this evaluation and recommended that the boy stay with his father and see his mother only in the company of a contact person. This was motivated by Mary's very strong despair, her repetitive interrogation of her son, and the strong hatred she expressed toward her ex-husband in front of the boy. We also recommended supportive treatment for the mother and psychotherapy for the boy.

Trying to Reach a Collaborative Working Relationship

At this time, Peter's father wanted Mary to accept psychiatric treatment for her difficulties because these difficulties hindered their ability to communicate. Although we could not give her such treatment, we offered to give her support in her parental role, which she accepted.

Mary felt she had been treated badly by the psychiatrist at the hospital and by the social agency during the last years. Under no circumstances would she let the psychiatrist take part in our work at the clinic. Instead, she sent us letters she had written some years ago. Her hope was that we would understand her constant worry that her son was being sexually abused by the father. Now Mary sent them to us with a covering letter (below) saying that she had got in her possession drawings made by her son at the day-care center he attended. They made her think Peter was sexually abused and she had nobody to talk to about those drawings.

> *There are two girls working at the day care centre and I cannot say one word to them. During the years 1986–1989 I was talking with the staff and of course with the head of the institution about my fears for my son. The only result of this was that Peter was treated badly. They told the father of my suspicion and after that my son had to suffer even more. Besides, the staff members were evil and scornful towards me. I have learned my lesson and now I know that the best thing is to keep silent in the interest of my son. Never again will I expose him to the evilness of other people. Yes, I think there are no worse people than those bloody hags. Not to talk about the social agency. Since 1986 they have done everything they could to break me and they still do. Only you at the clinic can save the life of my son.*
>
> *Best wishes,*
> *The mother Mary*

This is one of many attempts by the mother to be heard. We were reading Mary's letters during and between sessions with her. At this time we were not sure whether our contribution had any beneficial value. Mary, however, wanted to continue the discussions with us about her life with her children. We organized the sessions so that one of us did the talking and the other listened to the conversation. We listened to Mary and let her listen to and take part in our reflective talks. In every setting we tried to explore what Mary found meaningful to talk to us about at that moment.

During our conversations some themes recurred frequently. Essential was Mary's need to be heard. Other themes were, Who is able to understand? and, In what way shall we communicate? After recognizing these themes, Mary started to develop her own goals for our ongoing therapeutic relation:

- How she could make the best out of the meetings with her son together with Lottie (the contact person) and figure out "nice things to do." (Mary said that Lottie lived a sheltered life and was afraid of everything, even going for a swim.)
- To what extent should Lottie be near Mary and her son. Could they be in separate rooms in the apartment?

In order to increase the opportunities for reflective talks, Mary invited both her son and Lottie to the sessions. Peter's problem was how he could learn to understand his mother's anger as he couldn't imagine where it came from. Mary brought up the question of whom her son should be protected from. Herself or his father?

The themes of gender and poverty were also recurrent: "I am a woman, I'm poor, and I live in a community where women are extremely dependent on their men. That's my heavy burden," Mary said. She often expressed hatred toward women, so we decided to change positions during the sessions. We changed so that the listener (a female therapist) took over the talking and the interviewer (a male therapist) took the listening position. This change was supported by Mary. The shift brought up new issues:

MARY: You are afraid of me, you support the other women. But (*to the listening therapist, a man*) he understands me. . . . What's unique here is that I can say what I think without you mocking me or laughing. . . . You understand me.

Another recurrent theme is murder. When Mary gets too hard on us (i.e., demands that we accept her version as the whole truth), we set up boundaries regarding what we will listen to. We also try to move the conversation toward questions of today and the future. When discussions get polarized into "good and bad," we bring the conversation back to the issues agreed on, namely, how Mary can best be a support for her children. Mary thinks that nothing good can develop when you are forced to accept expertise opinion on what is right or wrong.

Sometimes the person in the interviewing position finds the mother's accusations (toward police, ex-husband, and social agency) to be killing monologues and is rescued only by the reflective conversation. This means that the third person in the room, who has been listening, suggests that we talk about these thoughts symbolically. Mary claims that nobody will listen to her even though she has evidence that someone close to her murdered Olof Palme (Swedish prime minister assassinated in 1986). We reflect on this as murder of herself and her human rights. In that way we move ahead quite a bit. We don't try to solve Mary's huge problems, but only to keep up the conversation about them. For instance, we might say, "Justice is done in courts. Here we can talk about your feelings and thoughts concerning those issues."

Partners in Conversation

We worked with reflective processes so we could exchange as much information as possible. Mary worked energetically in order to make every meeting useful to herself. The meetings took place every second month, always at Mary's initiation.

We (Peter, Lottie, the therapists, and Mary) are now partners in a conversation; we are no longer investigators. Mary is working on her old conceptions of reality. We are moving from suspicion toward curiosity; from victim to cooperating person; from not being heard to being heard.

Post-Office Receipt

The client's narrative talent inspired us to suggest correspondence between the sessions. This idea was offered by the therapist in the reflective position after Mary brought up the theme herself. Mary didn't comment on this idea during the session.

After some days, we received a letter from her:

> *I talk so much and I didn't have the time to answer all the questions that came up . . . about corresponding . . . it would be worthwhile . . . concerning transmission of the letters: I prefer post office receipts since it makes me feel secure.*

From that point on, we corresponded with the client between sessions. This correspondence widened the reflective process that takes place during the sessions when we meet.

An example from another letter:

> *Thanks for your letter. Its content was a big surprise to me. I've been suspicious toward you on account of your insistence on the result of your investigation of sexual abuse. The fact that you two nowadays sometimes have doubts concerning this, makes me feel good. You can admit that . . . in that respect you are unique. Nothing I am used to.*

We got so much information, especially written, that we wondered what to do with it. When we asked Mary to collaborate with us in writing a narrative about our work she was very positive. She wanted to tell everybody what can happen if, in a stressful situation, you are all alone with your thoughts for a long time, especially when you feel like a stranger in your own society. Mary described a friend whom she met in a mental hospital who was in a very bad state:

THERAPIST: Have you never had a period like that yourself?

MARY: No, never like that.

THERAPIST: But, you have been talking about the time when you had to take so much medicine that you didn't feel okay.

MARY: It was never like I was totally losing all control—but I had those hallucinations for three years and three months all around the clock. I thought I had invisible friends and I was practicing to speak without moving my lips. That's how lonely I was.

THERAPIST: You mean that you had secret conceptions?

MARY: Yes, it was secret. That's how crazy it can get when you are all alone.

THERAPIST: It sounds like science fiction.

MARY: Yes, it does.

THERAPIST: You should write a novel now when you have left this behind you.

MARY: Yes, it was awful at that time.

THERAPIST: You mean what was in your dreams, in your fantasies.

MARY: In the middle of the night I was sitting on a chair in the kitchen with a knife in my hand waiting for my ex-husband to come and kill me, but I was prepared. I could protect myself. Then there were those ghosts. I had pictures of my two sons on the wall above

> my head. Suddenly one of the boys seemed like a devil to me and his eyes were shining so I took the picture down and cut out his eyes with the knife. Five o'clock in the morning the ghosts went away. Yeah, I stood there in my nightgown, opened the door and they went out. I could feel them going out and knowing they were on their way to my ex-husband's house. I saw them going there but I did not see myself as mad. In the morning I couldn't go to my school, I phoned and told them I was ill. And these things I have never told anybody. I only told what my ex-husband had done to my boy and how he frightened us. That you have been strongly touched by me and my narratives is good. If this work could be used in a way that would help others I would be delighted. If so, my hell is not in vain . . .

Everyday Life

During the five years we have been meeting with Mary, she has fixed up her apartment and also slowly started to communicate with her mother, father, and siblings. She has made new friends. She has a baby daughter, whom she is taking care of. She's very happy about that. The baby helps her to be sensitive to other people and they respect her. For example, when she goes by bus, people are smiling at her and her baby. She sees Peter every second weekend, not just a couple of hours every Wednesday. She is also able to spend hours with her ex-husband together with the children. Peter, our originally identified patient, does not have any symptoms that require treatment and is doing rather well with his life at home, in school, and with his friends. Mary still meets with us now and then to discuss current dilemmas.

FINAL COMMENTS

Within the borders given, we try to shape a discourse that makes it possible for many different dialogues in the room to be listened to by the others, who in their turn will have another dialogue. This brings multiple realities into the room as a strong counteracting force to ascribing to others our own thoughts and feelings. What is talked about and how it is talked about becomes important. During the reflecting process, power and control are distributed among all the participants. Everybody, including the experts and authority officials, in this setting is entitled to and responsible for his/her own understandings and feelings. Working with reflecting processes is especially valuable in those situations in which strong feelings of anger, fear, or anxiety are held by the client, family members, and/or colleagues. Providing a safe setting for all concerned to present issues of violence, abuse, and fear makes it possible to talk about them.

Anything that diminishes the self-esteem of parents reflects back onto their children and makes the children feel bad and ashamed. Therefore we must be as respectful as possible. Shame-bound reactions such as withdrawal or aggressive acting out also tend to block communication. Being able to talk openly about difficult dilemmas, in a way that does not violate the integrity of the persons involved, seems to diminish these painful feelings and the reactions to them. The reflective setting provides a liberating opportunity to talk to each other without having to prove who is right or wrong. Instead of deciding how things should be, talking about how things are and how this affects all concerned creates a new understanding of oneself and others. These discussions, added to what's already known, make everyone more capable of dealing with their dilemmas. Seeing yourself either as a criminal, an alcoholic, a victim, or as a person who, among many other attributes, has been violent, drinks too much, or has been abused, makes a big difference. It also makes a big difference if you see yourself as an expert on curing mental disorders or if you see yourself as a professional who creates an atmosphere for conversation and communication among all parties who comprise the problem defined system (Anderson & Goolishian, 1988).

We feel comfortable with this shift: from being caught in preconceived meanings to being free to make new meanings.

REFERENCES

Andersen, T. (1991). *The reflecting team: Dialogues and dialogues about the dialogues.* New York: Norton.

Anderson, H., & Goolishian, H. (1988). Human systems as linguistic systems: Preliminary and evolving ideas about the implications for clinical theory. *Family Process, 27,* 371–394.

McCarthy, I., & Byrne, N. (1988). Mistaken love: Conversations on the problem of incest in an Irish context. *Family Process, 27,* 181–199.

CHAPTER 3

Treating Psychosis by Means of Open Dialogue

Jaakko Seikkula
Jukka Aaltonen
Birgitta Alakare
Kauko Haarakangas
Jyrki Keränen
Markku Sutela

A NEW KIND OF psychiatric system has been developed since the beginning of the 1980s in the western Lapland province of Finland. The new system is based on the active participation of the families in treatment. In the beginning, we attempted to have all families involved in family treatment, but in 1983 we realized that our methods were not effective in connecting us with all these families. In fact, of the total number of 350 patients referred to the Keropudas Hospital, only 20 were actively engaged in family work. This result was a function of a treatment team that viewed the patient and his/her family as objects of treatment rather than active participants in the planning and implementation. The treatment team gathered information from the case records and individual interviews and imposed a treatment plan upon the family.

Based on this information, we changed our methods in 1984 and started to invite all the families of the referred patients to discussions before any plan was made to begin family therapy or any other treatment. The conversations in these treatment meetings began without any preplanned notions of themes or topics for discussion. All discussions were organized to maximize team work. For instance, the doctors and psychologists no longer had a separate dyadic interview with the patient; instead, admission interviews were conducted as a more public forum including the whole ward team. The family and the professionals who had previously been involved with the patient were also invited to these discussions. Thus, a new system was organized emphasizing joint treatment meetings.

In the beginning we had two rules for ourselves in order to accommodate to the change in working style: (1) we were allowed to speak confidentially with the patient only for a good reason (e.g. in an individual psychotherapy session), and (2) we were allowed to speak about the issues concerning the patient only when he/she was present and to make decisions concerning the family only when the family was present.

In our early work, the boundary around the treatment team was a closed one in that the team made the treatment decision according to its own analysis; now the boundary was opened in the way that allowed all the involved parties to participate in the treatment discussion. An open dialogue was started among all the participants in the treatment process.

This shift in treatment organization led to confusing experiences. On the one hand, we were openly discussing all the issues in the treatment process; on the other hand, the "old healer" inside us (i.e., the traditional way of doing family therapy) often emerged and led us again to try to change the family (Seikkula, 1994; Seikkula & Sutela, 1990). This led to case experiences where we had to change our behavior if we wanted to progress in the treatment.

CASE: THE MAN WITHOUT A WIFE

During a one-year period a pattern developed between a male patient and the safety ward (closed ward) team. Although the treatment plan was repeated over and over again it had not been successful. The patient had been abandoned by his wife and after that he began to drink heavily and was admitted to the hospital in bad physical condition. He also was very fearful of people. The plan was to treat the patient by means of family discussions with his primary family (i.e., his mother and sister). After two weeks, he decided to leave the ward, before the treatment plan was implemented. Two weeks later he returned to the ward in the same condition as previously described. The same plan was implemented with hope of a long inpatient treatment, but the patient left the ward again. This sequence was repeated many times during the year so that the treatment periods got shorter and shorter and the periods outside the hospital got shorter and shorter, too.

Once, on a Friday afternoon, when the members of the ward were going to leave for the weekend, he returned to the ward following a three-day discharge. The members of the ward team began to discuss their frustration with the treatment process. The ward treatment team members told the man, "We can't do anything more for you. The only alternative would be to prescribe a compulsory treatment for you, but it won't succeed, because you are not psychotic. In order to become psychotic you would need to drink more, but it seems that your body does not tolerate that amount of alcohol. So we can't make any new plans; we'll see you on Monday morning."

To everyone's surprise, this discussion (or, should we say, the unloading of this frustration) facilitated a change in the relationship between the ward team and the patient. The patient stayed in the hospital for a six-month period and both family and individual discussions proceeded. The best treatment seemed to come out of the planning process. Earlier, we thought we first had to devise the treatment plan and then implement it; by opening the boundaries of discussion, the joint process itself started to determine the treatment, rather than the team itself or the treatment plan of the team.

From this type of experience the very first rule of dialogical discussion emerged: There cannot be any subject or object in dialogical discussion; all participants are in a mutual coevolving process so that the treatment team is also changing all the time. In order to emphasize the importance of this finding, we termed this process the "system of boundary" (Seikkula & Sutela, 1990); the most important issues in the treatment did not occur *within* the ward but *between* the ward and the patient's family or "on the boundary." In the beginning we did not fully understand this situation; however, the works of Mikhail Bakhtin, Valentin Volosvinov, and Lev Vygotsky helped us to understand the dialogical nature of language (Seikkula, 1993).

After beginning the open discussion with all the participants in the treatment process, rapid changes in the treatment organization began to occur. We considered the fact that patients often had to wait a week or more at the ward before the treatment was started because of delays in the first treatment meeting. Therefore, in 1986 we started to organize admission teams whose task was to organize the first meeting before the decision to admit the patient was made. This way of working was recommended by the Finnish national schizophrenia project conducted in the 1980s. In 1987 the polyclinic team was organized to take charge of these admission meetings. One or two members of the polyclinic team organized staff members from the inpatient ward, from the mental health outpatient clinic, from the general practitioner, and so on. They also asked the family to invite those people they wanted to participate in the discussion.

This way of working rapidly changed the incidence of hospitalization in the psychiatric treatment. Several studies (Keränen, 1992; Seikkula, 1991) noted that 40% of the total number of referred patients were not admitted to the hospital. Instead, an outpatient crisis intervention was organized by the same team. According to the results of the research, the admission meetings often were held at the patient's home because the resources of the families were more evident in their home setting. After such meetings it was no longer a question of admission to the hospital but of crisis intervention work in general. When the need for hospital treatment decreased, the need for hospital staff also decreased, and those resources from hospital were transferred mainly into the outpatient context for crisis intervention work. In total, six mobile crisis intervention teams were formed.

The need for hospital beds drastically decreased for the western Lapland province from 320 inpatient beds to 63 currently. Almost all treatment of acute psychosis now takes place as outpatient crisis intervention, and 90% of those admitted are long-term patients. This development does not mean that patients are being abandoned or homeless. Special mobile home treatment and rehabilitation teams for long-term patients have also been organized.

FROM MONOLOGUE TO DIALOGUE IN THERAPEUTIC CONVERSATION

The shift from the old system to the new one can be illustrated by means of the metaphor about monological and dialogical language. The old system is an example of monological language because all the considerations and plannings and decisions were made by the team, within the treatment system, and the family did not have any place in that process. The new system is dialogical in the sense that a joint process is established from the very beginning of the therapeutic discussions.

Dialogue and dialogism can be seen as a general definition of language, whereas monologue is a specific part of dialogue or, as Markova (1990) stated, "monologue is unequivocally dialogical in nature" (p. 9). The monological forms of culture and the forms of interaction between people can be understood in this general sense as a part of dialogism, not as an opposite to it. This general dialogical principle becomes true in those circumstances where the monological utterance can be seen as an answer to some other discourse (Hirschkop, 1986). An example of this is a political debate in which each participant sees his own side of the discourse better than his opponent's because his aim is to negate or defeat his opponent's case. In the monological dialogue the utterances are closed circuits, which does not open a new flow of questions but always shuts down the discourse. Because the monological utterances are either acknowledged or denied, there is no possibility of producing any combination or integration of them.

Another example of a monological dialogue is the diagnostic interview of a physician where the physician has to be in dialogue with his/her patient in order to receive information about the symptoms. The physician asks questions about the symptoms in order to be able to accept or reject in his/her inner dialogue the alternatives of different illnesses. The map for this monological dialogue is within the physician's head because the physician knows better than the patient the context in which different symptoms can be understood. However, as long as the physician searches for answers only in order to accept or reject his/her own hypotheses, the interactional context stays monological. Both Bakhtin (1981) and Volosvinov (1973) consider dialogism a presupposition that the language can gain some inner meaning. In a consultation with a physician, only the physician has the possibility to determine the actual meaning of the symptoms the patient describes. Unfortunately, the interview with a psychiatrist also often takes this form, because the psychic symptoms or other problems create an internalized sense only on the doctor's side when the doctor has the diagnostic map inside his/her head. The psychiatrist could change this monological context by commenting personally on the answers of the patient. Language becomes true between oneself and the other speaker in a social reality. When monological utterances are used, they do not gain any internal meaning or understanding because, according to the ideas of Bakhtin and his coworkers, understanding always presupposes dialogue (Volosvinov, 1973). When answering in a dialogical way, for instance, by commenting personally on the patient's story, the psychiatrist could evaporate internal understanding about the problems as Vygotsky (1970) states it.

Bakhtin (1984) discovered this form of dialogism in Dostoyevsky's novels. According to Bakhtin, the characters cannot be examined as a complement to each other, as parts of one plot or narrative; instead, they are in irreconcilable conflict with other characters, and therefore they cannot be examined as a part of dialectical evolution. The dialogue takes place between these contradictory characters when every character speaks his/her own word. One's word is not, however, an answer to another's word in the sense that some entire understanding of one plot would emerge. Only an understanding of each subjective language can exist. There are as many plots and stories as there are speaking subjects in the text. While the monological language speaks about the already spoken and already seen world, the dialogical language speaks about the world that is open, not ready and makes the unspoken spoken: a definite answer or unity, however, is never gained. In dialogical discussion, every utterance is an answer to the previous utterance, which, again, waits for a new utterance as an answer to it. This chain is never completed in the sense that some definite final outcome is reached. New meanings arise whenever conversation is started and the discourse becomes true at the very moment it is spoken. After that we are already in a different situation, which follows one after another in a never-ending flow.

Volosvinov (1973) says that in dialogical conversation, the answer is built in the dialogical utterance: It waits for an answer because without answering words the dialogical utterance cannot be completed. The understanding in language is originated in the dialogue and without answering words the understanding of the speaker and the interlocutor cannot expand. Understanding strives to match the speaker's word with a counterword, or every word calls for a reply (Lacan, 1981; Patterson, 1988). In dialogical conversation the language is constructed between the speaker and the interlocutor and the meaning of the themes under discussion belongs to a word in its position on the borderline between the speaker and the listener (Volosvinov, 1973). Markova (1990) talks about a three-step process as unit of analysis in dialogue where the third and the most important step for the creation of meanings is taking place between the interlocutors.

In therapeutic conversation the meanings of the patient's experiences and his social network (or, also, the meanings of the incidents inside the ward) are constructed in the first place between the therapist and the client, and these discourses can obtain an internal, constructive meaning for the psyche if they expand the already spoken reality or open new perspectives on reality. In the dialogical dialogue with the patient we can also respond directly or give advice, which also achieves therapeutic importance if we think that it can help to generate dialogue.

OPEN DIALOGUE IN CLINICAL PRACTICE

Understanding these dialogical principles has "forced" us to change the organization of the treatment system. Now the crisis intervention facilities, rather than the hospital, are the most essential sites for this kind of work. The guiding principle of the mobile crisis intervention teams is to organize the first meeting with the patient and his/her family and other social network during the first day after the contact. If there is a question of hospital treatment, the admission meeting is arranged before the decision to admit (voluntary cases) or during the first day of inpatient treatment (for compulsory admissions). The patient, relative, or referral agency contacts our mobile crisis intervention team, which then initiates the first meeting. Any members of the treatment staff—both outpatient and inpatient staff—who have previously participated in the patient's treatment will be contacted and will join the team if possible. The admission team could, for example, consist of a clinic worker as a family therapy specialist, a mental health outpatient clinic worker as an individual therapist, and a nurse from the inpatient ward. This team takes charge of the whole treatment sequence regardless of whether it takes place at home or in the hospital. The hospital boundary thus becomes flexible in two ways: (1) the team consists of both inpatient and outpatient staff and (2) the team continues its work after treatment in the hospital has ended.

As this approach is applied in every case referred to the hospital or in other crisis situations, it is impossible for the psychiatrist of the clinic or the ward to participate on every team. The psychiatrist should participate in the initial meeting, when decisions on admission are made. If the psychiatrist does not attend this meeting, the team consults with him/her about the decision, and if the psychiatrist, for instance, disagrees with the team about the decision, a new joint meeting is organized at which the psychiatrist and the admission team discuss their different views. If they do not achieve consensus, the psychiatrist makes the decision and team members can offer their opinions.

Similar crisis intervention projects have been reported in England (Martin, Cermignani, & Voineskos, 1985) and in the United States (Langsley, Pittman, Machotka, & Flomenhaft, 1968; Rhine & Mayerson, 1971; Rubinstein, 1972). However, our practice differs in that the hospital staff is involved in the system organizing the treatment from the first day. It is not only family therapists or crisis intervention workers who take part. Such involvement can prevent resistance among other hospital staff (Rubinstein, 1972) and because outpatient crisis intervention staff are also involved, it can also prevent the needless use of hospital beds (Martin et al., 1985). The new element in our work is that family therapy work is not conducted by specific family therapy teams only; rather, all staff members participate in family discussions in treatment meetings.

Our goal in treatment is to create an interaction between the family and the hospital so that the symptom-perpetuating behavior becomes unnecessary. Anderson and Goolishian (1988) have argued that problems are created linguistically by naming some aspect of behavior as a problem, and that this begins to construct the family's behavior. In family therapy a conversational network is created that is partly determined by the naming of the problem. The aim is, through conversation, to give new meanings to the behavior defined as a problem. The conversation (i.e., the construction of a new language) about the problem dissolves the problem-determined system (Anderson & Goolishian, 1988).

In constructing the new language, the treatment meeting has three important functions: (1) to create the space for joint experience by gathering information about the family's life and the events that led to the hospitalization in such a way that all the team members participate in the interviewing; (2) to define relationships within the family, in the ward team (e.g., different opinions about the treatment), and between the family and the team; and (3) to contain difficult feelings the problem may evoke in team members, because by discussing different ideas arising during the conversation, the team can make dangerous issues less dangerous for themselves and for the family (Seikkula & Sutela, 1990). The aim is to improve understanding about the problem and its context. All discussions and decisions are made together simultaneously with the family and within the staff.

We consider that all participants in the meeting have their own truths about the theme under discussion and that every utterance has an equal value in building up a polyphonic truth; we must not aim at one truth or solution but at generating a dialogue between the different voices (Bakhtin, 1985; Seikkula, 1993). The task of the meeting is not to decide which opinion or voice is the right one but, instead, to generate dialogue between the different voices and thus make joint understanding possible.

Andersen (1991, 1992) sees the reflective process as a transition between listening and talking. When talking to a listener we are in outer dialogue; while listening to someone's talk we are in inner dialogue with ourselves, which is the prerequisite for change. Therapeutic conversation creates a place for that kind of reflective process where the participant can proceed with his/her own process. One part of the reflective process is the team's internal discussion, which gives the family members a chance, in their inner dialogue, to see their problematic situation in different way.

At the treatment meeting (where patient, family, team, other authorities, and social network are present) the dialogism and the double- or multivoiced discourse become the coordinating factors of our clinical practice (Seikkula, in press; Seikkula & Sutela, 1990; Seikkula et al., in press). In the context of a conventional systemic family therapy session monological discourses often occur because the therapy team defines the actual context and the actual subjects—the family is an entity that is the object of the therapeutic action. The treatment meeting differs linguistically from that kind of situation because both (or all the) parts accommodate their own behavior to the behavior of the other part. The monological aspects of the discourse are not so much in focus because the interaction of the participants is always based on what was previously expressed by one participant. In the treatment meeting, one participant coordinates its action according to the answer of another, and thus the conversation at the meeting becomes open and endless. The team does not plan the themes of the discussion or the way of acting in advance without the family but in the actual situation and driven by the "pressure" of the family.

The reflective idea has been put into practice in training and in consultation situations by organizing the audience into different voices of the treatment system. For instance, our family therapy training program is made up of seven person groups, one or two members taking care of the discussion with the clients and the rest of the group divided into "voices"; one voice listens to the dialogue within the voice of the mother, the other one within the voice of the child, the third one within the voice of the team member, and so on. With bigger audiences in consultation situations, small groups are generated, representing each important voice of the system. After the team–client dialogue the trainer/consultant begins the discussion with the audience voices by soliciting each one's perspective on the discussion previously heard. In the last phase, discussion is allowed between these audience voices. This kind of consultation is also used when there are no clients present. The consultant initially inquires about the persons in the story the consultee is going to tell and then divides the audience into small groups representing each of these voices. The audience listens to the story silently and afterwards the consultant asks for their ideas. Often these different voices are such new perspectives for the consultee that no conclusions by the consultant are needed. Instead, the discussion and listening to the different voices help the situation to become unstuck.

LIVING IN COEVOLUTION

Because everything lives in coevolution with the patient and his/her network, the team is only a part of the new story. In some cases this means that there is no recovery at all, in some cases it seems impossible to construct new, more secure conversation. Frequently in these cases the conversation is so unclear and confusing that it is impossible for the team to construct a reflecting language that could open new perspectives (see the case discussed next). In the coevolving process the team becomes entangled with the family's functional structure and the same story continues. In Seikkula's (1991) study he noticed that if the coevolving process did not start well at the first treatment meeting, it was difficult to change in the course of the treatment.

The therapeutic process happens in discussion that often seems to be very ordinary daily conversation. The following sequence consists of first comments in a first-episode psychotic case. The patient is 22-year-old Sakari, who contacted the mental health outpatient clinic on Monday morning. This meeting took place the same afternoon. Sakari is alone and the team consists of two nurses and a psychiatrist.

NURSE 1: Where should we start?

SAKARI: The whole . . . I can't really remember anything.

NURSE 2: Has it been that you can't really remember anything for a long time now?

S: Well . . . I don't know if it has been that way since midsummer. I do remember whether I've been in contact with someone. . . . But then when I leave my place, I don't know if I was even there, only suddenly come into sight and find myself here and so . . .

N2: With whom are you living?

S: I've been living by myself but now I've gone to my parents'.

. . .

N1: Whose idea was it that you came here?

S: Well . . . mother's.

N2: And what was mother worried about?

S: I don't know if I've been talking with her. I can't remember really anything. I have a feeling that I have even hit someone, but I can't even remember.

N2: Has someone said that to you?

S: No . . . I am paranoid and one thinks that something has happened.

N2: What about father? Is he worried about some specific issue?

S: I don't know but yesterday evening when we were looking at TV he went to bed and in the morning he had gone to his job.

N2: And what was the situation then?

S: I was afraid, I was quarreling well with that type of guy. They have a key into my place and them. . . . They were fucking the asshole on July and did all this kind of things.

N2: In July?

The discussion begins with Sakari's comment and the team continues his theme, the team members adapt their questions to Sakari's utterances. Instead of having some specific method for interviewing—

circular questioning, for instance—the team strives to catch Sakari's experience in his terms. The space for joint experience is under construction. It is important to start every discussion with the client's words in order to have the client's experience as the basis of the dialogue. In our working style there seems to be, on some occasions, a danger that the team's inner reality captures the discussion and creates a reality of its own, which does not include the patient's experience.

Sakari's case is also a good example of coevolution, of how the patient's and his family's language begins to live within the treatment team. Sakari's story becomes more and more violent and simultaneously the structure of the sentences dissolves, which can be seen as a sign of Sakari's overwhelming fear and confusion. In the beginning the team asked very concrete questions about Sakari's life and the story was coherent and understandable. As the interview progresses, the story becomes more and more threatening and psychotic and the team's confusion grows in the course of discussion. One way to gain control of the situation could be the team's internal reflective discussion, but Sakari's way of describing his terrible experiences seems to inhibit this. Each one acts independently from the others, which leads to a situation in which Sakari is dominating the conversation. As Luckmann (1990) and Linell (1990) have noted, the patient can gain the initiative in conversation by telling such strange stories that the nurse or the doctor has to listen to him.

At the end of the admission meeting it was agreed that the next meeting would take place at Sakari's home, where his parents and his sister would be present. This session was like a continuation from the first interview. Both mother and father had an opportunity to tell their stories about Sakari's problem. These stories, however, were more like descriptions about some story that did not concern them; no emotions were present. It was a story about how to handle Sakari's problem and not about belonging together and suffering together. In coevolution, as mentioned above, this often means that the team will have difficulty in constructing a deliberating and reflecting atmosphere in discussion. This seemed to happen here. The team did not discuss and define anything with each other.

The treatment process began with closely spaced meetings. Sakari calmed down in the beginning so that he stopped speaking about his fears; however, at the same time he also stopped leaving his home and little by little began to keep himself apart from his friends and others. In the course of treatment, the family's problems rapidly emerged. Father left his family, as they tell it, "for Sakari's sake." Slowly the family began to hint about the father's drinking problem, which had not, up to this point, come into the open. After a half year's treatment, the process was stuck so that referring Sakari to the hospital was seen as the only alternative. After a one-week period in hospital, a treatment meeting was organized at which the family, the treatment team, and the ward team were present. At the end of the meeting a discussion began about the difficult situation of both the family and the treatment.

After this long meeting, it was agreed to have a new meeting the next day. The discussion was now dialogical, with joint understanding being constructed together. When someone said something, he/she formulated the utterance so that a response was necessary; without the response, the dialogue could not proceed. This is the definition of the dialogical utterance (Bakhtin, 1981; Lacan, 1981). However, the interaction within the family was so difficult that even within this dialogue permanent solutions to the problem could not be found. It was not possible to bring the conflicts into the open through discussion. The only alternative was for the father to leave home.

Patterson (1988), in comparing the ideas of Bakhtin and Levinas, has stated that dialogue includes the risk of vulnerability, because one's own utterances are open to the other's comments. During the course of a dialogue the speaker, in a way, takes off his/her clothes and is naked while waiting for the interlocutors to do the same. Both parties need each other, as they create the context and content talked about. While listening to the reflective discussion between team members the others have a possibility within their inner dialogue to consider the danger of the subject. As Bakhtin (1981) stated the spoken issues become dialogical when they are personified in such a way as happened here.

Sakari went home but returned to the hospital very soon because his fears and stories had become even more furious. For instance, he described how Manfred Vörner's (Secretary General of NATO) agents are after him and that two nuclear warheads are directed toward the hospital from northern Norway and most of the people outside the hospital have been killed.

At the ward we had a lot of discussion with Sakari about his fears. However, these discussions did not calm him but, instead, got him more agitated so that one day he assaulted a doctor on the ward corridor. Sakari said that this doctor was a Russian agent who wanted to kill him. During the two-and-a-half-month period that he stayed in the hospital Sakari began to calm down a little, but he still spoke a lot about his fears. He also began taking a neuroleptic medication, which did not, however, have any rapid effect on his fears. Sakari continued talking about powerful external threats. The family discussions were continued and father began to talk about his drinking problem. He became very depressed and began to talk about suicide. After this episode the family's situation began to improve so that the parents decided to buy a larger residence in order to move back together and have Sakari at home. Sakari was discharged from the hospital and at this phase the first noticeable movement toward a more secure reality occurred. Sakari rapidly began to calm down and to visit his friends. During the following months, he talked about his fears every now and then and visited the hospital for a two-week period after a big quarrel with his parents and younger sister. Two years after the outset of treatment, Sakari is living at home with his family without noticeable psychotic ideations. The family discussions continue.

As a summary, the nature of this coevolving process and the quality of the participants in it can be described. Both Sakari and his family began the discussions in a very neutral or cold manner so that there was no anxiety present even if they discussed terrible fears. This became more understandable when the very conflictual situation within the family, and especially between the parents, was openly defined. This also made the team's disengaged way of working more understandable; with a disengaged family it often is impossible to construct lively reflective discussion because it is too unusual for the system. The reflective, open discussion became possible only after a six-month treatment process. It was important to take into account all the issues within the family, not only Sakari's problems.

NEW VIEW ABOUT PSYCHOSIS; NEW VIEW ABOUT PSYCHIATRY

"On the boundary"—between the team, the patient, and the family—a unique process is formed in the treatment of every case. The crucial skill of the treatment team becomes its ability to generate dialogue between the different parts (or voices) so that the potential resources of the patient and his/her nearest social network are utilized. Different opinions about psychosis and different therapy methods are voices of the treatment process and these voices are stressed in each process according to the needs of the particular case.

The patient and his/her family bring their own way of interacting according to their own structure (Seikkula, 1991) and this system begins to exist within the boundary system between the treatment team and the family. In this context, psychotic problems can be seen as a varying way of behaving in each treatment process that begins to live on the boundary and, in that way also, within the dialogue and behavior of the treatment team. Psychosis is no longer seen as some independent quality in the patient but as one voice of the therapeutic interaction taking place at the moment.

Volosvinov (1973) describes the relationship between the form of language and social context. Each sign, as well as each meaning of each sign, is formed in social organizations of human interaction, which means that each social organization creates its own language in its own special context. All patients bring with them their own way of acting in therapeutic conversation, and this type of discussion can be understood as functional rules controlling the way of acting at the beginning of conversation in each special situation.

In treatment meetings (Alanen, 1993; Seikkula & Sutela, 1990; Seikkula et al., in press) the treatment system and the patient's system begin to coevolve, a process that creates a new mutual system across the boundary between them ("system of boundary"); a system from which the stories creating joint understanding derive their meaning. When the patient acts according to his/her functional rules, his/her psychotic experiences also begin to exist in this coevolving system. The nature of the coevolving dialogue determines whether the patient needs psychotic stories, as the terror that causes psychotic behavior is always embedded in the actual conversation. If the patient answers psychotically, the conversation about these themes is at the moment too dangerous for him/her. The "reason" for psychosis can be understood in the present interaction rather than in the analysis of past experiences. Because the team can only change its own behavior, it can (e.g., by reflectively discussing with each other) construct new language that makes the world more secure for the patient and for his/her social network. A Finnish newspaper, *Helsingin Sanomat,* interviewed one patient about her first psychotic episode. She was surprised that the team members had little interest in her childhood but, instead, focused on present issues in her life and in her family's life.

Because growth of understanding goes hand in hand with dialogical conversation (Bakhtin, 1981; Volosvinov, 1973), the most important skill of the treatment team is its ability to generate dialogue. Research (Seikkula, 1991) indicated that the team's understanding grew on the basis of the amount of the team's internal reflective discussion, not so much on the basis of the knowledge that was gathered by interviewing. In conversation, the problem-defining stories of the patient and the family begin their existence in relation to the treatment team, which shares these stories. The team coordinates its own behavior to each process so that coevolution becomes possible.

Beginning with the admission meeting, the quality of the coevolving process between the team and the family determines the treatment (Seikkula, 1991). The best way of coordinating team behavior with family behavior seems to be reflective discussion within the team. In this reflective discussion the integration between the family's psychotic story and the team's professional ability can begin.

THE STUDY OF ACUTE PSYCHOSIS IN THE NEW TREATMENT SYSTEM

Some studies (Keränen, 1992; Pattison & Pattison, 1981; Seikkula, 1991) have noted that the psychotic problem is not the same after the first hospital visit. The Finnish national project IATAP (the Integrated Approach to the Treatment of Acute Psychosis) consists of first-episode psychotic patients who have not had any psychotherapeutic treatment or medication before this contact. This project has made it possible to follow the coevolution of psychotic behavior with the treatment system when there have been no prior contacts.

IATAP has six research centers. In western Lapland—the location of one of the six research centers—the specific task has been to avoid neuroleptic medication in the beginning and to treat most of the cases in outpatient settings. Table 3.1 describes the IATAP material from a follow-up period of two years.

Of 30 cases seen, a great majority were treated in an outpatient setting, and only 9 of them had more than 31 hospital days. Nine of the cases were in the hospital for some time (between 1 and 30 days), which often means that referral was nonvoluntary referral or there was a need to guarantee safety for both the patient and his/her family during some critical days of the crisis. Over one third have had no hospital contact at all.

During a two-year period, the treatment was completed in 20 cases; in three cases there have been relapses, thus the true number of completed cases is 17. In the rest of the cases treatment continues. These cases can be seen as the most difficult. Neuroleptic medication was used in nine cases. In six of these the medication has been discontinued. Thus, neuroleptic medication was avoided in most cases, and if it was used, on

TABLE 3.1. First-Episode Psychotic Patients (4/1/92)

		Medication				
Inpatient days	Number of patients	Antidepressant	(D.)	Neuroleptics	(D.)	Treatment completed
0	12			2	2	11
1–10	6	2	1			6
11–30	3			1	1	2
> 31	9	2	2	6	3	1
Total	30					17[a]

Note. Follow-up period 2 years. D. = Medication discontinued.
[a]20 completed –3 relapses = 17.

some occasions, it has been possible to stop it. Most of these cases are in the hospital treatment group, which means that neuroleptics have probably been used in the most difficult cases. However, a question arises as to whether medication is too automatically used in an inpatient setting, without enough consideration of other alternatives in the handling of psychotic outbursts. In two of the cases, violent behavior became a problem in the ward and in three cases at the patient's home. In some other cases there was a fear of violence.

At a two-year follow-up of the 30 patients it was found that psychotic symptoms are not present in 20 cases and are mildly present in 7 cases; 3 still have quite severe psychotic problems. The "discussion treatment" used in this study seems to have an effect on the psychotic symptoms, although it is not aimed at a rapid removal of the symptoms from the start. In about half of the cases (in the 17 in which the treatment has been completed) the process was over quite rapidly, but in the rest of the cases the therapeutic process has taken longer. It seems that two or three years of active therapeutic work at treatment meetings with the social network and/or in individual therapy (in some cases) is an adequate approach for this work. Relapses happen—as in the 3 cases of 20 in this material—and in a few cases there is probably a danger for chronicity.

A two-year follow-up interview of Sakari and his family indicates that Sakari is one of the nine cases with more than 31 hospital days and one of the six with neuroleptic medication, which will be discontinued in the near future. He has his own therapist whom he visits every second week. Family meetings take place every second month. Most often the father is absent from these meetings. Sakari is viewed as one of the most challenging and difficult cases in the research project.

In the follow-up interview, his mother said that she felt supported and relieved during the first half year's treatment at home. The father said that he had suggested some more radical procedures to the team but the team did not listen to him. Sakari did like the home treatment more than hospitalization, but now, in hindsight, he considers the hospitalization necessary. When asked why his father is often absent from the discussions, his mother says that they have such different attitudes that the father does not like to participate in the meetings. The father says that he feels uncomfortable in the discussions, but he has decided to participate more in the future. They all are optimistic. Sakari is seeking a job, has a girlfriend, and has not been frightened for a year.

The preliminary results of the new project illustrate the dramatic change in the whole psychiatric inpatient and outpatient organization in western Lapland. Whereas the traditional psychiatric treatment emphasized controlling psychotic behavior and rapidly removing psychotic symptoms by means of medication, the new system of "discussion treatment" emphasizes working together with the patient and his/her social network. The need for hospitalization and the number of "chronic patients" has decreased, according to official Finnish state statistics.

CONCLUSION

The fact that our team has had the same members for many years allowed us to experience a profound reorganization of our way of working. Most of us have experienced both the old, controlling psychiatric treatment as well as this new one. Since the reorganization of the work started, there seems to have been no end to the changes; the process itself seems to determine the new outcomes and our task is to adapt continuously to the new situations. The more we can trust in the power of open dialogical discussion with the patient and his/her social network the less we need controlling interventions. For instance, when the new project with acute psychotic patients was started, we thought that at least a short hospitalization would be needed in almost every case, that at least one third of the cases were going to be chronic, and that about half or more of the cases would need neuroleptic medication. But none of this has been true. We continually have had to accept new basic assumptions for our work. It has become increasingly important to reflect on our own position within the treatment system and within the coevolving system in which we are only partly subjects of the whole process. The resistance for changing has not been in the family or in the patient but, rather, in our way of organizing our own thinking.

Although we are very enthusiastic about this new system, it is not psychiatric utopia. There still are many problems and failures in the treatment process and probably there always will be. However, in analyzing these failures we have learned to concentrate most on our own behavior rather than on the patient's behavior or on the family's qualities. This presupposes open dialogue.

REFERENCES

Alanen, Y. (1993). *Skitsofrenia: Syyt ja tarpeenmukainen hoito.* Juva: Wsoy.

Andersen, T. (Ed.). (1991). *The reflecting team: Dialogues and dialogues about the dialogues.* New York: Norton.

Andersen, T. (1992). Relationship, language and pre-understanding in the reflecting processes. *Australian and New Zealand Journal of Family Therapy, 13,* 87–91.

Anderson, H., & Goolishian, H. (1988). A view of human systems as linguistic systems: Some preliminary and evolving ideas about the implications for clinical theory. *Family Process, 27,* 371–393.

Bakhtin, M. (1981). *The dialogic imagination* (M. Holquist, Ed.). Austin: University of Texas Press.

Bakhtin, M. (1985). *Problems of Dostojevskij's poetics.* In K. Hirschkop (Ed.), *Theory and history of literature* (Vol. 8). Manchester, England: Manchester University Press.

Hirschkop, K. (1986). A response to the forum on Mikhail Bakhtin. In G. Morson (Ed.), *Bakhtin: Essays and dialogues on his work.* Chicago: University of Chicago Press.

Keränen, J. (1992). The choice between outpatient and inpatient treatment in a family centred psychiatric treatment system [Summary]. *Jyväskylä Studies in Education, Psychology and Social Research, 93.*

Lacan, J. (1981). *Speech and language in psychoanalysis.* Baltimore & London: John Hopkins University Press.

Langsley, D., Pittman III, S., Machotka, P., & Flomenhaft, K. (1968). Family crisis therapy—Results and implications. *Family Process, 7,* 145–158.

Linell, P. (1990). The power of dialogue dynamics. In I. Markova & K. Foppa (Eds.), *The dynamics of dialogue.* London: Harvester.

Luckmann, T. (1990). Social communication, dialogue and conversation. In I. Markova & K. Foppa (Eds.), *The dynamics of dialogue.* London: Harvester.

Markova, I. (1990). A three-step process as a unit of analysis in dialogue. In I. Markova & K. Foppa (Eds.) *The dynamics of dialogue.* London: Harvester.

Martin, B., Cermignani, P., & Voineskos, G. (1985). A short-stay ward in a psychiatric hospital: Effects on the hospital caseload. *British Journal of Psychiatry, 147,* 82–87.

Patterson, D. (1988). *Literature and spirit: Essays on Bakhtin and his contemporaries.* Kentucky: University Press of Kentucky.

Pattison, E., & Pattison, M. (1981). Analysis of a schizophrenic psychosocial network. *Schizophrenia Bulletin, 7,* 135–143.

Rhine, M., & Mayerson, P. (1971). Crisis hospitalization within a psychiatric emergency service. *American Journal of Psychiatry, 127,* 1386–1391.

Rubinstein, D. (1972). Rehospitalization versus family crisis intervention. *American Journal of Psychiatry, 129,* 715–720.

Seikkula, J. (1991). Family–hospital boundary system in the social network [English summary]. *Jyväskylä Studies in Education, Psychology and Social Research, 80.*

Seikkula, J. (1993). The aim of therapy is generating dialogue: Bakhtin and Vygotsky in family session. *Human Systems Journal, 4,* 33–48.

Seikkula, J. (1994). When the boundary opens: Family and hospital in co-evolution. *Journal of Family Therapy, 16,* 401–414.

Seikkula, J. (in press). From monologue to dialogue in consultation with larger systems. *Human Systems Journal.*

Seikkula, J., Aaltonen, J., Alakare, B., Haarakangas, K., Keränen, J., & Sutela, M.

(in press). Living in co-evolution: From family therapy to treatment meetings. *Journal of Systemic Therapies.*
Seikkula, J., & Sutela, M. (1990). Coevolution of the family and the hospital: The system of boundary. *Journal of Strategic and Systemic Therapies, 9,* 34–42.
Volosvinov, V. (1973). *Marxism and the philosophy of the language.* New York: Seminar Press.
Vuorio, K., Räkköläinen, V., Syvälahti, E., Hietala, Aaltonen, J., Katajamäki, J., & Lehtinen, V. (1993). Akuutiin psykoosin integroitu hoito. II: Uusien skitsofrenniaryhmän psykoositapausten ennuste ja hoitoa ohjaavat kliinisest tekijät. *Suomen Lääkärilehti, 48,* 582–588.
Vygotsky, L. (1970). *Thought and language.* Cambridge, MA: MIT Press.

CHAPTER 4

When Patients Somatize and Clinicians Stigmatize

OPENING DIALOGUE BETWEEN CLINICIANS AND THE MEDICALLY MARGINALIZED

James L. Griffith
Melissa Elliott Griffith

"YOU DON'T KNOW what it is like for a doctor not to return your phone calls, then to pretend like his staff didn't give him the messages. . . . If the disease doesn't kill you, that will. I feel like a stepchild."

These words, spoken by a woman with chronic pain whose frequent consultations with physicians had brought little relief, are typical for many patients whose bodily symptoms cannot be explained by modern medicine. During the years of our work with those labeled in the medical system "somatizers," we eventually concluded that the problems from which they most suffer are to a great extent the same as those of other persons and populations that are marginalized within the culture in which they live.

A woman married to an anxious patient who had an unusual tremor said with exasperation, "It finally dawned on me that his doctor thought he couldn't function on the job because we had family problems. Any family problems we have are from living with an illness and not knowing whether it will ever get better, or whether he will be able to keep his job, or whether we will be able to pay the note on our house." Such patients and their families feel that they do not belong to the health care community on which they are vitally dependent. Sensing that their concerns and protests are invalidated, they fear being extruded from our medical care system by a referral to a mental health clinician for a bodily illness that is "all in your head." For this reason, many alienated patients and families angrily refuse to meet with mental health clinicians when referred by their physicians. This is the dilemma often faced by clinicians such as us, located in general hospitals and teaching hospitals where we are consulted to evaluate patients and families considered by medical, surgical, and nursing colleagues to be "resistant," "hysterical," "treatment failures," "help-rejecting complainers," "addicted to a sick role," "drug seeking," or "personality-disordered." So the mental health team enters, accountable to but often uninvited by the patient and family, accountable to but often constrained by the perspective of a referring colleague, and facing a complex and puzzling symptom. Thus, it can be tempting for these team members to close their own circle defensively by talking among themselves, pathologizing the patient or family, and widening the gulf between team members and the patient with their family even before the relationship has begun.

We have struggled with many of these dilemmas over the last 11 years, but the way we deal with them changed significantly in 1988, when we encountered the work of Tom Andersen and his Norwegian colleagues (Andersen, 1987, 1991, 1992). Their open, democratic approach, operationalized in the reflecting team, provided a structure for communication that could enable dialogue even when the conversational participants felt embattled, humiliated, unheard, or devalued. Since that time, our clinical work, supported by research data, suggests that a reflecting team consultation can open a fruitful dialogue between clinicians and medically marginalized persons who have been labeled "somatizers" (Griffith & Griffith, 1992a; Griffith, Griffith, & Slovik, 1990; Griffith et al., 1992).

THE PROBLEM OF SOMATIZATION

Contemporary medicine considers a somatizer to be a person who presents a bodily symptom for which there is, in the clinician's judgment, insufficient medical evidence to account for either its occurrence or its severity. In the psychiatric nomenclature, those patients with headaches, backaches, seizures, vomiting, gynecological complaints, weakness, or dizziness are categorized, largely out of a psychoanalytical tradition, into somatoform disorders (those whose bodily symptoms are thought to be produced by unconscious mechanisms), factitious disorders (those who fabricate the appearance of medical illness but whose motivation for doing so is considered to be unconscious), and malingering disorders (those who with full awareness fabricate the appearance of illness for gain, such as money or drugs) (American Psychiatric Association, 1994). Somatization is considered to be a serious problem in our health care system because of the suffering it brings to patients and families, the frustration it brings to health care providers, and the wasted health care dollars spent on unneeded medical treatments (Griffith & Griffith, 1994).

Some of the most troubling forms of somatization are "by proxy," in which a parent repeatedly brings a child to a physician for treatment of medical symptoms even though medical investigations repeatedly fail to show evidence of disease within the child's body (Griffith, 1988; Meadow, 1982, 1985; Schreier & Libow, 1993). In severe cases of somatization by proxy, it may be discovered that a parent has been fabricating the appearance of illness by contaminating laboratory specimens or surreptitiously giving drugs to the child. In less severe cases, somatization by proxy is termed "doctor shopping," in which a parent, acting on a conviction that a child has an untreated or undiagnosed illness, takes the child from one physician's office to another, even though each sequential medical investigation fails to show concrete evidence of disease (Woolicott, Aceto, Rutt, Bloom, & Glick, 1982).

There is compelling evidence that a pattern of somatization by proxy is destructive for many of the children involved. Among the severe cases, children have been harmed or killed by parent-induced illnesses or inappropriate diagnostic tests and treatments. In other cases, children continued to live an invalid lifestyle through adulthood, despite an absence of medical disease (Meadow, 1982, 1985; Schreier & Libow, 1993). The harmful effects of somatization by proxy on the mother are almost never acknowledged. The parent most often involved, her life has been largely undeveloped due to her commitment to get medical attention for her child. Somatization by proxy is poorly understood and difficult to recognize in our fragmented health care system and even more difficult to treat with the psychiatric and psychotherapeutic methods currently available.

A CULTURAL UNDERSTANDING OF SOMATIZATION

Although the dominant medical perspective views somatization as the expression of an individual's psychopathology, cultural anthropology offers a different perspective that holds more therapeutic possibilities (Kirmayer, 1984, 1989; Kleinman, 1977, 1986). Based on cross-cultural studies, Kirmayer (1989) argued that personal distress is always manifested simultaneously in both verbal and bodily expressions. But cultural practices and other social forces can effectively silence verbal expression, leaving the bodily expression as visible evidence of distress. Kleinman (1986), for example, showed how neurasthenia, a disorder of generalized weakness and fatigue, was frequently diagnosed in China during the oppression of the Cultural Revolution, when speaking about one's experience of distress was physically dangerous. As such, somatization is a bodily idiom of distress, a language of the body that dominates when talking is forbidden or unsafe (Griffith & Griffith, 1994; Kirmayer, 1989).

This understanding shifts attention from the psyche of the patient to a surrounding social context that suppresses talking about personal distress. In our clinical work, we assume that a bodily symptom in the absence of disease is a signal of hidden distress. By the same token, our attention in somatization by proxy is shifted from the psyche of the perpetrating parent to the hidden systemic distress. We assume that the parent is bound in an unspeakable dilemma and the kind of conversation needed to resolve it cannot take place. However, we can learn about the dilemmas in which our patients and families are bound only if there is a situation safe and comfortable enough for dialogue about matters that are too frightening, embarrassing, or guilt producing to be discussed in ordinary conversation (Griffith & Griffith, 1994).

THE CONTEXT OF OUR CLINICAL WORK

From 1985 through 1994 our setting was the University of Mississippi Medical Center, a tertiary care medical center organized as a teaching hospital for the state medical school. The medical director, psychiatry resident, psychiatric nursing specialist, social worker, and family therapist for an inpatient Behavioral Medicine Unit worked together as a family therapy team conducting reflecting team consultations from 1988–1993. Consultations were made for patients admitted to the Behavioral Medicine Unit; to related psychiatric services, such as the Inpatient Psychiatric Unit and the Sleep Disorders Laboratory; and to the hospital medical and surgical services. The team had a unique structure due to the dual roles of several of its members, who were often related to the same patients through traditional hospital medical, psychiatric, nursing, and social worker roles, as well as members of the systemic family consultation team. Hence, the content of their reflecting team conversations were often drawn both from observations in the therapy session and from the whole of their daily contact with the patient and family members.

During these years, there was ongoing collaboration between our program and clinicians working with reflecting teams at the University of Tromsö in Norway. Consequently, our clinical model closely followed the structure originally described by Andersen (1987, 1991, 1992). In practice, the forms of our reflecting team consultations have included the following: (1) One or more reflecting team members entering the therapy room for a conversation among themselves while the therapist and the family members observe from the reflecting position; (2) one or more reflecting team members entering the therapy room to converse with the therapist while the family members observe from the reflecting position; and (3) the therapist and family switching locations with the reflecting team and then observing the team conversation from the observation room.

Because ours is a training and research program, we have had the economic freedom to experiment with different consultation configurations, employing several therapists within a single session as team members. Due to lack of reimbursement in private practice settings for clinicians other than the primary clinician, we typically employ only a single reflecting consultant in our private practices and often for only the initial session or particular requested consultations. Such consultations have proven so fruitful for establishing a productive frame for the therapy that we have considered their use justified on a regular basis, even though this has often meant reduced reimbursement for each clinician in our fee-for-service system.

Creating a context for conversation about the broader social and family contexts of somatic symptoms is often a daunting task. Through reflecting team consultations, we have been able to initiate therapeutic conversations that might otherwise be slow in developing, or even impossible, as illustrated by the following story of a mother who came to our sleep disorders laboratory with her daughter "doctor shopping" in a pattern of somatization by proxy.

A MOTHER'S SEARCH FOR MEDICAL CARE

Mrs. Hillman called to arrange an appointment for her 15-year-old daughter, Jane, in our Sleep Disorders Center. Jane, she said, had been so sleepy throughout the day that she could not get her school work completed. Mrs. Hillman had read about sleep apnea in a health magazine and worried that Jane might be showing its symptoms.

Due mainly to Mrs. Hillman's description of symptoms, the lab had conducted a polysomnogram, an examination in which many physiological measurements—the electroencephelogram, heart rate, blood oxygen, muscle tension—are made while the patient sleeps. The findings appeared definitively to rule out a sleep disorder as a diagnosis. But the laboratory clinicians were concerned about what they learned during their contact with Jane and her mother.

During the diagnostic evaluation, Jane was nearly noncommunicative. Mrs. Hillman described her daughter as a homebound invalid with rheumatoid arthritis and a number of other health problems requiring regular, intensive medical care. But medical records obtained from Jane's physicians did not fit this story. The physicians were skeptical whether Jane had rheumatoid arthritis. It appeared that they agreed to see Jane so frequently because they worried about her emotional well being as an isolated, homebound teenager with her divorced mother. Evidently, it was her mother's conviction that Jane was ill, not Jane's complaints of illness, that fueled their intense involvement with doctors.

When clinicians at the Sleep Disorders Center reported their findings to Jane and her mother, Jane seemed detached and unconcerned. Mrs. Hillman seemed more worried than before, stating her certainty that something was the matter with Jane, whether or not their tests could show it. Concerned about this interaction, the clinicians asked Mrs. Hillman and Jane to return the next week to meet with the family consultation team.

During the family consultation, a family therapist, Lu Ann Fischer-Bross, interviewed Mrs. Hillman and Jane, while the team members observed the interview by closed-circuit television from an adjacent room. A reflecting team consultation was conducted after the first half hour of conversation between Lu Ann and the family. Ten-minute transcripts of the interview immediately before and after the consultation show its impact on the therapeutic process of the session. As the session began, Mrs. Hillman repeated the story of her concern about her daughter's possible apnea, while Jane sat silently. After listening respectfully until she finished, Lu Ann sought to expand the conversation to include the broader family and social contexts of Jane's symptoms:

MRS. HILLMAN: It just seems there are more and more problems all the time. Every time we take her to see a different doctor, they find new things wrong with her.

LU ANN: Could you tell me the rest of Jane's medical story? Starting from the beginning?

MRS. HILLMAN: Well, when she was a small baby . . . up until she was about five years old, she had pneumonia. And I tried to take care of her and keep her warm and everything. I would take her to work with me in the beauty shop, and I feel like that spray and stuff maybe brought on a lot of it. But then she started hurting. I noticed when I would pick her up, I would try to be real easy with her. If I would change her clothes, she would cry, like it hurt her, you know. I got to where I would carry her on a pillow, and I was taking her to the doctor all the time. And he was telling me there was nothing wrong with her, or that she was just a little sore, or that maybe she had been handled too much. She had these older brothers and sisters. They were like 14, and the twins were 16, and her brother was 17 when she was born. I just got so worried about her. I was taking her to Dr. Jones, and he finally told me he reckoned she had rheumatoid arthritis. We took her to the hospital here and made an X-ray when she was in the sixth or seventh grade. She fell at school—I think she passed out— I got a call from the teachers. It scared the teachers, and they said come to the school house and talk to them. They suggested we put her on the Homebound Program and let her be taught at home. She is not even able to do her work at home right now.

LU ANN: That was in the sixth or seventh grade. Jane is 15 now?

MRS. HILLMAN: She's in the ninth grade this year. But about a month, or six weeks ago, the assistant principal and the school counselor came out. They are aware of what I'm doing with her and come out to check on her. They said as smart as Jane is, it is not going to hurt her to miss a few months of school. With her headaches and all—until she gets her problems straightened out—she can miss school.

LU ANN: What has changed most recently—in the year, or the last couple of months with her school?

MRS. HILLMAN: Her teacher who came out to the house quit and they have not found a replacement for him. I had been picking up her work at school, letting her do it, and taking it back. They said she was doing fine. And then she started having headaches and the trouble with her vision and all. Dr. Jones said he thought she was on the verge of a nervous breakdown, and he put her on Tranxene. She doesn't take them all the time, just when she feels like she needs one. She does hate for me to bring her to the doctors, but I love her and I need to get help for her.

LU ANN: About how many doctors are you visiting now? How many different clinics and how many doctors?

MRS. HILLMAN: There are the ones here at the university, and the ones at the Children's Rehabilitation Clinic. And, of course, if she has a cold, I take her to Dr. Jones.

LU ANN: How has the situation with the school checked out?

MRS. HILLMAN: Well, I have her books back at the house. They said wait and see how Jane feels. And if she feels like doing some work this summer, they will grade it and pass her on. That's what they did last summer. Jane doesn't like me to say this either—she is a real smart child. She started taking computer in the seventh grade, and as they said, smart as she is, she can pick it right up.

LU ANN: What do you think a solution for all this difficulty might be?

MRS. HILLMAN: I thought we might find something that could ease her pain. There is a fine arthritis specialist in Jackson. He suggested one time that we fit her with braces. He wouldn't suggest surgery at her age, and I don't know what else to do for her.

LU ANN: You are looking for answers to a really complicated problem. As a young mother, you took Jane to the doctors many times because you knew something was wrong. The doctors finally told you she had arthritis. She has done exceptionally well for a child with juvenile arthritis. How did you all come through that as a family?

MRS. HILLMAN: I didn't let the girls handle her too much. Her older brother helped with her more than the girls did. We just handled her real easy.

LU ANN: You have always been very protective of her?

MRS. HILLMAN: I don't know. I let her have things and do things like other kids. She had a bike. I let her ride it until the doctor said no more bikes. I let her go onto the playground with the other children. Of course, it made her pain worse. But the doctors said they wanted it that way. It was better to see her hurt a little bit than to give up. She went out last Friday night and Saturday night, but she came in early both nights. She is in a lot of pain today.

JANE: (*sits with arms crossed, silent, looking away*)

LU ANN: I guess it's difficult both to take care of her and to let her grow up normally. It is different being the parent of a young child with medical problems and a child in the teenage years. Jane, are you going out more now in your teenage years?

JANE: (*looks down*)

MRS. HILLMAN: Well, I have always let her go. Her older brothers and sisters always wanted her to go with them a lot. Her brother would take her home for days at a time, and he would keep her until she didn't want to come home.

LU ANN: Who lives in the house now?

MRS. HILLMAN: Just the two of us.

LU ANN: How old are her brothers and sisters now? Do they live near?

MRS. HILLMAN: They all live nearby in Greenwood. My daughter next to her is 25 years old. And the twins are 28 and her brother, 32.

LU ANN: Jane has been a very special child for you.

MRS. HILLMAN: Yes, she really has been good company. We do a lot of things together. I try not to discipline her too much. I'll say, "If you do that again, you'll have to stay home a certain number of days!" (*laughs*) But then I'll give in.

LU ANN: I wonder if our team has any ideas at this point that it would be helpful to hear. Would you like to hear from them?

MRS. HILLMAN: Certainly.

[Mrs. Hillman, Mother, Jane, and Lu Ann move from the therapy room to the observation room, swapping places with the four team members who take their place in the therapy room. The reflecting team members are James (Griff) Griffith, the medical director of the Sleep Disorders Center who is overseeing Jane's care in the hospital; Hodges Martin, the psychiatry resident conducting Jane's sleep disorders evaluation; Jenny Freedle, the clinical social worker from the inpatient unit where Jane was admitted for her evaluation; and Melissa Elliott Griffith, the family therapy coordinator who, until now, had not met Jane. The family and therapist now observe a conversation among the members of the family consultation team.]

GRIFF: One thing I was wondering was whether Jane and Mrs. Hillman feel that they are getting anywhere, or whether they feel like they are running in place.

JENNY: With the sleep disorders evaluation turning out normal, her mother is still very concerned. I was wondering what she is thinking. She still sees a problem. Perhaps she has some thoughts about why it did not show up on the sleep evaluation.

GRIFF: Uh huh. I wondered whether they feel that they are getting answers, or finding solutions. . . . If they aren't then I wonder whether we should try something different, a different kind of solution, another angle on it. I am puzzled, but maybe Jane has some thoughts about what that might consist of.

HODGES: We know from the sleep disorders exam that her brain is normal. But there are lots of reasons why persons can have unusual sleep problems besides neurological problems. Perhaps Jane or her mother might think about what other reasons there might be, and how they fit into the everyday life of the family. For example, it is common for a college student to come home from college depressed and go to bed and sleep 15 hours straight, while her worried parents gnaw their fingernails off to the bone.

GRIFF: That was one thing that I did go over with Jane and Mrs. Hillman earlier. While she was here, Jane did complete a scale for evaluating depression and she scored quite highly on depression.

HODGES: That means what?

GRIFF: Based on Jane's responses in the lab, she had a score that would suggest that she feels quite depressed. Depression is something that can lead to excessive sleepiness.

MELISSA: What strikes me about the idea of depression is that it is a lot like running in place and not getting anywhere. Depression is something that slows you down. If that is the case—that depression is something that slows you down like running in place—what would that mean for Jane? Where would she want to be moving? What is "slowing down?" I read a description someone wrote who said his experience of depression was like "getting shot in my legs so I wanted to run but I couldn't move." So I wondered, if this were to have meaning for Jane, where would she be wanting the movement to be? And if there is movement that Mrs. Hillman wants for her own life, where would that be? And I was struck by the dilemma her mother described: Wanting to let Jane go out on the playground, but knowing she would hurt if she did. And that Jane goes out with her friends, but knowing she will have pain if she does. I wondered how they weigh those decisions about what is worth the pain. They must have felt like playing on the playground was necessary for Jane's development, but . . .

HODGES: How much pain equals how much development?

MELISSA: Yeah. She seems to be willing to have a lot of pain. . . . What do they believe might be the next step developmentally for her, if she weren't slowed down?

JENNY: It must be frustrating too for her mother. As a mother, you want to do for your child when they are not feeling well, and you'll go to almost any lengths—anywhere—to find someone to help your child. And as the child gets older and is a teenager, as Jane is now, she rebels against that—it's natural to rebel. And I can appreciate being tired of all that, although I can also appreciate what it must be like for her mother, obviously trying to keep her child functional. It is a hard dilemma, balancing it out, to where a mother and a daughter are both able to communicate with one another and it won't be so upsetting.

HODGES: Because you do have some chronic pain—headaches and extremity pain. This is a greater problem than you normally have raising teenagers while they are pushing the limits and the parents are saying, "Should I pull them back or let them go?" Here you have an added factor.

GRIFF: Why don't we hear some more of their ideas?

[The reflecting team members rise and walk to the observation room. Lu Ann, Mrs. Hillman, and Jane return to the interview room]

LU ANN: Were there any new ideas you heard expressed by the group, or was there something said in a different way by the group?

MRS. HILLMAN: No, I don't think so. . . . (*pause*) It is just that we both have problems that haven't been touched on today that have more to do with this than just Jane's medical problems. And that may have a lot to do with Jane's depression.

LU ANN: I appreciate your telling me that. . . .

MRS. HILLMAN: No, it's not anything that I mind discussing. It's just that . . . as far as I feel about Jane going out, I let Jane do what she feels. In the afternoons, I had rather that she stay at home, because I don't believe she feels like doing anything. But her friends will come by and want her to go riding. She goes out with Shauna, her best friend, and Shauna's parents love Jane to death.

[Jane still has not spoken, but looks more animated, head up and smiling.]

And I feel like, out there at their house, Jane has the sense of being in a family. They include Jane in their family dinners and everything, and Shauna's daddy—he loves Jane to death, and, well, her mother does too. I have some medical problems. And they have wanted Jane to talk to me and let them have custody of Jane. You know, but (*looks at Jane, and they exchange smiles*) I'm not about to give Jane up!

JANE: (*speaking for the first time*) But they don't think of it nearly as much as Momma does.

LU ANN: When did this idea first come up?

MRS. HILLMAN: Oh, gosh! It's been going on a long time—ever since they first met her. I used to let her spend a lot of time out there—spend the night and everything—but since she's had this sleep problem, I don't like for her to spend the night. I like for her to stay home with me.

LU ANN: You mentioned that you have some medical problems?

MRS. HILLMAN: Yes, I do. She loves going out there, though. And I understand it. It's different at our house, with just the two of us. I know she needs a father image. I tried the remarriage bit. She thought an awful lot of him. . . .

JANE: But not one to live with. . . .

MRS. HILLMAN: I didn't get married for the right reasons. So I couldn't handle it.

JANE: I don't like having more than one parent. I don't like having more than one person telling me what to do. I don't like being told what to do at all (*laughs*). But they said something about depression—you know, I don't stay depressed all the time. A lot maybe, some days all day. But maybe some days, never. Some days I do, you know, when I'm stuck at home and can't get out and go anywhere. Like when me and Momma go shopping or something, it's okay. I just don't like to stay at home.

MRS. HILLMAN: She thinks that sometimes I should go out more, but I don't really care about it. There really is nowhere to go in our town.

JANE: But she has got a lot of friends. She's got more friends than I do. And she's got a car and a driver's license, and I'm not old enough to have my driver's license yet. I don't ever get the car. But still I get to go out and have fun, and she doesn't go out. And then she'll say, "I always have to stay home." So I tell her, "Well, you are feeling sorry for yourself. You stay at home then, but I'm not going to stay at home with you if you are not going to go. Because you've got a car and you can go if you want to." And that's the truth!

MRS. HILLMAN: (*smiles*) But sometimes Jane feels guilty. I tell her not to. I can find somewhere to go if I want to go.

JANE: She thinks she should stay at home, so, in case something happens to me, they can bring me home. But I always know where she's going to be. If she weren't there, I would go where she was. She thinks I am going to get sick and have to come home. She's afraid I might fall down and break a bone, or something. (*laughs*)

MRS. HILLMAN: She has cracked her foot twice since October.

JANE: (*starts to speak, but stops*)

LU ANN: Were there ideas of the team that matched more with some of what you were thinking than other ideas. Because they mentioned several different things.

MRS. HILLMAN: Well, so far as the Sleep Disorders Lab is concerned, I feel a little relieved over the test. . . . But I still wonder, you know, if. . . . We didn't know anything about SIDS [Sudden Infant Death Syndrome] when Jane was a baby, but she would stop breathing on me. But then, after I learned about SIDS, I was sure Jane must have had it, too. I wondered if this could be after-effects of SIDS, or some connection with it.

LU ANN: SIDS is really a childhood disease. Even if she had it as a hereditary problem, she has grown up past the critical age, since an immature neurological system creates the problem. Because she is older than three years of age, she has really grown out of the risk period. Adolescents and adults don't have that kind of sleep disorder. I don't know if that will allay your fears. . . . I can understand that you would be very worried about it.

MRS. HILLMAN: I feel better since these tests have been done.

JANE: (*giggles aloud*)

MRS. HILLMAN: (*looks at Jane and smiles*) But we have other problems right now. We are having financial problems, which I am sure is depressing to Jane. That reminds me, her main concern is getting her driving license in June and getting a car to drive.

JANE: One of my problems is that I am realizing all my friends are older than me. This summer they are going to be moving out and going to college. (*laughs bitterly*) And I don't even have a car yet. I've just started realizing that now, that this school year is over, and they are getting ready to leave.

MRS. HILLMAN: She has occasionally threatened suicide. And that has me concerned.

JANE: (*again exchanges smiles with her mother*) I wouldn't ever do that. You know that.

MRS. HILLMAN: (*smiles and giggles*)

LU ANN: So you are very worried about what they said about depression, and if she might need some other treatment?

MRS. HILLMAN: I think most of her threats are just verbal. . . .

JANE: I don't care what you do to me, just don't put me in Charter Hospital! I've got two friends that came out crazy after they've been up there.

MRS. HILLMAN: The reason I am laughing—I know suicide is no laughing matter, threatened or otherwise—is that I had told her one night that she couldn't go somewhere or something. I told her she should never have gotten that upset over it. She told me later that she had tried to kill herself. She had gotten three different knives. And I had to laugh at that, because, I told her there wasn't a knife in our house sharp enough to cut her wrists! (*laughs*) I told her she would have to take one of those steak knives and saw for a while! It wasn't anything serious.

JANE: That was pretty funny. (*laughs, while rubbing her wrists*)

LU ANN: (*pauses*) I have a dilemma right now myself, not knowing where to go next with the family. There is this sleep lab evaluation that you came for, then there are the things the team brought up and the things you are talking about now. . . . I don't want to force counseling on you.

MRS. HILLMAN: No, if there is something you want to touch on, ask. Because I really don't know what to tell you either. Nothing they said. . . . It was pretty much what I was feeling and thinking about already. But I don't know about Jane.

JANE: What?

MRS. HILLMAN: What they said. What the team talked about while we were in there listening.

JANE: My brain was very tired. Very tired today. I don't remember what was said.

MRS. HILLMAN: Well, you feel relieved over your test results, too, don't you?

JANE: Yes, ma'am.

MRS. HILLMAN: (*to Lu Ann*) So, like I said, if there were any things you want to touch on, go right ahead.

LU ANN: I guess I was wondering about some of the things that go on at home that might help her grow up. If you can do some of the things at age 15 similar to what you did at age 3, having her do whatever she was capable of doing.

MRS. HILLMAN: We've already talked. Jane knows that she needs to see someone for counseling. And she has even said that she would need some private sessions. And that is fine with me. I have told her to tell whatever she feel . . . because nobody is going to be able to help her unless she brings it all out into the open. There might be something that she doesn't even realize is bothering her that somebody trained can find.

LU ANN: So you wouldn't have any objections to working on it together, as a group, the three of us sometimes?

MRS. HILLMAN: Or if she feels like talking to you by herself, I don't mind. I just told her she is going to have to be open and honest about her feelings if anybody is going to be able to help her. We talk about things at home. We have a good relationship. She comes to me with her problems. But it has got to the point where I can't help her anymore. She needs professional . . .

LU ANN: I guess I would need to meet with Jane sometimes alone. I would like to meet with both of you sometimes, and sometimes just you alone. Would that be okay?

JANE: Okay.

MRS. HILLMAN: Whatever you feel is necessary.

OPENING CONVERSATION ABOUT UNSPEAKABLE DILEMMAS

When asked whether the reflecting team had offered any new ideas, Mrs. Hillman responded, "No, I don't think so . . ." but then matter-of-factly related the terrible binds she and Jane lived within—the threat of another family "adopting" Jane, the loneliness of Mrs. Hillman's envisioned future without Jane, Jane's isolation after her friends leave for college, financial problems, and Jane's depression and suicide threats. It is quite possible that Mrs. Hillman's statement was literally true, that she had considered all the perspectives and ideas offered by the reflecting team but that there had been no suitable place—including her physicians' offices—where they could be talked about with safety and discussed without shame.

How did the reflecting team consultation elicit such an immediate shift in the conversation when an empathic, supportive inquiry by a face-to-face therapist had not yet done so? We have regularly noted such therapeutic shifts following reflecting team consultations with patients and families presenting somatic symptoms (Griffith & Griffith, 1992a; Griffith, Griffith, & Slovik, 1990). These clinical observations are supported by our empirical study of patients referred for psychiatric evaluation of a somatic symptom. We utilized the Structural Analysis of Social Behavior, a well-validated system for the research coding of communications, to code family communications 10 minutes before and 10 minutes after a reflecting team consultation during initial family interviews. Family communications coded as "loving and approaching" significantly increased, as communications coded "watching and controlling" and "belittling and blaming" significantly decreased (Griffith et al., 1992).

With Mrs. Hillman and Jane, there were two therapeutic outcomes that we consider related, at least in part, to the reflecting team. The first occurred within the process of the session: greater openness about relationship issues that might be perpetuating the medical consultations, more vocal involvement by Jane, and greater comfort in the conversation indicated by the warm laughter and smiles of both mother and daughter.

The second outcome was that Mrs. Hillman and Jane chose to return to work in therapy with Lu Ann for a series of sessions focused on the relationship issues broached in this initial session. Although their involvement with doctors did not cease, it did decrease when they had having a place where their concerns reliably would be heard and carefully considered, a move toward integration rather than fragmentation of their health care.

There are a number of explanations that can be offered as to why a reflecting team consultation can have such effects. In our understanding of our work, we highlight two aspects of the reflecting process that we consider critical for its usefulness in our work contexts: how the reflecting position creates a physiological readiness to perceive the world in a different way, and how the reflecting process deconstructs professional knowledge in a way that rebalances power relations between the clinicians and the patients with their families.

THE REFLECTING POSITION AND EMBODIED KNOWLEDGE

Biologically, emotions represent a bodily predisposition for action. With fear, the body is readied to flee; with anger, the body is readied to attack; with shame the body is readied to hide. Each readiness consists of shifts in the distribution of blood flow between muscles and internal organs, in heart rate and blood pressure, in the glucose level in the blood, in release of stress hormones, and in many other physiological changes that reconfigure the body so it can move quickly and efficiently along the anticipated path of action. Concomitantly, there are shifts in cognition. Attention is focused so it can be maximally vigilant for signals of threat (fear), of provocation (anger), of scorn (shame). Behavioral repertoires are readied for rapid response to signals of threat (Griffith & Griffith, 1992b, 1994).

We term these integrated configurations of body readiness and cognitive readiness for action as "emotional postures" (Griffith & Griffith, 1994). The kind of physiological and cognitive mobilization to defend or attack that occurs with emotional postures of fear, anger, and shame preclude the kind of creative reflection needed to find novel solutions for intractable problems. However, there are emotional postures of tranquility, such as listening, playing, grooming, musing, and daydreaming, in which vigilance to threat is low, attention is inwardly focused, and the body rests in physiological quietude. Effective work in therapy usually occurs only during emotional postures of tranquility. The trick for a therapist is how to foster emotional postures of tranquility, rather than mobilization (Griffith & Griffith, 1992b, 1994).

Cross-culturally, a look into the face of the other heightens the emotional intensity of the encounter (Kirmayer, 1991). In some contexts, such as love making, this meeting of gazes amplifies tenderness and passion. But when there is a potential threat and the nature of the encounter is ambiguous, the meeting of gazes may place each of the parties on guard. For example, British soldiers marching through hostile territory during their colonial era followed the Dragoon Rule not to look directly into the eyes of local citizens lest the look be taken as either a challenge or a threat. We intuitively expect face-to-face conversations to be different from those in which we listen in from the side, as indicated by the often stated wish, "If I could only be a fly on the wall. . . ." Philosopher Emma Fiumara (1990) has noted the difference between face-to-face listening and listening from the side: "The bewitchment of authoritative voices appears to persist as long as they address us directly. . . . When the voice 'speaks' to someone else and we perceive the interaction [from the side], an inner awakening recreates a critical distance" (p. 58). Similarly, Mrs. Hillman and Jane had been given the same findings from the sleep disorder and depression evaluations in a face-to-face encounter with their clinicians. But they heard it differently and experienced relief only upon hearing it, from the same clinicians, from a reflecting position.

Due to stigma associated with somatization in medical settings, patients and family members typically reside in emotional postures of mobilization during clinical investigations. We propose that a reflecting team conversation effects openness and trust in dialogue largely because it structures a social encounter in which its participants can listen in freedom from the bodily mobilization that is so easily amplified by face-to-face conversation (Griffith & Griffith, 1994).

THE REFLECTING TEAM AND THE POLITICS OF THERAPY

Traditionally, a clinical team, including the therapist, would have met without the patient or family members in a separate conference room, pooling their data and puzzling over the data until a unified conclusion was reached that could be delivered to the patient and family. The delivery of the recommendations, usually by the psychiatrist team leader, typically would be conducted from a stance of authority, all the more so for the consensus reached among the experts on the team.

But with Mrs. Hillman and Jane, the clinicians puzzled and meandered and spoke of the data but presented them for the family's consideration, not as a conclusion. On the reflecting team, the social worker's voice was heard as clearly as the chief psychiatrist's voice; the women were heard as clearly as the men. There were no major disagreements on this team, but, had there been so, they would have been heard as well. Team members spoke in the same breath of medical and psychological tests and of family and developmental concerns.

Mrs. Hillman and Jane had been accustomed to receiving politely the recommendations from their medical caregivers, often in reassurances such as "Don't worry so much!" Yet their worries had only increased, leading them to make more appointments with more and different doctors. When the puzzling among the experts was conducted in their presence, the process of the clinicians' thinking became clearly visible, deconstructing the professional knowledge and practices. The use of the reflecting position in this sense is in essence a political act whose function is to distribute power among all the different voices in the discourse, dominant and nondominant, among members of the treatment team and between clinicians and patients with their families. The clinician thereby renounces a monopoly that is implicitly conferred by society upon the clinician, as a professional, to dominate the therapeutic discourse exclusively. The gain for the clinician is in the fertile ground that is laid, where the melding of perspectives can bring forth a new reality in which the body of the patient is freed from its binds (Griffith & Griffith, 1994).

REFLECTING TEAMS IN MEDICAL SETTINGS

Mental health professionals increasingly work on interdisciplinary treatment teams and as consultants for primary care clinicians. Usually, however, professional roles have evolved out of traditional medical care models that are hierarchical and tend not to include patients and families in discussions that negotiate how the reality of the clinical problem is to be considered. Such social structures are poorly suited for dealing with problems of somatization, where marginalized patients and families are already sensitized to issues of having a voice in the clinical conversations. Creative employment of reflecting team consultations can provide an important counterbalancing to processes of marginalization, thereby opening new possibilities for therapeutic dialogue.

REFERENCES

American Psychiatric Association. (1994). *Diagnostic and statistical manual of mental disorders* (4th ed.). Washington, DC: Author.

Andersen, T. (1987). The general practitioner and consulting psychiatrist as a team with "stuck" families. *Family Systems Medicine, 5,* 468–481.

Andersen, T. (1991). *The reflecting team: Dialogues and dialogues about the dialogues.* New York: Norton.

Andersen, T. (1992). Reflections on reflecting with families. In S. McNamee & K. J. Gergen (Eds.), *Therapy as social construction*. Newbury Park, CA: Sage.

Fiumara, G. C. (1988). *The other side of language: A philosophy of listening.* New York: Routledge, Chapman & Hall.

Griffith, J. L. (1988). The family systems of Munchausen syndrome by proxy. *Family Process, 27,* 423–437.

Griffith, J. L., & Griffith, M. E. (1992a). Speaking the unspeakable: Use of the reflecting position in systemic therapies for mind-body problems. *Family Systems Medicine, 10,* 41–51.

Griffith, J. L., & Griffith, M. E. (1992b). Owning one's epistemological stance in therapy. *Dulwich Centre Newsletter (Australia), 4,* 5–11.

Griffith, J. L., & Griffith, M. E. (1994). *The body speaks: Therapeutic dialogues for mind/body problems.* New York: Basic Books/HarperCollins.

Griffith, J. L., Griffith, M. E., Krejmas, N., McLain, M., Mittal, D., Rains, J., & Tingle, C. (1992). Reflecting team consultations and their impact upon family therapy for somatic complaints as coded by Structural Analysis of Social Behavior (SASB). *Family Systems Medicine, 10,* 41–51.

Griffith, J. L., Griffith, M. E., & Slovik, L. S. (1990). Mind-body problems in family therapy: Contrasting first-order and second-order cybernetics approaches. *Family Process, 29,* 13–28.

Kirmayer, L. J. (1984). Culture, affect and somatization. *Transcultural Psychiatric Research Review, 21,* 159–188.

Kirmayer, L. J. (1989). Cultural variations in the response to psychiatric disorders and emotional distress. *Social Science and Medicine, 29,* 327–339.

Kirmayer, L. J. (1991). The place of culture in psychiatric nosology: Taijin kyofusho and DSM-III. *Journal of Nervous and Mental Disease, 179,* 19–28.

Kleinman, A. (1977). Depression, somatization and the new cross-cultural psychiatry. *Social Science and Medicine, 11,* 3–10.

Kleinman, A. (1986). *Social origins of distress and disease.* New Haven, CT: Yale University Press.

Meadow, R. (1982). Munchausen syndrome by proxy. *Archives of Diseases in Childhood, 57,* 92–98.

Meadow, R. (1985). Management of Munchausen syndrome by proxy. *Archives of Diseases in Childhood, 60,* 385–393.

Schreier, H. A., & Libow, J. A. (1993). *Hurting for love: Munchausen by proxy syndrome.* New York: Guilford Press.

Woolicott, P., Aceto, T., Rutt, C., Bloom, M., & Glick, R. (1982). Doctor shopping with the child as proxy patient: A variant of child abuse. *Pediatrics, 101,* 297–301.

CHAPTER 5

Reflective and Collaborative Voices in the School

Susan Swim

HISTORICALLY, THERAPY in the school setting has taken place within modernist frameworks that place problem definition, diagnosis, and treatment in pathologizing categories. Such categorizing labels focus on eliminating mental deficiency or illness. This chapter offers my experience with an alternative approach that transcends modernistic views and presents the possibility of a quite different therapeutic stance. This postmodern posture creates room for a collaborative, egalitarian relationship in which the "voices" of the client and related participants (teachers, peers, and parents) join with that of the therapist. The result: a new discourse that generates new meaning and options for change.

In 1984, I began experimenting with a collaborative group format to work with school-age children, defined by the school staff as "emotionally disturbed" with "severe behavioral problems." Due to their "pathology," these children were removed from the mainstream of their peers and placed in self-contained behavioral classrooms. "Sally," an 11-year-old fifth-grader who was placed in such a setting, will be used to exemplify how alternative approaches utilizing the works of Harlene Anderson, Harry Goolishian, and Tom Andersen (Andersen, 1991, 1992, 1993; Anderson, 1993; Anderson & Goolishian, 1992) impact on therapy in the school environment.

My first attempts to utilize a group format to provide therapeutic services incorporated the brief therapy concepts of the Mental Research Institute and the Milan approach, along with the unique style taught at the Galveston Family Institute in the early 1980s. At that time, as it continues today, the primary population I worked with in the schools were children diagnosed with "severe behavioral problems." I put such modernistic terminology in quotations because of the constructed generalized definitions, which in my experience do not adequately define the child or the problem system.

At school these children were viewed as emotionally disturbed, and psychotherapy was seen as ineffective due to the severity of the children's mental deficiencies. The children were placed into self-contained behavior modification classrooms. Prior to my involvement, psychotherapy consisted of seeing each child individually for counseling sessions to diagnose and treat each one in accordance with his/her "individual pathology." Teacher participation was limited and the therapeutic relationship between the teacher and therapist held a history of conflicts. The teacher and therapist, due to unsuccessful outcomes, appeared to diagnose and pathologize each other in their attempts to understand why these children did not improve.

Parental involvement was not utilized due to the perceived "pathology" of the families and the inability to involve the parents in treatment planning. Previous therapeutic interactions postured themselves with hierarchical diagnosis and intervention based on the voices of theoretical paradigms that often ignored or invalidated the voices of the children and parents. Therapeutic intervention was viewed by the participants (teachers, children, and parents) with skepticism and fear of worsening the already difficult contexts.

The goal of my participation with these groups was to create space for voices that had extensive histories of marginalization. I began to have conversations not only with the children, but with other participants in the problem defined system. Teacher, student, and parents began to have conversations with each other. The voices that emerged created a shift from constricting labels and narratives of pessimism, to new dialogues opening options for change.

CURRENT PHILOSOPHICAL POSTURE AND PURPOSE OF THERAPEUTIC RELATIONSHIP

Since the early 1980s, my theoretical and clinical ideas have evolved in a postmodern direction. My primary agenda in any therapeutic context is to generate and facilitate conversations that cocreate and discover new more freeing, self-action narratives. The therapeutic relationship is one of cocreating conversations that generate new meaning, and set the stage for the evolution of new solutions and options for change. As Gergen and Kaye (1992) write:

> The client's voice is not merely an auxiliary device for the vindication of the therapist's pre-determined narrative, but serves in these contexts as an essential constituent of a jointly constructed reality. (p. 174)
>
> Psychotherapy may be thought of as a process of semiosis—the forging of meaning in the context of collaborative discourse. (p. 182)

These ideas reflect the philosophy in which we work at the Houston–Galveston Institute, as developed by Anderson and Goolishian. Therapy is a process of creating collaborative and egalitarian conversations that permit new understandings, new opportunities, and options for change to occur. These conversations are client- not therapist-driven. From this posture, the therapist takes a position of "not knowing." Anderson and Goolishian (1992) describe this process as follows:

> [the] therapist [exercises] an expertise in asking questions from a position of "not knowing," rather than asking questions that are informed by method and demand specific answers. (p. 28)
>
> Not-knowing requires that our understandings, explanations, and interpretations in therapy not be limited by prior experiences or theoretically formed truths, and knowledge. . . . Meaning and understanding are socially constructed by person in conversation, in language with each other. (pp. 28–29)

The therapist's preknowing (personal beliefs, theoretical paradigms) does not define the problem or the direction of the therapeutic conversation. Questions and content areas to be explored come directly from a curiosity to understand the client's meaning and to share with the client the co-construction of new discourse.

For me, this approach to therapy is a process that encourages competency for self-solution rather than hindering the client or client system in preheld beliefs, theoretical paradigms, right or wrong thinking, or right or wrong actions. Self-solutions or the capacity for them is then familiar and a natural occurrence of the sharing of the dialogical experience (self-tailored) and not perceived by the creators as too unusual or counterfeit. Instead it is constructionally representative of one's history and interest. Shotter (1993), in discussing counterfeit narratives, states:

> And by having not been properly aware of the power of language, of the power of storytelling to "lend" a sense of reality to wholly fictitious worlds, we have allowed ourselves to have been talked into accepting a counterfeit version of our social lives together—where what I mean here by the term "counterfeiting" is the appropriation and use by individuals for their own

purpose of certain special, communally constructed and sustained resources, which (like money) are the resources in terms of which the community in fact maintains itself as a community . . . money has no reality except as a medium of exchange . . . also with language. (p. 138)

REFLECTIONS WITH MULTIPLE VOICES

The collaborative conversational approach that I utilize in the school setting incorporates of the reflecting perspective as developed by Tom Andersen. I had the privilege of watching Tom Andersen participate in reflecting teams several years ago when the Houston–Galveston Institute was still called the Galveston Family Institute. What I particularly remember witnessing was his gentleness and caring posture and the participant's conversations and reflections, and the newness that flowed from these conversations.

I utilize my interpretations of this reflecting format when working with client systems: families, training groups, workshops, school groups, or any context that includes multiple participants and multiple voices.

The primary concepts I use in the reflecting process are (1) focusing on how the participants wish to utilize the time we spend together, thereby allowing collaborative problem definition; (2) creating a space for multiple voices and multiple new understandings to occur; and (3) promoting all participants to actively dialogue about concerns of self in a manner that is respectful and caring.

Andersen best describes these positions:

There are very few rules to follow. The rules are all about what we shall not do: We shall not reflect on something that belongs to another context than the conversation of the interview system, and we must not give negative connotations. (1991, p. 61)

A problem creates a system of meaning; it is not that the system creates the problem. When these meanings are appropriately different, the various holders of the meanings might listen to each other and discuss the various meanings. Under such conditions new ideas might emerge. (1993, p. 310)

THE SETTING: MULTIPLE VOICES AND AGENDAS

As part of my private practice I consult with various school districts in a 30- to 60-mile radius. In this consultation I provide group therapy for children diagnosed as "emotionally disturbed" and placed into behavior modification classrooms. For the purpose of this chapter, I chose a school district that I feel provided unique services in a way that demarginalizes the voices of children.

Harry Goolishian would often state that therapists have created a context in which deficiency labeling has created voices that are marginalized, and which are viewed only within their deficiency labels. I find this valid, especially when a child is labeled "emotionally disturbed," when most of his/her emotions, thoughts, dreams, goals, and narratives are viewed as pathological. Teachers in these settings often read psychological profiles before meeting with their students, and these profiles lend to, as Andersen states, *vor-verstehen* or preunderstandings and prejudgments, that envelope perceptions and actions (p. 303).

When a teacher or therapist engages in communicative action from a preheld belief system (e.g., treats a child as if he/she is deficient), this is an action that is often not respectful of the person and can reflect a position of dominance and subversion. Such a relationship can create a reciprocal loop of teacher and student in conflict with each other vis-à-vis respect. As with most hierarchical systems, this is not a win–win situation for either student or teacher.

The classrooms for these children are often devoid of any pleasantries; instead rules on behavior are set up at child eye level to enforce "behavioral cues." Often the children are seated in cubicles that do not allow for any view or interaction outside the cubicle walls. Sometimes I wonder to myself how these children are able to learn in this isolated context.

Interaction in these structured environments is limited to short intervals because of the understanding that "these" children "cannot" engage in normal interactions or play.

To enter into these structured environments, the children must have had a history of unsuccessful behavior in mainstream classrooms. Concurrent with these histories, behavioral plans to modify their mainstream classroom behavior were consistently unsuccessful. With the emergence of unsuccessful behavioral plans, the students are given psychological evaluations, tests, and diagnoses. With the appropriate diagnosis, the child is placed into a structured modality, separate from the mainstream population of his/her peers.

The voices of the parents and children are often outweighed by these evaluations and the narratives of the school and school personnel. Because of these variables, the school and families quite often view each other with suspicion and distrust, with multiple voices and agendas rising out of chaotic contexts.

The school personnel fare no better. The teachers are expected to follow behavioral guidelines for student behavior with students who do not want to be in the controlled settings and who have extensive histories of distrust and dislike for the teaching population. The parents, who feel marginalized, are frequently antagonistic toward the school hierarchy. Conversations with teachers and other school personnel included narratives of perceived harassment and potentially dangerous actions (i.e., threats of bodily harm or harm to the school) by both the students and parents. Turnover rate is high for these teachers.

In Sally's school, I was contracted to provide therapeutic services for the children, teachers, and parents. The school administration requested therapeutic group therapy for the children (to help the children "obey" so that learning could ensue), teacher consultation (to aid in supporting the teachers and guiding them toward effective methods of relating to these children), and parent groups (to ensure parent participation and help the parents to overcome their "dysfunction"). In Sally's classroom there was the additional goal of evaluating Sally's teacher, whom the school felt was ineffective in managing classroom procedures.

Because there is no one agenda but a progression of conversations where new agendas arise and others dissolve, or are no longer of particular interest to any of the participants, new agendas are always in the process of developing. New agendas that arose during the conversations with Sally's teachers during the school year included helping the teachers and teacher's aide network with higher-level school administrative personnel, helping mainstream teachers cope with students entering their classrooms (after some modified behavior on the part of the student), and helping to troubleshoot situations as they arose between sessions.

The teacher with whom I consulted in Sally's classroom had a 20-year history of educating children. She stated that she felt marginalized from her department and was unsure whether my participation would be of benefit. Her initial reaction to my participation was based on her prior experiences with school therapy. This experience was perceived in a negative light because she felt inadequate when processing the children's actions with the previous therapist; not because of the therapist's critiques, but because she was insecure with the psychological terminology and fearful of the appropriateness of her own actions, especially in regard to managing her classroom and redirecting the student's behavior. She viewed the previous therapist as "coddling" the children instead of making them adhere to classroom rules. In her paradigm, all psychological factors for the children (divorce, stepparents, abandonment, low self-esteem, etc.) were secondary to her need for tips on how she could competently handle the class.

STARTING THE CONVERSATION: RESPECTING AND ENCOURAGING VOICES

My first step in participating in a therapeutic group format in a school setting is to initiate conversation with the teachers, as the participatory effort will be held in their domain. Because I am a visitor to their classroom, I hold for them the same respect I would for a new acquaintance whom I was visiting in his/her home. Our initial conversations focus on how my participation will be of benefit to them and their students. I attempt to provide a dialogical space, to provide an environment in which they can express their conflicts and desires. My posture reflects collaboration and respect. Working in this manner not only allows for the codevelopment of new understandings and narratives but sets the stage for a respectful climate, which I feel is necessary for any therapeutic conversation.

In this preliminary meeting, I invite the teacher and the teacher's aide to coparticipate in the group therapy format. The teacher and the teacher's aide come to take a position that eventually leads to the role of a cotherapist.

After the initial meeting with the teaching staff, I proceed to initiate "group therapy." My first meeting with the children is similar to my meeting with the teaching staff, to provide them with space for a multitude of voices that are not marginalized or pathologized. Often this is the children's first experience in being asked what kind of group they would like to own and how our participating together can be of benefit for them. As with the teaching staff, they are invited into participation.

Our voices become blended to provide a context of how to proceed and form our group. In this first group meeting, we decide about the participants who may be invited in the future (i.e., parents, other teachers, and additional administrative personnel). We compile "rules" for the group. Because they are already in a structured format, we comply with "school rules" but add such individually tailored features as promotion of respect and caring, confidentiality, no fronting, no slamming, no showboating (no unfair criticism, no bragging, no making up stories to show off), and no gossiping. In the setting I describe an opportunity was created for the participants to meet in a context of respect and caring. Our meetings become a place for brainstorming and support and an avenue where internal dialogues are made public, leading to tailored understandings, new meaning, and change.

CONVERSING WITH SALLY: CASE ILLUSTRATION

Initially Sally was not excited about participation in group therapy. She stated that she did not "like" me and wanted the prior therapist who brought treats, and with whom she had a five-year history. Sally had a close bond with the previous therapist, a bond she in greatly valued since her mother's departure several years ago. We had a conversation about this as it was imperative for me to be informed of her understanding and concern before further conversations could take place. As our discourse progressed, we decided that I would be able to be in dialogue with the previous therapist and that the previous therapist could resume contact with her outside the group format when the chance arose. Thus, I was not replacing but adding to.

In this first meeting, other student participants voiced their concerns and initial agendas. In future conversations the initial agendas were replaced by new ones. I did not attempt to draw on any theoretical paradigms in this first meeting. My primary agenda was to allow collaborative problem definition to occur, to create a space for multiple voices, and to promote an atmosphere of respect for self and the ideas of others. I wanted to learn about the dilemmas of self for all the participants.

The children were eager to voice opinions and directions. One would expect that the teachers, because of their history of hierarchical relationships, would experience some frustration with the allowance for the varied voices. In my experience, because the teachers were included as important participants and observers in the development of these groups, because they, too, were given power in their voices, and because initially we had cocreated the format and the initial direction for the orchestration of the group conversation, teacher involvement was cooperative and participatory. If, perchance, an issue arose that they felt was not appropriate or relevant, once again we would have a conversation about it in the group, often leading to different perceptions and comfortable understandings.

An example of such a situation occurred in the second session when the teacher and students wanted to come up with some new ideas about classroom participation, especially in regard to Sally, as she was viewed as the most "uncontrollable" student. We discussed Sally's history and her behavior in the classroom context, which produced much frustration for her and her teacher, as well as the teacher's aide, who also attended the groups and participated in classroom discipline.

In this conversation, an item of particular interest for me was the consequences for Sally for her misbehavior, Sally's perception of her misbehavior, and the teaching staff's (teacher and aide) perception of Sally and themselves in regard to this context. Sally's misbehaviors were reported to happen continuously. To the degree that little academic content was able to be presented due to this "acting out" behavior, the first mode of teacher interaction was to reason with Sally—to attempt to coerce "good choice and alternative behavior." If this was unsuccessful, which most of the time it was, the next step was to attempt to call her parent on the telephone. As Sally's father (the parent with whom she lived) was at work during the day, Sally stated that she often ignored this consequence because there was no immediate punitive action by a parent. If this alternative did not work, Sally was then literally "sat on" by the teacher or teacher's aide until she could acquire more controlled, "subservient" behavior. After we dialogued about the first two alternatives in detail and explored the perceptions of the teachers, Sally, and the other students, we tackled the subject of being sat on and being the sittee. I was informed in detail of how it was to be sat on, an action that Sally feared and the staff disliked. By the end of the conversation I had many beginning ideas of what it was like to be in Sally's position and also a clearer sense of the teacher's perceptions around this behavior modification technique. What was so wonderful to watch was the new understanding that Sally and her teachers were developing for each other in the course of these conversations. Sally (as with most students in this program) would get her "feelings hurt" by teacher critiques of her behavior (e.g., "don't do that, Sally") and would also feel embarrassed by the negative attention being called to her activity. Because of these perceptors she would feel devalued and feared that more devaluing would occur by the teacher's actions (e.g., more conversations about her negative behavior or teacher consequences). Toward the end of this session, all parties decided that alternate methods might be more useful. We agreed to draw up some beginning ideas to help in this situation.

One idea that developed from the conversation was that Sally was intent on making the teachers miserable if she felt her feelings were hurt by redirection activity. Once she felt threatened, she would disregard the consequences in order to retaliate. Often in this process she would wait to back down, but she "knew" her behavior had escalated to the sitting process. At that time, she felt her only recourse would be an offensive one and getting the first "lick" before she was "attacked." Sally, in "hearing" the process of her thinking in regard to the previous "spontaneous" actions, decided along with the other students to develop new actions in regard to the teacher actions (i.e., exploring and finding alternative thoughts and meaning before the escalation to the sitting alternative). Among the options voiced were voluntary "time-outs" to aid in deescalation. The students and teachers began exploring various dialogues about future behaviors and actions, both for the students and for the teaching staff. The teachers had a new understanding of Sally's need for affection and her low tolerance for her self-perceived negative input from her teachers. Sally saw how uncomfortable it was for the teachers to be watchdogs and policing activity.

The other students (four in all) also participated in the narrative of finding alternative pathways for themselves. Initially, when Sally got into trouble, they viewed her actions as amusing and sought to participate in what they viewed as a "free-for-all," a time, like recess, where they could act wild and crazy and cheer on Sally and her "defensive moves." From the conversation, it became apparent that these actions were not too helpful in the course of Sally's "winning" in this situation, and they felt very sad to see the final consequences for Sally. The remaining students, Sally, the teacher, and the aide reflected alternative roles for the students one by one. It was decided that possibly the teacher's aide could work with the other children on some "relaxing and pleasurable activity" when tensions mounted between any teacher and any student.

These uniquely collaborative alternatives or self-solutions were finely tailored and they were cocreated out of the immediate conversation. One could say that these were "interventions"; some modernistic viewpoints would add that these types of solutions (voluntary time-outs, removal of the nonescalative children) could be used in any classroom and obtain similar results. I strongly disagree with such of descriptions or explanations. First, these opportunities for self-solution were developed by the coevolved narratives. We could have talked about similar issues with similar participants and, because of differences in perceptions and narratives, come up with vastly different alternatives. These types of self- solutions are neither my solutions nor those of one of the student's or the teacher's. The narrative alternatives come directly from the conversations at hand and are finely tailored to the participants who are in the process of dialogue.

CONTINUITY OF NARRATIVES

Before I provide in more detail about the reflections of the participants, I would like to address the issues of continuity of these narratives outside the therapeutic sessions. In my view, therapeutic conversations arise in the therapy sessions but are in continuous process of dialogical action and revision *outside* the therapy room. We would be in danger of being overly ambitious if we were to conclude that participating with someone or a group of people for one hour per week accounted for therapeutic change.

The therapeutic conversation is just one conversation that participants have in coalescing around problem and solution definition areas.

A multitude of conversations occur between meetings in regard to my school consultation. Even though the group is organized to meet on a weekly basis, I do not assume that problematic areas raised in the previous week need to be addressed in subsequent conversations. For example, if I attended the next session with this school group and expected narratives about the same content areas but found little evolved dialogues about these issues yet proceeded to inquire along these lines, my conversation participation would be therapist-driven and I would be participating outside the parameters of the therapeutic conversation.

As it happened, in the next session we did dialogue on the experience of "experiencing no-sittings" for the previous week and how that was for all the participants. It is not that miraculously no infractions or frustrations occurred, but the participants felt they had created a new "beginning," a new system with which all felt comfortable. I use the term "beginning" because I do not believe that these alternatives are a curative action. New actions may need to be added or deleted depending on the narrative actions of the participants.

SELF-SOLUTION AND CHANGE

In the process of conversing with Sally and her school group, Sally's behavior dramatically improved to the point that she was able to move out of her structured special education setting. In order to understand the dramatic change, I would like to discuss the narratives that evolved from conversations with Sally and her teachers. I have saved this discussion for the latter part of this chapter to cut down on *vor-verstehen* (Andersen, 1993).

Sally was an 11-year-old fifth-grader. She had been diagnosed "emotionally disturbed" since she was in kindergarten. The school perceived that she could not follow normal classroom rules, and could not learn without a structured environment. In my experience, once a child is placed in this restrictive environment, filled with rules and facilitated by teachers whose primary role is somehow to enforce these rules, the chances of being mainstreamed are low. The children in these settings often form a peer subculture where the prevailing thought is to defend against the hierarchy. The peer relationship becomes very strong due to their marginalized voices. Once admitted into these programs, the children most often no longer participate in play or learning contexts with their mainstream peers, so that most peer interaction is with other pupils who share their negative perceptions of school, learning, and teachers and who respond to negative situations with active forms of "defiant" behavior. In Sally's case, she had proceeded in school with a group of peers and had little peer interaction outside school. The classroom was viewed by Sally as one form of play, except that the teachers often prevented "play" from occurring. In conversations with students in these settings, they do not see the serious repercussions of their marginalization. They do not participate in school sports, dances, physical education, lunches, parties, and so on. Indeed they do not "know" what they are missing from the mainstream population. They do know, however, what it is like to be perceived through labels.

Sally's parents had separated when Sally was three. For many reasons she had limited contact with her mother, although this was a relationship she held in high esteem. Her father had multiple relationships and Sally held no esteem for these female role models. Her mother was in another relationship that had produced a brother, whom Sally felt was overcoddled and had worse behavior than herself. She had not visited her mother for the last few years because of her relationship with her mother's significant other and the tensions that arose between herself and her mother's new family. At first, when I began conversing with Sally and we would talk about family issues, she was reluctant to discuss these areas because of the pain involved. If one were to be prejudiced by Sally's history, one would think about "depression" or find other psychological perjorative terminology to describe Sally. But in conversation with Sally, one could see fiery strength, a great sense of humor, a passion for life, and great survival skills—she could hold her own.

As this group evolved, the participants developed much affection for each other. The teachers and students found new ways to relate and work with each other in a fashion that led to mutual respect and caring. As Sally's behavior and that of all the participants changed, the teacher and the teacher's aide became role models and mentors. The days were not filled up with rules but with lessons on academics and life. The other students (all of whom were at least two years younger than Sally) began to view Sally as a trailblazer and role model and the last one to ever be sat on. As she began to be mainstreamed into non-special education classes, she would report back to the group on her trailblazing and how to combat marginalization, specifically how to fit into mainstream classes. With the occurrence of all these positive events, she flourished. At the end of the school year, Sally was entirely mainstreamed, and although she often was not present during the last few group meetings, she popped in and informed us of her experiences and progress.

In the group we talked about a multitude of issues: parents, parents' significant others, peers, academics, peer pressure, life events, world topics, and so on. Each content area for each session was decided on by the participants and agreed on by the participants. Usually the content areas or issues were driven by experiences between meetings. There were no quick "fixes," but there was an ongoing puzzling of issues, boundless curiosity, evolution of new meaning, understandings, ideas, new self-solutions, and new directions to build on. We simply talked and reflected and talked and reflected more, opening some options and closing others. There was never a "wrong" view or advice given. Through this collaboration, we became respectful and caring of each other.

These reflections were never produced the same way twice. In some contexts, all participants would share how the week had progressed. Everyone always had a voice and ownership in the group. Sometimes an important issue had just arisen or occurred that the members had saved for the group. Often students and teachers would listen as if they were a parent, peer, or teacher and reflect on their understandings and positions. Often they would listen as themselves and share ideas and issues. A theme could be elected and then it was the process of the group to think and one by one share thoughts. In this manner of listening—conversations and reflections (and more listening, conversations, and reflections)— new meaning occurred, as well as opportunities for new self-action. As Andersen (1991) states in the process of reflections, "it invites one perspective then another, it becomes a way to embrace the possibility of both . . . a co-evolutionary view rather than a more fixed problem focus" (p. 100).

In my work I often invite "visiting" participants, including teachers or parents. The decision of whom to invite is created out of the dialogues between myself, the teachers, and the students. In my work with Sally, her "new teacher" participated in a couple of groups prior to her mainstreaming and thereafter. I attempt to have parent groups every month. At these groups, parents, teachers, and students sit with each other and have conversations. These conversations lead to coevolved issues and new actions. There is a dissolution of marginalized voices and the teacher, parents, and students become collaborators. Sally's father was not able to attend parent meetings due to his work schedule, but often he was in conversation with the teacher and would write notes to the group on particular themes of interest for him.

REFLECTIVE AND COLLABORATIVE VOICES IN THE SCHOOL

As an example of how the reflecting process worked, a composite of conversations during one session is offered:

THERAPIST: Well, Hello Ms. P, Mrs. K, I noticed the door. You sure do have some great artists around here.

MS. P: Yes. We are getting ready for the holidays a little early this year. Okay, guys, put up your work. It's time for group.

THERAPIST: Hi, guys, how have things been going?

MS. P: Sally has some new news to share.

MRS. K: Yes. Sally, would you like to let Ms. S know about the new news?

SALLY: Okay. I'm getting a new stepmom! And a new baby brother!

EDDIE: Oh that's not new. You told us yesterday.

ANN: Yeah, and sometimes little babies are a pain in the petutie. I have one at home you know.

SALLY: I know, I have one, too, from my mom. But this one is different. He is soooo sweet and I get to feed him and change his diaper! (*sounds of "yuck, gross" from the participants*)

THERAPIST: Well, Sally, it sounds like you're happy about this new addition to your family. How did it come to be that you are getting a new stepmom and a baby brother at the same time?

MS. P: We found out this week when her dad sent a note to us. He was a little worried about how Sally felt about this, especially, since the addition of her mom's baby was kind of hard on Sally before.

SALLY: Oh, but Ms. P, this is different. My new stepmom just loves this baby, but she also says she loves me, and she loves the way I take care of the baby. I know this baby won't turn into a brat the way that Jason has. Anyways, if the baby cries or something, Jan, my new stepmom, knows it's not my fault!

THERAPIST: So, Jan is the name of your new stepmom. What is she like?

SALLY: Well, she is real pretty and she has hair like mine. She likes to fix my hair, too. She and my dad have been dating only a little while so I don't know her too well, but I think she is nice. She washes my clothes, helps me with my homework, and does my chores before dad gets home, so I don't get into trouble.

THERAPIST: Oh, she's a lot of help then?

SALLY: Yeah! But sometimes I feel bad about liking her so much because I have a real mom . . . like sort of guilty.

THERAPIST: Well, Eddie, you had a new stepmom a few years ago. Did you ever feel that way?

EDDIE: Not really. Well . . . maybe.

THERAPIST: So, Eddie, how was it for you having a new stepmom?

EDDIE: Well, at first she was real nice and then after a while she got real comfortable and started making up rules. Then, after she and my dad had my younger brother, he got all the attention. But it's better now after we had family therapy.

THERAPIST: So, Eddie, how do you think family therapy helped?

EDDIE: Well, the therapist told my stepmom she wasn't paying enough attention to me and then she started being nicer and things got better.

THERAPIST: Well, did you ever feel like Sally then, you know sort of feeling guilty about your real mom?

EDDIE: Not really.

THERAPIST: Well, Eddie, I bet you're glad about that. How about you, David? Have you ever felt that way, like Sally?

DAVID: I don't have any stepparents.

THERAPIST: Oh yeah, guess I forgot. Well, what do you think it would be like?

DAVID: Well, hmm. I guess it would be like if you made a new friend and your best friend moved away. You would miss your best friend, but at the same time you would like your new friend, and maybe you would think about your old friend when you were with your best friend and that would make you sad.

THERAPIST: Hmm. What do you think Sally?

SALLY: Yeah, that's kind of what it is like. I think I miss my mom more now, even though I missed her a lot before, because I have a stepmom now who acts like a mom and so, like Eddie said, I think I miss her more now. It makes me kind of sad.

ANN: Maybe Sally could call her mom.

SALLY: My dad wouldn't let me.

MS. P: I am really proud of the way Sally has coped with all this new change and I am happy she has a new family.

THERAPIST: I think we're all happy for Sally. What if each of us thinks for a few minutes to see if we have any ideas that would help Sally? If you were Sally, what kind of things would help?

ANN: Getting a new puppy. Puppies are adorable!

THERAPIST: Okay, that's an idea. A new puppy. That sure cheers people up! Well, let's sort of add everybody's comments first before we ask Sally for any comments.

DAVID: Well, since she doesn't have her mom's phone number, she could write her mom a letter and tell her mom that she loves her and will always love her, even if her stepmom is a good mom, too.

THERAPIST: Okay, David. So a letter is another good idea. Who's next?

EDDIE: Well, she could talk to her dad about it and see if he has any good ideas.

THERAPIST: You guys have such good ideas! Hmm. I wonder what Ms. P and Mrs. K think?

MS. P: Well, I think it is normal for Sally to feel this way in the beginning. If I was to get a new stepmom and I had not seen my real mom in a while, I would get sad sometimes, too. Maybe it would help if Sally could talk about it with myself or Mrs. K. Sometimes talking about it helps. I bet that both mothers would be pleased to know that Sally is such a caring daughter!

MRS. K: You know, that made me think my son Tom had the same kind of ideas when I married Mr. K. Maybe I could ask him tonight about what kind of things helped him and then I could share these with you this week. I think also that if you need to talk about this, we're here for you.

THERAPIST: Okay, Sally. We have lots of thoughts. What kind of ideas have they given you?

SALLY: Well, I'd like a puppy, but we have a rotweiler that doesn't like any other dogs or anybody but my family. I didn't think about talking to my dad about it. I was worried I might hurt his or my stepmom's feelings or make them mad. Maybe I could talk to my dad about it and maybe I could write a letter, but I don't know my mom's address. Maybe my dad could find out.

Sally went on to ask her dad about this. Sally's dad helped her to send a letter to her grandparents, who were aware of her mom's location. After the holidays, I questioned Sally as to whether this was still an issue. It was not, and she appeared curious as to why it would be. I had not been in conversation with her for weeks, subsequent conversations with her dad and teacher had put this issue to rest. Sally and her biological mother did start conversing.

What I hope these voices imparted are the collaborative coevolving process of multiple ideas and multiple solutions that are created through the therapeutic conversation. All ideas are valid and Sally was free to evolve which idea fit best for her. Guilt changed into sadness and sadness held the opening of new possibilities for solutions.

PARTICIPANTS' FEEDBACK: REFLECTIONS ON THE EXPERIENCE

The groups often start out with little support except for the school administrative personnel. With time, dramatic changes in collaborative conversations appear, and group ownership and a spirit of positive thinking develop. Students and teachers alike are famished for voices and power in their voices. When I enter into a classroom, the climate becomes one of mutual respect and caring. Not all students change as dramatically as Sally. But students are eager to engage in conversations that help each other and promote positive alternatives. It feels good to talk about resolving issues. It builds hope and relationships based on respect and caring. The students make such comments as, "Can you come everyday," and, "These are things we have talked about before, but when we talk with you it is different and easier to learn good choices." Teachers report feeling respected for their ideas. In one recent conversation one teacher made the comment, "Our ideas blend so well, I feel that you and I share the same thoughts and I find myself questioning the same ideas or finishing others for you." Teachers attempt to attribute change, either positive or negative, to my services. I attribute the change to the participants since I have expertise in creating a space and process for the conversations, but they have expertise through living daily in these contexts.

A crucial component is parental involvement. Often this is not possible due to work schedules. When we are able to incorporate parents into the process, the options are boundless. Parents report feeling valued for the first time in their relationship with school personnel. Parents report feeling invited and valued into their roles as parents versus feeling blamed or pathologized for deficient parenting skills. Parents "make time" to become involved in classroom projects and report feeling collegial with the teachers.

Administrative feedback often comes from department heads (e.g., directors of programs and principals) appreciative about their "lack of involvement": Less time was required of them, because teachers, students, and parents were actively problem solving. Typical statements have been: "No longer do I receive telephone calls from teachers about a crisis in the classroom." "Complaints from students or parents never reach my office since resolutions occur in the classroom." "We can't believe these are the same kids." And, "since the groups have started, most of my interactions in the classroom have become pleasurable experiences."

CONCLUDING THOUGHTS

I believe that providing therapy in this manner is significantly cost-effective. The group format decreased the amount of time spent providing therapeutic services both in number of sessions and in billable hours. Because the teachers can contact me to help "trouble shoot" issues, other school personnel are not required for these services and can attend to their other duties. In the school described in this chapter, the administration decided to collapse the self-contained structured settings and opted to mainstream the "emotionally disturbed" population. The cost-effectiveness of this step is outstanding considering the financing of self-contained classrooms, and the price that restricting and marginalizing children cannot be measured.

In preparing the children for this process of mainstreaming, we would role-play potential situations. We would create conversations of their ideas or what they would like to see happen—how they could "fit in" and form a sense of community with other students and teachers. One year later the children are mainstreamed and reportedly doing well. My involvement finished when mainstreaming was completed.

As I work with other school districts where diagnostically emotionally disturbed children continue to be placed into self-contained units, I look forward to a time when children performing "differently" from the mainstream population are not removed from their peers and attached to labels. As one student recently (and wisely) stated, "We need to be treated as individuals and not statistics, to be seen and believed for who we are and not through the eyes of books or diagnosis."

REFERENCES

Andersen, T. (1991). *The reflecting team: Dialogues and dialogues about the dialogues.* New York: Norton.

Andersen, T. (1992). Reflections on reflecting with families. In S. McNamee & K. J. Gergen (Eds.), *Therapy as social construction* (pp. 54–68). London: Sage.

Andersen, T. (1993). See and hear, and be seen and heard. In S. Friedman's (Ed.), *The new language of change: Construction collaboration in psychotherapy* (pp. 303–322). New York: Guilford Press.

Anderson, H. (1993). On a roller coaster: A collaborative language system approach to therapy. In S. Friedman (Ed.), *The new language of change:*

Constructive collaboration in psychotherapy (pp. 323–344). New York: Guilford Press.

Anderson, H., & Goolishian, H. (1992). The client is the expert: A not-knowing approach to therapy. In S. McNamee & K. J. Gergen (Eds.), *Therapy as social construction* (pp. 25–39). London: Sage.

Gergen, K. J., & Kaye, J. (1992). Beyond narrative in negotiation of therapeutic meaning. In S. McNamee & K. J. Gergen (Eds.), *Therapy as social construction* (pp. 166–185). London: Sage.

Shotter, J. (1993). *Conversational realities: Constructing life through language.* London: Sage.

CHAPTER 6

A Spell in the Fifth Province

IT'S BETWEEN MESELF, HERSELF, YERSELF, AND YER TWO IMAGINARY FRIENDS

Imelda Colgan McCarthy
Nollaig O'Reilly Byrne

> And what was strange was that there were times when I didn't know if the things I did see were real or was I imagining them. I seemed to be living on a borderline between fantasy and reality.
>
> —*Friel (1994, p. 58)*

IRELAND HAS A LONG oral tradition. For particular historical and geographical reasons this practice survived as a prominent feature of an earlier Celtic civilization. With colonization, the special bardic class of storytellers, poets, and musicians was disbanded and, over time the language itself has for the most part disappeared. What has survived in the culture, however, is an elaborate affliction for story telling and a polysemic language remarkable for its overflow of ambiguity, exaggerations, and evasions. Everyday language bends under the weight of its own display, submitting wherever possible to poetic license.

The story we tell is in this tradition. It is a story that exists in that "borderline country" between myth and reality, a speaking and listening at the margins of "reality." The spokespersons in this story include "Paddy" and "Molly" (a young couple requesting help) and a novice systemic team (the authors and Philip Kearney). The couple expound a fatalistic vision based on a legacy of "madness" and suicide against which they construct a desperate vigilance and isolation. The team as an audience for the couple's story is powerfully drawn into an embodiment of the dilemma of themes of myth and reality, connection, and isolation. The fear of contagion was the moving point describing a familial plague from which Molly and Paddy were trying to escape. Metamorphosis[1] was their unique escape route, providing an isolated state cut off from social contact and the grasp of a contaminating madness in the repudiation of a familial lineage.

The isolation of a sealed-off home became the location for their unique metamorphosis. The team was attempting a metamorphosis from a linear world of individualism to the embodied mind of a systemic team. In contrast to the couple, we envisioned that our attempt to reflexively connect the biographies of clients with our own personal responses to them and to each other might be the self-conscious measure of this metamorphosis. Inspired by the Milan model (Hoffman, 1981; Palazzoli, Boscolo, Cecchin, & Prata, 1980), our goal was to stake out a process and a politics that reflected a systemic view.

Nothing could have prepared us for the journey we were about to embark on in this search for an embodied team identity. Implicating Paddy and Molly in our account has exposed them to a special scrutiny on one occasion. On this occasion an unfriendly audience confirmed their "borderline"[2] status and recommended a firmer treatment. Happily a collegial audience in the systemic field has guided us to see that the contour of our story was etched on theirs, a play of responses in an endangered space. Initially, the designation "borderline" was offensive to us. Here we usurp the term and invite you, the reader to enter this borderline country with us. This story is our re-membering[3] and retelling of our own participation. Transcripts from sessions will give readers an opportunity to position themselves as audience to the clinical encounter and to enter somewhat into the power of its original telling. The dialogue in the excerpts illustrates a fifth province approach, which we (ICM and NO'RB and Philip Kearney) have been developing since 1981. Nowadays, this team is referred to as the Fifth Province Associates.

THE SHADOW OF LOSS

Some events cast a long shadow. Untimely death surely does. Somehow the suicide of someone close by ushers in a reality of overwhelming

[1]Metamorphosis refers to a change of form whether by magic or natural development.

[2]Borderline in this instance refers to diagnostic criteria according to the fourth edition of the *Diagnostic and Statistical Manual of Mental Disorders* (American Psychiatric Association, 1994).

[3]Hyphenations are used to highlight the polysemic (multiple) meaning of terms.

confusion and anxiety beyond the horizons of expectation and imagination. One is faced with such questions as, "Is this the ultimate outcry in the face of an unendurable life, or the ultimate risk compelled by the belief in a further shore?" Such a death builds for itself an abode within us, cross-joining gaps of memory into an impermanent understanding. Desolation and outrage are often camouflaged by the obsessive pursuit of reasons, and in time explanations, knowing why, soothe the disbelief. Here the elaborated discourses aim to mute and seal off the event, hiding it from view in the ordinary passage of our lives. This reputed knowledge by the community of the event becomes the immunizing factor warding off fear flowing in its wake. But can we be so easily immunized by rational explanations? Fear is the great propeller of imagination, turning the banal and the ordinary into coded forebodings and predictions.

The death of a beloved colleague was a cloud that darkened over our decision to form a team. Now, with time, it has become an elongating and shifting shadow that follows, precedes, and hovers over us, overdetermining our existence as a professional group. It draws us back to our beginnings and encloses our continuity in the shadow it casts. Her death, our own early and fragile team formation, and experimental clinical work drew together a simultaneity of resonant connections into a fateful coherence. It was as if the baleful motifs of contamination and contagion winged their way unsuspectingly from the confines of the clinical situation into our own professional system. We have asked ourselves over and over again, how did it escape so? What was this strange convergence of events that reflected each other on either side of us and foretold an unseen death? At this time it appeared that in this interpenetrating world of meaning, events coalesced into a nuanced phantom network of signification. The footholds and handrails of the customary were no longer in sight in this "borderline country." Our playful pretense of inventing connections was shattered. When we recalled our conversations with Molly and Paddy, sharing with us the ghostly outline of a generational trajectory, we imagined there an embedded warning, a sign, that some danger was in the air. But on first hearing we had listened without understanding. We had not made the connection that we were also trying to allay our own fears of what might happen in our engagement with the unfolding of Paddy's and Molly's story. This story is pockmarked with the immodesty of our fearlessness. "Nobody has to die here." Words were fun, playful things to be bent and shaped into an ethereal whimsy. A story appeared to be just that—a free-floating exposition devoid of any substantial truth. However, we were to find out that on the contrary, some stories have roots and limbs. They are the spiritual markers of the social landscape that ordain our attention and reflection.

THE FATE OF PADDY AND MOLLY

Perhaps it was Paddy's comportment that lured us into fanciful relief. He epitomized the ambivalent Irish attitude to life—a mixture of comic detachment (Hederman & Kearney, 1977) and a certainty of predestination. Paddy said that we, the team, were their "last hope." Despite his efforts and myriad professional involvements over a three-year period, Molly, his young wife, could not be cured. "You can see for yourself, she is a lovely little thing, but she does be upset all the time." However, he had a stolid indifference to the professional help Molly sought out against his better judgment. When she was in the hospital, where she sometimes felt better, he urgently requested her to return home. During the recent hospitalization, which preceded their referral to us, in an uncustomary release of caution, she confessed to a junior staff member that her husband "was driving her mad." This little aside generated enough confusion about her diagnosis to have Paddy and Molly catapulted into marital therapy.

Paddy's hold on his marriage was ambiguous from the start. He was more surprised than anything when Molly accepted his reckless proposal. She stated that she had hoped that life with Paddy would have been her escape from the confines of an "overprotected" girlhood. When Molly's pregnancy was confirmed, Paddy remained unconvinced about the evidence right up to the delivery date. The maternity hospital eventually located him and prevailed on him to visit his wife and newborn daughter. As the son of his mother, however, he was never in any doubt about his filial attachment and was drawn closer to her by her deepening unhappiness and confusion. Subsequent to his mother's abandonment by an alcoholic partner she spent long periods in a psychiatric hospital, keeping her children in nervous attention. As with his siblings, the grief of separation, present since childhood, demanded a bewildering pursuit of attachment to a mother now existing in the thrall of "madness." This "mad woman" (Paddy's mother) resolutely adored her children but included the young Molly in her list of enemies. In various rituals of harassment, mainly by telephone, she addressed Molly with obscene epithets and accusations. Paddy, lost in confusion, doubted Molly's version.

Paddy's mother was dead for three days before the alarm was raised. Ironically, it was Molly who agreed to identify the decomposing body, as members of her family, including Paddy, could not face this sad task. This ordeal confirmed Molly's ambivalent participation in the tragic events and their aftermath. Nothing in her life had prepared her to face that day. From that point on, the tragedy had transformed her, leaving her to doubt her own sanity. Paddy, however, could not hold back his conviction that Molly had entered into his mother's affliction, "gone funny," the destiny of motherhood.

When we first encountered Paddy and Molly, some great tragic distortion was afoot between them. It appeared that they were condemned to exile, isolation, and suffering. They unfolded with us a spellbound narrative shaped by archetypal fears of madness, isolation and predestined death. This narrative was premised on the lineage of a family, described by Paddy as "royal and mad." It was a lineage in which the legacy of madness and suicide as a result of childbirth was handed down over three generations. Our initial dilemma was whether to resist or follow into this endangered space? We followed in the hope that we and they could break out of our joint Celtic legacy of superstition. But superstition has deep and enduring roots less easily repudiated in times of crisis. The invasive claims of rational boundaries cannot so easily denature a potent affective mythology. To be open and affectively attuned to their story required that the team move beyond the restraints of psychiatric description. Paddy described Molly's fearful preoccupations thus: "No I didn't think she was crazy. I personally thought she would wake up one morning and her mind would have snapped. I thought that she'd know at that point that she didn't care if she wanted to live or die."

This comment, at once so unsure and so certain, features metamorphosis as a guiding premise. In Paddy's description, Molly's invalid state is that of brittleness, a disposition to sudden fracture. Here madness and sanity and life and death were but serial instances of dilemmas, breaking points as it were, in human experience. Molly was not yet mad, but Paddy's obsessive surveillance of her movements, her facial gestures, and her commentaries was his measure with which to identify its moment of arrival. Chameleon-like, Molly appears to have become an heir to Paddy's legacy. Sanity and madness exist along borderlines easily passing into each other. Like his grandmother, mother, and sister, Molly too "had gone funny" after childbirth. In our following of this story our fifth province approach became both our life-line and our guide.

TWO CELTIC MYTHS: THE FIFTH PROVINCE AND THE CHILDREN OF LIR

In our teamwork we use the metaphor of the fifth province as an insignia for our systemic practice. In the words of our first woman President, Mary Robinson, the fifth province is a symbol for that "place within each of us that is open to the other" (Robinson, 1990). However, it is the saga of "the Children of Lir" that is the allegorical lodestone[4] for our

[4]Lodestone is a guiding principle.

early developments. The story of the Children of Lir is one of three famous Celtic sagas, now referred to as "the three sorrows of Erin" (Jacobs, 1972). The structural motif is that of metamorphosis, that Celtic desire and belief in a change of substance in which the drama of banishment and isolation is played out. The tale recounts the fate of the four children of the sea-god Lir who were placed under a spell by their jealous stepmother, Aoife. The spell transformed them into four swans, retaining human speech and cast them into exile for 900 years. In retribution, King Lir transformed his wife, Aoife, into a demon of the air, in which form she was to live eternally. The suffering of the four children is not mortal death but that of exile from humankind in another form beyond imaginable human life spans. In the Christian retelling of the saga there is a recurrence to their human form and inevitable mortality with the claim of redemption and spiritual afterlife.

A FIFTH PROVINCE APPROACH

A fifth province approach takes its name from the ancient Celtic myth of the fifth province and its orientation from the work of two Irish philosophers, Richard Kearney and Mark P. Hederman (Hederman, 1985; Hederman & Kearney, 1977; Kearney, 1990).

The fifth province may or may not have existed. There are many versions. Some say it was a nonplace, a province of imagination and possibility, alongside yet different from the four geographical provinces that continue to make up modern-day Ireland. Another story cites the fifth province at the center of Ireland where the four provinces met. At this center kings and chieftains are said to have come to receive counsel and resolve conflicts through dialogue with Druids.[5] Today the only remaining trace of the fifth province is in myth and in the Irish language where the word for province, *cuaige,* means fifth.

However, in the work of Hederman and Kearney, the fifth province has come to represent a dis-position toward openness. In our own work we have used the myth of the fifth province as a metaphor for the embracing of social and linguistic domains that are saturated with ambivalence and ambiguity; opposition and contrast (Byrne & McCarthy, 1988; Byrne & McCarthy, 1994; Kearney, Byrne, and McCarthy, 1989; McCarthy & Byrne, 1988).

Celebrating language and storytelling, the metaphor of the fifth province guides us in imagining an ambivalent dialogical field constituted

[5]Druids were Celtic priests, soothsayers, and magicians in ancient Ireland.

by the reciting and resiting of many contrasting, diverse and often conflicting stories. The ambiguous discourses engendered in such domains may not be symmetrical. Some stories are recognized as embodying greater social privilege and the marginal story is everywhere vulnerable to erasure and silence. Paradoxically, in not re-cognizing privileged or dominant stories (e.g., of mental health in a given time and society) there is a greater danger that the recitation and elaboration of the marginalized stories (e.g., madness) will be further disqualified. A prime example occurs when the mental status examination usurps a personal account.

To aid us in the construction and deconstruction of narratives in clinical encounters we have devised a four-way diagrammatic schema. We refer to these schema as diamonds (see Figure 6.1). These diamond forms depict two intersecting axes of thematic pairs which oppose and relate. The diamond re-presents a domain of connections where emotional, ideational, and behavioral contradictions may be held together in creative tension of "both–and" rather than dichotomized into "either–or" categories. The tension engendered in this juxtaposing is envisioned to "pull taut the nerves of insight" (Le Brocquy, 1981, p. 136) and to avoid unnecessary imposition. In our construction a forum is created for the telling and witnessing of diverse and conflictual stories.

The free play of contradictions, by way of their elaboration and exaggeration, avoids the premature capture and resolution of opposing elements (e.g., myth and reality). Standpoints or speaking sites are

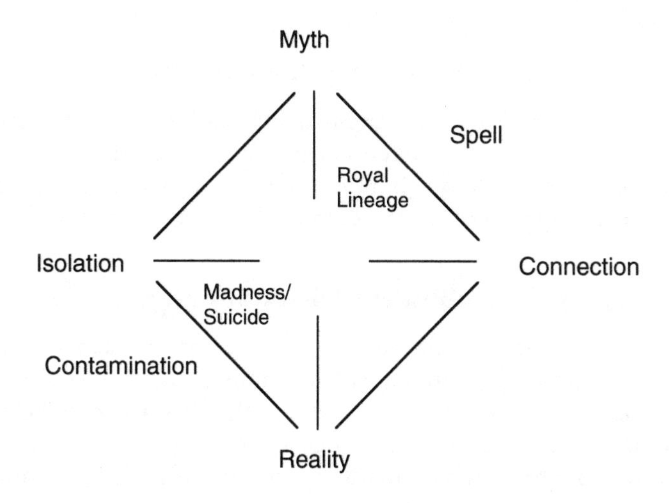

FIGURE 6.1. Spell-binding fearful dilemmas.

elaborated not as endpoints in themselves but as reflexively connected elements, now transformed in their exaggerated encounter. This structural principle is suggestive of a linguistic coherence. However, that is but part of the picture. It also re-presents a celebration of openness to difference, to dissensus. It is, as it were, a nonplace of consensual dissensus. The following transcript of our 10 sessions with Paddy and Molly highlights a narrative–dialogical approach wherein the Milan systemic method was enlarged to constitute what we refer to as juxtapositioning, re-membering, questioning at the extremes, and ambivalent dis-positioning (Colgan, 1991; Hydén & McCarthy, 1994).

Juxtapositioning

Juxtapositioning refers to a cognitive, affective, and discursive process of holding together contrasting and opposing themes. It is operationalized in the team's insertion of a question or statement proposing a contrary view together with the questioning of those with contrary views in each other's presence. The diamond is our aid in visualizing, constructing, and deconstructing juxtaposed contradictory and contrasting views.

Re-membering

Re-membering includes the emotional and ideational responses of therapists and clients; the imagined viewpoints of different participants in the minds of other participants and the imagined views of absent/silenced parties or topics.

Questioning at the Extremes

These questions address the extreme manifestations of the logical frames of participants or re-membered participants within the conversational system. It is the method whereby opposing viewpoints are stretched (elaborated/exaggerated) to the extremes of their own logic.

Ambivalent Dis-positioning

Ambivalent dis-positioning refers to a therapeutic stance that holds together contrasting, contrary, and/or conflictual views/positions. This may be done through posing questions that juxtapose opposites and tolerating in imagination simultaneous opposing viewpoints without attempting to introduce a premature clarification and/or closure. Rather, it has been our experience that it is within the interweave of juxtaposed stories and their exaggeration that solutions present themselves. They emerge "under one's hands and not because of them" (Le Brocquy, 1981, p. 146).

"Is There Anybody Listening?"

The question-posing mode outlined in this story was invited by Paddy himself:

PADDY: It was the junior doctor who was dealing with her of course. And he was talking to me for about an hour and he just said, "keep talking." Well, if he had asked me questions I could have explained it better, but seemingly he was quite happy. He took his own meaning out of the way I was trying to express myself. Now to me, I tried to express myself to the best of my ability but if someone could ask you, say twenty questions, I am not saying they would be the right questions, but you might be able to elaborate a little further on what you are trying to say. But to actually talk about it, I found it difficult, not to talk but to express myself better by just "keeping talking."

Here, Paddy appears to be invoking the formal dialogical process of a Socratic inquiry as one way to disrupt the enclosure of a monological nonwitnessed narrative. In fact, it may well be that such words in the mouth of Paddy were the significant utterances that enchanted the team into an animated audience. As an apparent mouthpiece for the team, one of us, (NO'RB), embarked on such an enchanted course with Paddy and Molly.

"Do You Know the Story?"

As a long-standing protector of his beloved mother, Paddy remains divided between two accounts, either an unhappy marriage or the unhappy fate of childbirth. Paddy was the second child.

NOLLAIG: *(to Paddy)* Do you know the story?

PADDY: Well, there are so many versions to that story you don't know which one is true.

MOLLY: You hear one thing from one side and another from the other side . . .

PADDY: (*simultaneously completing Molly's sentence*) . . . another from the other side. You know, my father said my mother was mad and she said he was mad.

NOLLAIG: Yes, so there was some doubt about whether each or both of them were crazy.

PADDY: (*laughs*) Well . . . doubt amongst themselves.

NOLLAIG: In *your* mind who was the crazy one?

PADDY: Well, my mammy committed suicide.

NOLLAIG: Yes.

PADDY: And I would say with all the unhappiness that my father put her through that . . . but he reckons that after the second or third child, my mammy went funny.

The audience is now in place. Wholeheartedly embracing the questions, Paddy introduces the story. His mother killed herself. In his mind this is the tragic irrefutable evidence of his father's accusation. Still protecting his mother, he introduces the ancestor who was instrumental in separating the children from their parents. He goes on to recount how as children they were sent into residential care, their mother being "crazy" and their father astray. Questioning at the extremes leads to the resurrection of this exaggerated ancestor and themes of madness are juxtaposed with those of badness.

"She Was an Old Jinnet Anyway."

NOLLAIG: Who was involved in the decision to send the children into care?

PADDY: My mammy.

NOLLAIG: Your mammy. And who helped her to make that decision?

PADDY: My granny, but she was an auld [old] jinnet anyway. [A jinnet is the infertile female offspring of a horse and donkey.]

[Paddy and Molly laugh and incline toward each other. Paddy looks pleased.]

NOLLAIG: (*to Molly*) Do you know her?

PADDY: No. She is dead, the Lord have mercy (*looking upwards*). Thanks be to God and I hope she stays there.

NOLLAIG: Is there any chance of her coming back?

PADDY: No. Well, I don't want to see her anyway. (*continues to laugh*)

NOLLAIG: (*to Molly*) Did you hear that one before, that granny was an auld jinnet?

MOLLY: (*laughing*) I did, I did.

NOLLAIG: So this granny somehow influenced your mother to send you children away?

PADDY: (*raises both arms and exclaims*) Yes, you see what it all comes down to . . . it was a clash of two families.

[Paddy's maternal grandmother is here cited as the central site of malignancy. However, such a hypothetical influence of lineage appears insufficient as Paddy proceeds to make connections between two semantic domains—the mad and the bad. This reflects not only his experience of marriage as the warfare of clans but also his literacy in the broad field of semiotics as well. Madness is now given a royal parade in a questioning that pursues the myth.]

"Maybe It Is True": More Royal Than Mad?

PADDY: All of my mother's family were mad. I could tell you stories of what they have done. It's unbelievable.

NOLLAIG: Mad in an interesting way or just mad?

PADDY: One of my mother's sisters was sold off to a man in marriage for thirty shillings.

NOLLAIG: Thirty pieces of silver.

PADDY: Yes, and another one of them, for example, phoned up and said his wife was dead. (*Molly laughs.*) They all went up to the funeral and she opened the door:

MOLLY: (*laughing*) Jesus, they were really crazy. But on the other side, they were always fighting.

NOLLAIG: They were just fighters, eh?

PADDY: Fighters, yeh.

NOLLAIG: But you think your mother's family was mad?

PADDY: Ah well, the things they did. They all thought they were somebody special. They all had high positions and they put titles on themselves that didn't exist. (*Paddy and Molly laugh.*)

NOLLAIG: Like they were all counts and countesses, kings and queens?

MOLLY: Ah, yes.

PADDY: Yes. Like there was royalty in the blood and everything.

NOLLAIG: And where was this royalty coming from?

PADDY: I don't know. France or somewhere.

MOLLY: On the grandmother's side.

NOLLAIG: France? They thought they were descended from a French line?

PADDY: From a French line of royalty.

MOLLY: Royalty.

NOLLAIG: Of course. Maybe it's true?

PADDY: Well, that's the trouble . . . I believed that and then . . . (*All laugh.*)

MOLLY: (*inclines toward Nollaig*) I made him disbelieve it.

NOLLAIG: What a shame . . .

PADDY: . . . and then an aunt on my father's side turned around one day and said, "Ah, yes, she was Queenie Ryan," from Annalivia Mansions [a fictitious slum area in the inner city] and so I don't know. (*Everyone laughs.*)

MOLLY: Imelda and Philip must be having a great laugh on the other side [of the mirror].

NOLLAIG: Maybe it is a true story. Maybe these people were royalty that weren't acknowledged. I'm serious . . .

MOLLY: (*laughs uproariously*) I didn't think I was going to get this good a laugh today.

NOLLAIG: It could be a true story.

PADDY: Well, I'm not sure if it is, but it doesn't matter anyway. I don't know how we got talking about this.

NOLLAIG: They may have fled France at the time of the Revolution or something. (*Molly continues to laugh.*)

[With a sham-comic air, Paddy gives further evidence of the madness surrounding him. The royal legacy, however, is ambiguous and holds the risk that belief makes one party to a delusional discourse. Sensing this dilemma, Nollaig stepped inside. In juxtaposing myth with reality by way of questioning at the extremes, fantastic constructions fall away on their own account. In the fifth province, deconstruction best proceeds by way of exaggeration. Thus the activity of demolition is absent in deconstruction. Given enough time any blown-up construction of doubtful premises weighted with many stories finally topples.]

"She Will Never Come Out Now": Fear of Contamination

PADDY: What did not help my mother was my granny.

NOLLAIG: Oh. They were very close?

PADDY: They were very close and she was a bad, ill pill, that one.

NOLLAIG: The jinnet?

PADDY: And I am glad she is where she is today. God forgive me.

NOLLAIG: Where do you think she is?

PADDY: The only thing I used to say, I hope they put ten tons . . . (*Molly laughs and begins to interrupt.*) No. Let's be serious now . . . you shouldn't be laughing . . . ten ton of Readymix [concrete] on top of her and she will never come out now. (*Molly and Nollaig laugh.*)

NOLLAIG: But what about her soul?

PADDY: Pardon? (*speaking with great emphasis*) She hadn't got a soul. She was too bad. She was a bad, ill person, that one, you know.

NOLLAIG: And you think that the bad things that have happened in your family have come from this old lady?

PADDY: Well, I would say she wasn't much of an influence on it anyway.

MOLLY: A good influence.

PADDY: She wasn't much of a good influence.

NOLLAIG: But somehow in your mind she is more responsible than your parents or anyone else?

PADDY: Well if they had a row, he always had a door to knock on and go in.

MOLLY: He would go to his sister's.

PADDY: And my mother always had her mother to take her in. Whereas if people at the beginning had said, "No, go on, go back and sort it out yourselves," things might have been different. I am not saying they would, but they always had too many doors open to them.

[In this embracing of Celtic metamorphosis (jinnet) and repudiation of religious resurrection (under 10 tons of cement) a permanent literal extinction for grandmother is called for. However, to remain on the safe side, Paddy implores forgiveness from God for his revenging wish. To lay waste to an exceptional seam of influence is now his passionate hope for the future of his lineage. Incarcerated in a concrete metaphor and beastly simile, the ancestor is banished beyond the reach of mortal return or spiritual afterlife. This humorous castigation is the distracting subtext, which rises up to offset the grief for so many casualties, with more to come. Prophesy becomes the order of the day and is carried through contaminating maternal matrices.]

"I Would Say He Would Be Next."

NOLLAIG: And how long after did your mother kill herself (*referring to the death of mother's partner*)?

MOLLY: Three years.

PADDY: About three years afterwards.

NOLLAIG: I see.

MOLLY: She did not do it straight away.

PADDY: She did not do it straight away, but then she did do it and that was the end.

NOLLAIG: And how soon after that did your sister succeed?

PADDY: About nine months.

MOLLY: Oh no.

PADDY: Was it not?

MOLLY: Your mammy will be four years dead on March 22nd, your sister was only a year dead in October.

PADDY: Sorry, two or three years . . . she died. But she did it differently.

NOLLAIG: How did she do it?

PADDY: She jumped out of a window, eight or nine stories up. I think she fell a hundred, seventy or eighty feet and when Mammy did it, it was with tablets. My sister just jumped, that was it.

NOLLAIG: And was anybody surprised?

PADDY AND MOLLY: No. Not really.

NOLLAIG: You knew it was coming?

MOLLY: She used to always say this . . .

PADDY: Well, you would never know it was coming. But then it did happen . . .

MOLLY: They were that kind of a family.

NOLLAIG: You can predict?

PADDY: Well it did happen. I would say my brother, he will probably be . . .

NOLLAIG: . . . next?

PADDY: I would say he would be next now.

NOLLAIG: And after that?

MOLLY: Especially now when it comes up to the time Mammy died.

NOLLAIG: He might do it?

PADDY: Well . . .

MOLLY: When his sister was alive, she used to send flowers for the anniversary, for her mother's anniversary to his brother. You see she was in England. She used to send flowers and mass cards and bouquets and what have you and this used to upset his brother. I don't think his brother would have gone near the grave very often, if it had not been for the sister. She would send the flowers and he would have to make the journey to the grave with them. An aunt used to say it was the sister who used to trigger him off. He would not think much about it or about his mother. The fact of having to go to the grave used to upset him . . . and shortly afterwards he would take the tablets or throw himself from O'Connell Bridge [bridge over river Liffey in the center of Dublin].

[Contrary to grandmother's fate, the mother's sad death is not an extinction but a calling home to the children separated from her. Fearfully the team wondered whether Paddy and Molly might not also be responsive to this calling.]

"So After That We Closed the Door."

NOLLAIG: You talk about Paddy's family as an infective kind of family

MOLLY: Yes, definitely.

NOLLAIG: Infecting both of you . . . and you can predict what is going to happen, and you have some prediction about your brother. Could you say now, what other things you can predict?

MOLLY: Well, you see the last year or so we have kept away from them altogether, really kept away from them. When his sister died they used to come to our house, another sister and an aunt and of course once they came there was upheaval. Now there really was murder. Paddy took their side and I really did not want them coming in, you know, I didn't. I had so much of them, I was frightened of them to be honest with you, really frightened. A great fear. And as far as I was concerned when we moved from our old house nobody knew where we lived and that was it and I was safe. Then they got back in again, of course, when his sister died, they found out where we lived and came up. This aunt and sister are also troubled. His sister is like his mother, the Lord have mercy on her. It has rubbed off there too. But how and ever they came and there was more trouble. So after that we closed the door.

[The "closed door" policy of Molly and Paddy became the metaphoric counterpart of the "open door" policy of Paddy's family and indeed the team. The closed door on a contamination/isolation threshold generated the explanation for the incarceration of this couple in life from life. Whereas the open door admitted conflict, madness, death, and destruction across its threshold, perhaps the closed door might be a countering prophylactic metaphor. The couple were not alone with their dilemma.

The team also differed as to how this literal threshold might be freely traversed. Might we be digging a responsive vein where madness was only lightly dormant? Were our probes the puncture wounds drawing blood from their unspeakable isolation. A tension developed in the team to release us all from what now appeared as the stranglehold of extremes. Fearful, part of the team moved away from our ambivalent dis-position and attempted to seek a more moderate course. The following "strategic" address of our dilemma was our attempt to re-cognize our deepening embeddedness in the prophetic mythoreality of the couple.

In the diamond (Figure 6.1) we depict a fifth province version of the intersection of the couple's dilemma with that in the team. In the figure, the couple are connected by their fear of the spell and through Paddy's "crazy royal" heritage. Their social isolation results from their fear of the contamination of madness and suicide. We in the team likewise wanted to be connected by our transformation from individual identities to the enlarged identity of a systemic team. Our subsequent isolation and fear of contamination was only to emerge later.]

"Close the Door–Open the Door": The Team's Dilemma

NOLLAIG: Do you know I have two colleagues who sit behind the screen and instruct me in various ways, so our way of seeing this is often . . .

PADDY AND MOLLY: different . . .

NOLLAIG: And perhaps the experience of being in here is different to the experience of being out there. And I just want to say what my experience of it is, that I am totally captivated by what you talk about. You talk about this in terms of it being located in one person, some tremendous force that comes out and touches people in its good and its evil parts.

PADDY: When you say captivated, do you mean totally taken in? Is that what you mean?

NOLLAIG: Captivated in the sense of being fascinated.

PADDY: Ah, yes.

NOLLAIG: (*to Molly*) I think you are very fascinated by Paddy's family.

MOLLY: Yes, you could be right.

NOLLAIG: Fascinated in all sorts of ways but left with this worry that maybe it disrupts one's mind or one's view of things. Now you see, I think it is very interesting and should be lived through even though what appears to have been bad things have happened, like your mother eventually doing something incredible with this force within her, like killing herself so that it seems to go with her. But, of course, it does not go with her, it continues. And I think that is a good thing that it continues. My colleagues disagree with me and they think it is a very good strategy you have of keeping well away from it. They think that it is a very safe strategy, that in fact your fears are correct. That if you do not close the doors you will get contaminated and go mad or kill yourselves or kill each other. And I disagree with that. I think that maybe one can come up close to it and really experience it.

[Molly returns to the next session claiming to be more distressed. As if bearing witness to our dilemma, she came forth in the sudden transform of the infected victim.]

"Gone Mad"

MOLLY: (*patting the back of her head*) Oh, oh.

NOLLAIG: (*patting the back of her head*) And this craziness, you felt was in your head.

MOLLY: I often said to Paddy, "Stop, stop, leave me alone. Don't say anymore to me: There is a little man in there. He is there again. He is banging." (*laughing*) It is just like there is somebody inside my head.

NOLLAIG: (*to Paddy*) So you are worried about activating this little man?

PADDY: Yes. I do be. I don't want it activated, you know. (*Molly laughs.*)

NOLLAIG: What kind of man might it be? It is a man not a woman, eh?

MOLLY: Ah well, it could be a woman. No, that is just the way we put it. I just feel like somebody is hitting me on the back of my head with a hammer.

NOLLAIG: (*patting the back of her head again*) Now I will go and re-arrange the two little men in my head for a while and come back to you. (*joins Imelda and Philip behind the mirror*)

[Molly's transformation is convincing and she has a man in her head to prove it. Lured by these extremes, Nollaig has joined her with matching men in her head. Together Molly and Nollaig are on a wave of "madness," leaving Philip and Imelda on dry land with no substantive voices. Paddy, the only legitimate candidate, suffers in silence. Nollaig, sensing that there is no going back, is sticking with Molly. After cautious team discussion Nollaig gave the following account of the team's dilemma.]

"Some Crazy Part of Me"

NOLLAIG: Well, my two imaginary colleagues, one male, one female want me to emphasize two points. The man wanted me to emphasize how you, Paddy, are a very protective father and husband, taking care of Molly, taking care of the children, worrying about them, covering all the odds. He thinks that is a very significant contribution to your family and for yourself in terms of this experience which became more realized for you after the birth of your infant son. He says he has no doubt but that will continue. The point that my imaginary female colleague made was that she sticks with the idea that both of you had last time in terms of keeping the environment as . . .

MOLLY: Germ-free.

NOLLAIG: Germ-free as possible. Thank you, Molly.

PADDY: Germ-free.

NOLLAIG: And she is not sure about that, because being a woman she acknowledges that you need a . . .

MOLLY: A social life.

NOLLAIG: Yes, she acknowledges that there is a high price but she was thinking that just as how you physically sterilize things and there are times when you have lapses (*referring to routines of exaggerated hygiene*) and she is saying that yes, maybe you can break that rule but she couldn't say when or where. Now I will give you my contribution, which is neither male or female, very amorphous, coming from . . .

MOLLY: Just you . . .

NOLLAIG: . . . some crazy part of me. And my part is that I remain totally enchanted.

PADDY: Yes?

NOLLAIG: Absolutely, totally enchanted, ignoring all the reality factors of the right thing or the wrong thing to do. And I am totally enchanted that in this family, particularly between the two of you, you deal with the most significant issues that I think most people put out of their minds—those issues are the possibility of killing oneself, killing the other, going mad, where that madness comes from? does it touch us all in some way?—and I think that is quite extraordinary. And although I don't absolutely understand how you do it, I acknowledge that you do it through your own special communion; that with your words, whether it is coming home and taking out the insurance policy and saying, "Hey Molly, sign this, you might pop off [die] tomorrow or I might kill you" (*Molly laughs.*) . . . and I am totally enchanted with that, that you see life with this dimension to it. And I leave you today totally enchanted.

[In dis-spelling the myth of contamination shadowing the couple, the three members of the team were drawn into a battle of exorcist proportions. In staking the dis-position of openness on the vulnerability of the couple and team to submit to the affective power of disclosure, the borders between the couple and team were fractured.

The conflict in the team mounted as Philip and Imelda complained that where once there were two, now there were three captivated people drifting together. Fearful, Imelda and Philip began to plan a rescue. Finally, they realized that only another spell could disrupt the spell-bound trio and release their colleague back to them. In connecting the story of the family to a cultural archetype, its local hold on Nollaig was displaced. Here, the three members of the team became the storytellers, transforming Molly and Paddy into an audience. Thus, they offered Nollaig the story of the Children of Lir as an allegory for enchanted metamorphosis and human isolation. In this allegorical traversal of stories, story-tellers and audience moved each other in an affective metamorphosis. Nollaig left her perplexed colleagues and returned to the couple.]

"There Is a Way for You to Become Mortal without Dying."

NOLLAIG: (*to Molly*) You became excited and entranced by Paddy's nonworldly family. They weren't mortals like other people. We think that you joined that world, really very willingly and very enthusiastically and we think that this mental torture that you mentioned, that you felt came from the family and in through Paddy and somehow to you, was a result of joining a different kind of world, a world of nonmortals, gods, kings and queens. We are now thinking that it is that world that you want to leave, not the earthly world around us. But for you to leave it is worrying for both of you, to come out of it. Because both of you feel that your lives are directed in some way by Paddy's mother. It seems that both of you, although you Molly are the one who is talking about it, feel you cannot ever get away from that spell and we think that explains your solution [suicidal thoughts]. We think that explains many of the things about the way you live. You live very close together, you don't really deal with the outside worldly world that much except where you have to. And we think you are tired of it.

MOLLY: (*nodding her head in assent*) Yes.

NOLLAIG: Maybe Paddy knows it better because he is in it a longer time. However, I think there is a way for you to become mortal again without dying.

MOLLY: (*showing great surprise*) Is there?

NOLLAIG: And my colleagues who want to help me have sent me this story which I will read to you.

[Here Nollaig reads the story of the Children of Lir, of the stepmother's jealousy of the four children, whom she transformed into swans for 900 years. With their human voices they sang their lament and moved through three destinations until finally they resumed their human shapes, aged, and died. However, in the Christian tradition, the ending of 900 years in "death" brought with it spiritual redemption and eternal life.]

"It's between Meself, Herself, Yerself, and Yer Two Imaginary Friends."

NOLLAIG: What I hear from the two of you, who are extremely united and caring and protective to each other, is that I get this overwhelming sense of how frightened both of you would be to change anything. And I know it is very difficult and I know you feel very frustrated but it would seem that with that fear there that the only solution for now, I am not saying forever, is for you Paddy to continue to attempt to take care of these episodes when they come up and you Molly, living through them. Philip and Imelda have also asked if you would like to include Molly's parents in the next session?

PADDY: No, Molly is very attached to me like she explained.

NOLLAIG: Yes.

PADDY: She wouldn't like anyone to know that she wasn't well and all these things. It's between meself, herself, yerself, and yer two imaginary friends.

Their manner of recounting a family drama of tragic proportions was more jocose than lamenting. The cutoff initiated by Molly, as a gesture to diminish her own overwrought sensibility, became the template for Paddy's panic-stricken vigilance, where he was the magisterial sanitary officer. However, there was a pall of suspicion over Paddy on two counts. The legacy of madness might have already seeded its infection in him, confirming him as his mother's child. As his father's child, the sins of the father might be on his head, repeating the destruction of mother/wife, Molly. Or had Molly herself, the mother of his children, encountered the ambivalent destiny of motherhood, where the day opening to the birth had its balance forever fractured. Constrained into isolation and exile from the pressure of external madness, they were now generating a purer culture of love, attachment, and protection suffused with unspoken fears and self-doubt. Molly languidly passed her time in this exiled place. Hers was the role of an invalid enclosed in a traumatic narrative. Paddy was the anguished spectator in the unfolding narrative, glimpsing portents of a more dangerous closure. As Molly's lethargy and litany of complaints developed into a pervasive chronicle for the day, he helplessly marked time by frequent checks. At lunchtime he dashed home uncertain as to whether Molly might have done away with herself and their infant son. When he asked her to sign an insurance form to cover financial expenses for a funeral, in the event of her death, she began to think that he too had become unhinged in taking her complaints so literally. Then he confessed to us that he also had been forced to drive his car to a cliff top overlooking the sea and played with the idea that this too might be his destiny. Molly's saga marked times past, of events she had witnessed. As a witness to her retelling, Paddy fearfully believed that she was foretelling the future of a recurring tragedy. Here the borderlines between a doomed past and a terrorized future were implicating each other.

The saga of the Children of Lir is a lament for the experience of indeterminate punishment for crimes not of one's own making. As witness to the story of Paddy and Molly, we heard a lament, breached up by humorous exaggerations and distortions including our own. By featuring the Children of Lir as the allegorical evocation of the story now witnessed, we were attempting to enclose ourselves with them in a story already told. Here their suffering is seen as a spell of endurance, slowing being erased by the hopeful redemption of time. Comforted by this understanding, the metaphor of waiting displaced that of watching.

Somewhere between these two juxtaposed spells, the saga of the royal lineage and the saga of the Children of Lir, Molly returned to social contact and Paddy's conviction of a damaging and damaged womanhood was shaken. For a short time Nollaig also returned to her colleagues, much to their relief. It appeared that the spells were broken but then shortly after we began to wonder whether the nets of the old spell had merely widened. Four days later, it being the fourth anniversary of Paddy's mother's death, the intimation of death foretold struck in an unexpected place. Our friend and colleague died. Bereft and anchorless, the team fled in different directions for some months. Her death surfaced a sensibility of panic and fear of which we had been aware only confusedly. At the moment of impact, we signified the story of Molly and Paddy as the portentous danger on a broader canvas.

"Is There Anybody Listening?"

In the aftermath, this new sensibility fractured the borders of events leaving us, our students, and other professional colleagues exhausted and endangered victims without compass or direction. We had promised to watch over the endurance of Molly and Paddy, but with none to watch over us, with what we, too, were enduring, how could this be? On this surface of bewilderment, sadness, and recrimination, forces of disconnection and silencing muted the fragile solidarity of the team. Gone was the playful transgression of implicating our own formation in the stories told to us by clients. In its place was the fearful caution and vigilance of bereft individuals. Somehow we regrouped, perhaps with the intimation that her death could rejoin us together, albeit in the extremity of solitude. This was the spell watching over us, requesting our endurance. Although, reunited, we felt under a pall of isolation, shuttering our work off from public display.

> Bolt and Bar the shutter,
> For the foul winds blow:
> Our minds are at their best this night,
> And I seem to know
> That everything outside us is
> Mad as the mist and snow.
>
> —Yeats (1984, p. 265)

We stayed there until we too happened upon an audience who could listen to our story. In the life of the team, an audience emerged from the field of family therapy[6] who listened and encouraged a tentative exit from our isolated haven of self-imposed exile and social exclusion. Each in his/her own way nurtured the way back to social inclusion. Their witnessing foretold a continuity beyond endurance, of a death retained in memory not as a blotted ending, but as the poignant opening cherishing connection.

The couple, for their part, returned to tell us that they had reopened their shutters and rejoined the social world. Paddy complained about our long absence and that the story did not suit him. Rip van Winkle would have been more apt for his predicament being only a 40-year sleep. It was some time, however, before we realized that we had inherited the couple's solution to contamination. In our fear we had sealed ourselves off together in secluded isolation until our story could be told and acknowledged.

Distanced now in time, we offer this story as a cameo of intertwining events which briefly metamorphosed a borderline space, reversing the sites of captivation between the couple and the team. This account is both a faded witnessing of our participation and a spiritual evocation of the fourth swan, our beloved colleague, JD.

[6]This important audience included Monica McGoldrick, Lynn Hoffman, Gianfranco Cecchin, Mia Andersson, Ernst Salamon, Klas Grevelius, and Don Bloch.

> My borderline country is where I live now. I am at home there . . . well at ease there. It doesn't worry me anymore what I think I see may be fantasy or indeed what I take to be imagined may very well be real . . . external reality. Real—imagined—fact—fiction—fantasy—reality—there it seems to be. And it seems to be alright. And why should I question any of it any more? (Friel, 1994, p. 67)

ACKNOWLEDGMENTS

We acknowledge the contribution of Philip Kearney, who with us comprises Fifth Province Associates; the enormous support of our colleagues and students in the Department of Child and Family Psychiatry, Mater Misericordiae Hospital, Dublin; and, last but not least, Paddy and Molly.

REFERENCES

American Psychiatric Association. (1994). *Diagnostic and statistical manual of mental disorders* (4th ed.). Washington, DC: Author.

Byrne, N. O'R., & McCarthy, I. C. (1988). Moving statutes: Re-questing ambivalence through ambiguous discourse *Irish Journal of Psychology, 9,* 173–182.

Byrne, N. O'R., & McCarthy, I. C. (1994). Abuse, risk and protection: A fifth province approach to an adolescent sexual offence. In C. Burck & B. Speed (Eds.), *Gender and power in relationships.* London: Routledge.

Colgan, I. (1991). *The fifth province model: Father–daughter incest disclosure and systemic consultation.* Unpublished doctoral dissertation, University College, Dublin.

Friel, B. (1994). *Molly Sweeney.* Dublin: Gallery Press.

Hydén, M., & McCarthy, I. C. (1994). Women battering and father–daughter incest disclosure: Discourses of denial and acknowledgement. *Discourse and Society, 5,* 543–565.

Hederman, M. P., & Kearney, R. (1977). Editorial. *The Crane Bag, 1*(1), 10–12.

Hederman, M. P. (1985). Poetry and the fifth province. *The Crane Bag, 9*(1), 110–119.

Hoffman, L. (1981). *Foundations of family therapy.* New York: Basic Books.

Jacobs, J. (1972). The fate of the children of Lir. In M. McGarry (Ed.), *Great folk tales of old Ireland.* New York: Bell.

Kearney, R. (1990). The fifth province: Between the global and the local. In *Migrations: The Irish at home and abroad.* Dublin: Wolfhound Press.

Kearney, P. A., Byrne, N. O'R., & McCarthy, I. C. (1989). Just metaphors: Marginal illuminations in a colonial retreat. *Family Therapy Case Studies, 4,* 17–31.

Le Brocquy, L. (1981). Notes on painting and awareness. In D. Walker (Ed.), *Louis Le Brocquy.* Dublin: Wardriver Press.

McCarthy, I. C., & Byrne, N. O'R. (1988). Mis-taken love: Conversations on the problem of incest in an Irish context. *Family Process, 27,* 181–199.

Palazzoli, M. S., Boscolo, L., Cecchin, G., & Prata, G. (1980). Hypothesising—circularity—neutrality: Three guidelines for the conductor of the session. *Family Process, 19,* 45–57.

Robinson, M. (1990, December 4). Inaugural presidential speech. *Irish Times,* p. 4.

Yeats, W. B. (1984). Mad as the mist and snow. In R. J. Finneran (Ed.), *W. B. Yeats: The poems.* Dublin: Gill & Macmillan.

PART II

✻

THE REFLECTING TEAM
Hosting Collaborative Conversations

The therapist's job is . . . to create a context within which the client can generate his own possibilities . . . taking the action he needs . . . in his own inimitable way.

—*John Weakland*

People do not present pathologies that need to be removed through some scientific process. They share stories that need to be honoured. . . .

—*Charles Waldegrave*

CHAPTER 7

Offering Reflections

SOME THEORETICAL AND PRACTICAL CONSIDERATIONS

William D. Lax

HAVING PARTICIPATED IN many different types of reflecting process conversations, I have been delighted by the creativity that therapists and clients show in developing formats and in offering perceptive, innovative, and useful reflections. These conversations have occurred in a variety of contexts and settings with a broad range of clinical issues, including outpatient and inpatient therapy, home-based work, supervision, research, consultation, training groups, hospitals, organizations, presentations, and teaching (cf. Davidson & Lussardi, 1991; Gottlieb & Gottlieb, 1990; Griffith & Griffith, 1992; Lax, 1989; Lussardi & Miller, 1990; Miller & Lax, 1988; Prest, Darden, & Keller, 1990). The utility of the reflecting approach has been found to be overwhelmingly positive, as demonstrated by responses from both clients and therapists participating in reflecting process conversations (cf. Katz, 1991; Sells, Smith, Coe, Yoshioka, & Robbins, 1994).

However, I have also noted, consistent with the reports of other colleagues (e.g., Madigan, 1991), that in some instances the reflections themselves have not been useful.[1] Clients felt that reflections were too confusing, did not address their issues precisely, did not give them enough direction, were too long, or left them feeling misunderstood by the

[1]As Sells et al. (1994) point out, there is sometimes a disagreement between therapists and clients as to the usefulness of the reflecting process. Clients are more likely to rate the reflections as more useful than therapists do.

reflecting therapists.[2] Reflections sometimes had a "watered-down" feel or pretend aspect with reflectors repeatedly using words such as "struck," "taken by," "impressed with," and "touched" and then followed by an overly positive (and Pollyanna-like) remark. In addition, as Madigan has described, therapists found that these comments frequently did not seem to be as rich as the later conversations they had among themselves.

Several general and specific questions began to emerge for me in light of these experiences. What happens when clients or therapists feel that this process is not useful? How is it that they feel misunderstood and might this misunderstanding be useful at times? How many ideas are too many? Is it okay for therapists to disagree or even question one another? When should new ideas be delivered or should the therapist stick only to what was raised by the clients in the interview? What components make up "successful" reflections?

This chapter addresses some of these questions, brings together existing material on some of the "rules" and guidelines for engaging in reflecting conversations, and provides additional directions for therapists on both the form and content of reflections. The guidelines presented are drawn from a number of sources, principally the work of Andersen (1987, 1991), Madigan (1991), and White (1994). Consistent with these authors, I specifically emphasize how reflections might be shifted more to the level of a "conversation" paralleling the interview itself.[3] I will not attempt to codify reflections but merely to look at their general characteristics. I will provide a brief theoretical backdrop for the reflecting process by drawing on some recent developments in postmodern thinking, including ideas from the areas of hermeneutics, social constructionism, and clinical psychology. What follows is intended to serve as a *guide only,* not as a prescription: to do otherwise would violate the underlying perspective of the reflecting process.

INITIAL GUIDELINES AND QUESTIONS

As I reviewed existing work, I realized that Andersen (1991) anticipated some of these questions. His guidelines are directed to both the process

[2]Throughout this chapter, whenever I refer to a reflector or reflecting therapist, I will be considering therapists offering reflections in a variety of contexts. These include, for example, a therapist working alone, a cotherapy team in a room with clients, and a team of therapists observing from behind a one-way mirror.

[3]I will refer to this part of the interview as a reflecting conversation, referring to both the process of offering reflections during the interview and how this specific conversation takes place, regardless of how many times reflections may be offered in an interview or with whom.

and the content of reflections, and he offers the following questioning and advice to therapists.

> When the reflections are delivered, one might think of this, "Should they be given in a monologue's form or as part of an exchanging dialogue? Should one stick strictly to just one certain idea or offer many ideas? Is the talk of the standstill system more intellectual and 'cool' or a bit more artistic or 'flowery'?" That might lead the reflections to be more straight forward in the first case and a bit more in the direction of metaphor and images in the latter. What is the speed of the talk? (p. 59)

In response to his own queries, Andersen (1991) offers a few rules: "The rules we have are all about what we shall *not do*: We shall not reflect on something that belongs to another context than the conversation of the interview system, and we must not give negative connotations" (p. 61). This first injunction asks us to attend to what is presented to us in the interview. Often we have prior knowledge of clients from referring agents, colleagues, or even other clients. If this information is not introduced in the interview itself, it should not be included in the reflections. One way to address this issue is to tell clients what you have been told about them at the start of the meeting. The second pertains to the negative value and impact of blaming. As Griffith and Griffith (1994) point out, "Anyone who has accidentally overheard oneself discussed in a derogatory manner in conversation knows the power of the reflecting position for magnifying hurt" (p. 161). This rule is extended to not even participating in negative conversations after a session, as those feelings have a pervasive quality in redirecting one's energy. As Buddhists warn, we must guard the thoughts as they lead to actions.

Andersen's (1991) guidelines also address how reflectors might talk with one another: "When we first started working this way we often found ourselves giving monologues. Over time we have turned to much more *conversations among the team members*" (p. 61, emphasis added). This conversation is the sharing of different understandings, with reflecting therapists asking questions of one another and the subsequent exploring and expanding of one another's ideas as well as those jointly developed. One question may lead to another, each potentially generating more information within the system between the participating members.

Madigan (1991) elaborates on conversation among reflectors. He describes how his experiences on reflecting teams included numerous incidents of therapists merely offering their own individual ideas to clients. There was little discussion among the reflecting therapists in front of the clients, as this dialogue took place after the clients left the consulting room. Consistent with Andersen's (1991) guidelines, he suggests that therapists should *specifically* ask questions of one another in front of the client system shifting to a *conversation* among reflectors with the inclusion of questions in this dialogue.[4]

Madigan continues by describing how the therapist in the reflecting process has the opportunity to open him/herself to change. To view the therapeutic process otherwise is to perpetuate a subject–object dualism that privileges the therapist and implies that the therapist has no need for new learning. By omitting the therapist from inquiry, the reflecting conversation gives support to cultural myths and sends several covert messages to the clients: Therapists are "neutral" in their thoughts and there are no cultural contexts out of which these ideas arise; therapists "have it all together" or are more highly "evolved" than the general population; and therapists can really "see" into others what is best for them, maintaining a hierarchical position for the profession. On the contrary, therapists' comments are culturally very rich, like clients, and come from a variety of local discourses.[5] Therapists cannot escape context either, as everyone enters all therapeutic conversations with, as Gadamer (1975) has described, some "forestructure" or "prejudice" that influences our interactions.[6] To ignore context would maintain the modernist "one-sided structure of therapy" to which "we keep ourselves therapeutically trapped" (Madigan, 1991, p. 15). Thus, by the greater inclusion of the therapist in this questioning process, all participants are actually assisted in making a shift from a modern to a postmodern position in which multiple descriptions may emerge.

If we as therapists, as Madigan suggests, truly follow a postmodern position of opening up this process to include ourselves with greater equity, might we include the possibility of clients asking questions of us during the interview? Isn't it possible that their questions of us might lead to the development of new descriptions or avenues of conversation that we had not considered? When we show some emotional response (or do not and they think we should) couldn't the client ask something about our thoughts

[4]Madigan, drawing upon a narrative framework (White, 1989, 1992; White & Epston, 1990; Zimmerman & Dickerson, 1994), views therapy as directed toward the opening of new narratives and reflections highlighting, for clients, "sparkling new events" or "new domains of inquiry."

[5]I use "local" here in a manner consistent with that of Geertz (1973). This local is always in a dialectical relationship to a "global."

[6]Andersen (1991, 1992) also comments on this postmodern shift and the inherent bias or "preunderstanding" in the questions that a therapist might ask. In recognition of this bias, he suggests that the reflecting team members "follow the same guidelines as the interviewer" and respond/interact as one might do in the interview itself (1991, p. 59).

or feelings at that moment? At the end of a session, couldn't a client ask how this session or therapy has had an impact on us?[7]

ASKING QUESTIONS OF THERAPISTS AND REFLECTORS

In response to these questions, I would like to assume that the answers are "yes" and that clients can be offered some of the same opportunities that therapists take with them. In an overt attempt both to lessen the power differentials in therapy (they cannot be eliminated) and to further the clinical interaction, many therapists already ask clients whether they have any questions they would like to ask of the therapist. They will do this during the session and at the end, hearing their clients from a position of believing that the questions are grounded in their shared narratives and that the questions can redirect the conversation. They may ask the clients why they asked a particular question but will almost always answer the clients, providing it is not beyond what the therapists feel is comfortable and appropriate for them. By having clients ask questions of the therapist, several outcomes are possible: More of the therapist's perspective is elucidated, more of the client's agenda can be introduced, and/or a new direction or narrative can unfold. It makes us as therapists more "transparent" in our thinking and more accountable. We can no longer remain shielded by theoretical rhetoric that invariably gives us the upper hand. It also possibly leads us to examine the therapeutic process and poises us to deconstruct the practices that we hold sacred. It permits greater informed consent and disperses with therapists as neutral or blank screens. The client is given a backstage pass to the inner workings of a large society of professionals.

Following Madigan, this questioning process can be extended to the conversation between reflecting therapists (see Madigan, 1991; White, 1995). All the above advantages are extended to this reflecting conversation. This questioning does not lead to a modernist reductionistic process but actually allows for different understandings to arise and for novel thoughts to be expressed. Reflecting therapists are encouraged to ask one another questions about their comments and thoughts. This process allows therapists to situate their comments within both the conversation

[7]White (1993) comments on the impact of the client on therapists, and how often we do not acknowledge the "inspiration," "joy," "metaphors that we are introduced to," and "sustenance that we obtain in this work." To help attune himself to this acknowledgment, he will at times ask clients, "What impact do you think this [new development/unique outcome/surprise] has had on me?"

they observed and their own lives, making the experience more personal and bridging the subject–object gap. These questions may include some of the following:

- What in the interview triggered your ideas?
- Was there anything specific that you saw or heard that led you to make these comments?
- Are there any ideas or values that you hold that influenced your comments?
- Was there something about what was said that touched you personally?
- Were there any experiences in your life that may have led you to those thoughts and would you be willing to speak about these at this time?

This process of questioning also allows for a greater sense of the therapist's transparency to emerge (White, 1992, 1995). This transparency often fosters greater connection between therapists and clients, which many clients and therapists see as beneficial no matter what kind of therapy one does.

For some therapists this shift toward greater equity, transparency, and accountability to the client is "scary." What, then, would lead us to take this leap? Why should we challenge existing models of therapy when they work well as they are? Are there existing resources that we can turn to in order to aid us in this endeavor?

THEORETICAL CONSIDERATIONS

Self and Other: Narrative and Social Construction

Whenever one challenges or examines a therapeutic process, questions arise, and the questions only lead to more questions: What aspects of this work facilitate change? Does reflecting itself make a difference? Does it really matter *what* is actually said or *how* it is said? Why should the therapist divulge his/her thinking to clients? How is that useful to the clients who are there for their own problems, searching to expand their own horizons? In offering reflections, can therapists or clients really understand what the other is saying? Must they develop an exact or even close representation of the other's world to have change occur?

Some of these questions can be addressed more generically by a turn to the interpretive fields of narrative construction, hermeneutics, and social constructionism. These approaches describe people as living their lives in language, through narratives or stories (cf. Gergen & Kaye, 1992; Sarbin 1986; White, 1989; White & Epston, 1990). These stories are shaped and give shape to our lived experiences. The stories that clients bring to us are constructed through myriad interpersonal processes, including their current interactions with their therapists and others. In therapy, it is the stories that clients generate with us about themselves that change as well as the stories we have about ourselves as therapists. Therapy becomes a process of an intersection of stories that allows for new narratives or understandings to emerge.

Thus, stories are relational. These stories and relationships are situated within a local culture that carries numerous "norms" and standards for social exchange. Stories are not, therefore, neutral, as they always come from some social or political context (White & Epston, 1989). Change occurs within social interaction, as we are able to participate *with* our clients in co-constructing/creating/developing an alternative narrative that is more consistent with their lived experiences.

This striving for relatedness is central to the hermeneutic and social constructionist positions. As Chalsma (1994) has written in his discussion of trauma and the stories shared with him by Vietnam veterans, "The hermeneutic attitude entails a willingness to respond to otherness . . . no matter how vast the gap" (p. 63) between one person and another. It implies an openness to other experiences, with the assumption that each person may change through this process of inquiry and exploration. This striving for relatedness is a shift from the individual to the individual in relation to the other. The development of a narrative or story is something that we do in conjunction with others, and the self cannot arise without the other (Shotter, 1989, 1993). This is also the epitome of the social constructionist perspective (see Gergen, 1985).

The development of a self through conversation with the other accents a shift toward a dialogical process of self-definition and challenges the Cartesian duality as well the modernist perspective of the self (cf. Kerby, 1991; Penn & Frankfurt, 1994; Shotter, 1993). From the perspective of modernity, the development of self involves a disowning or even a violence toward the other (Sampson, 1993). The other is experienced as foreign and marginalized, as evidenced in our treatment of women and people of color in the Western dominant culture.

However, each individual has, according to Gadamer (1975), a horizon or vista from which we encounter the world of the other. The intersection of our vista and that of others can be a "fusion of horizons." This fusion of horizons is the space developed through a shared meaning-making process in which each participant has a stake. This space does not preclude differences or the prejudices or biases of self and the other but allows for them. It is in this fusion that joint narrative construction takes place.

This joint narrative construction is part of a circular process of shared meaning making between individuals. It is not, necessarily, an intersubjective process, as the subject actually is displaced into the shared realm of mutual understanding of the self–other. While we can attempt to try to understand the content, process, and context of another's life, we can never truly come to "know" another's world but can only construct a mutual domain in which there is a shared, but not identical, understanding. The development of understanding is a process that is derived from the sets of information that both therapist and client bring to a conversation. The data of these interactions can only be "our own constructions of other people's constructions of what they and their compatriots are up to" (Geertz, 1973, p. 9). Out of this process arises a new whole with its own encompassing parts.[8] To participate in this shared world involves the temporary relinquishing of any fixed notion of "self" and adopting a willingness to enter into the world of the mutual generation of understanding with another. Understanding cannot be in the domain of a single individual, as "understanding involves two distinct subjects" (Weinsheimer, 1991, p. 82). It can become, perhaps, what Gergen (1994) refers to as the relational sublime, where even spoken language is not needed for connection to continue and self and other are blended.

Understanding arises when individuals relate to one another through language. In describing the work of Richard Rorty, Hall (1994) says that "from the perspective of understanding, one person's language is little more than a vague supplement to the language of another" (p. 6). Understanding is not a reductionistic process, moving toward one truth. In therapy it is often the experience of one of the participants saying something that the other experiences as coherent with his/her own thoughts, feelings, or behaviors. It is an interpretation that fits for the other. Yet an irony occurs, as described in the work of Fish (1989) and Derrida (1982), that the best any two communicators can do is "act like they understand each other," treating, reacting, and not objecting to one another, as if they understand one another. Then they can "say that they understand each other" (Taylor, 1992, p. 181).

Understanding is not facilitated merely by repeating others' words. "Only as interpretation *in other words*" can we advance our understanding of another's position (Weinsheimer, 1991, p. 82). By presenting one's ideas

[8]This intersection of participants forms what can also be described as the "hermeneutic." It is a relationship between participants that includes their individual and collective histories, cultural and local knowledges, what is already known, and what is new.

in other words we offer the opportunity to have the individuals think in different ways. Therapists do not stop with their own words as the final words but continue on a search and examination for new words, narratives, and descriptions. Connection is brought about through both using a client's words and rephrasing in other words. This position is best exemplified in White's (Sykes Wylie, 1994) dogged inquiry into clients' unique outcomes and his scrupulous notation of the words they use to represent these outcomes. These words are then offered back to the clients in both their original form and in White's own wording based on his different understandings of them, which might include describing successful steps, unique occurrences, or resistance to the pull of the dominant cultural discourse.

These words are not intended to represent a "true" reality. They are always *metaphors* that take on meaning through social exchange. These interpretative words or metaphors are always open for reinterpretation by the participants. Metaphor "always asks to be translated into another discourse" and "metaphorical discourse remains suspended in a generative play of similarities and differences that does not of itself terminate in a univocal concept" (Weinsheimer, 1991, p. 66). The metaphor must, however, carry with it some connection to the language of the other, as the connection to the other is central to this process. If the language is too different it will not be understood. Hence, we are always dealing with an exchange of distinctions. The art of therapy is to blend these distinctions, offer a difference, and remain present to negotiate the unknown future as a new gestalt is formed through the expansion of each's perspective, cocreating a new view, experience, or description.

Thus, therapy becomes a "generative conversation" (Gergen & Kaye, 1992) through a continual interplay of ideas searching for alternative narratives that can offer new coherence to one's life, joining the past with the future. This is the offering of the reflecting process: a presentation of both similar and *other words* to the client's words and the opportunity to develop another understanding in the exchange between the two. These words that bring about understanding, not being representational but always being metaphors, cannot be "correct" but only pragmatic. We always run the "risk" of being misunderstood.

Misunderstandings

Recently a couple I had been seeing for several weeks came in quite delighted with themselves and the changes that they had made during the past few weeks. One of them said to me, "What you said to us last session was really right on and has had a tremendous impact on us." They then went on to explain what I had said. As it happened, and I think that this is not uncommon in therapy, I did not remember saying anything like what they remembered and actually thought I had said something else! In the time between meetings one or both of us had somehow "changed" the words and/or meaning that had been expressed. I realized that this was not a new experience for me. Many times either I or my clients have "misunderstood" what I thought I had said.[9]

A similar experience occurred during an interview that Lynn Hoffman and I were doing with a couple. The clients had talked about "butting" heads with one another, and Hoffman thought that they had said "budding." She offered some reflections including an idea about the budding of new ideas in their relationship. The couple commented on this misunderstanding but were quite taken with the idea of budding rather than butting. The misunderstanding allowed the conversation to take a shift in a more positive direction, including their giving several examples of times that they indeed were budding into new experiences and exchanges.

These experiences are further supported by the work of Levine (1991) in his dissertation comparing post-Milan thinking with the Mutual Regression Model (MRM) (Gianino & Tronick, 1988).[10] The MRM addresses itself to the interaction between infant and caregiver and how they regulate their intersubjective interactions. This research highlights a participatory role in the development of communication between the infant and caregiver. This communication is developed through both a "match" and "mismatch" of interactions between the two, not regulated by either one or the other, as earlier research tended to describe. Levine (1991) likens this interaction to a dialogue or conversation. He noted that interactions include multiple misfits between two participants where there is a progressive (sometimes continuous, sometimes discontinuous) movement toward a consensual exchange or "fit" between the two. This state of attunement (Stern, 1985) is neither the product of one nor of the other but a new reciprocal arrangement with each as a participant in its construction.

I wonder about these misunderstandings or mismatches. Even if we could reconstruct "exactly" what was said in an interview, (e.g., by

[9]These misunderstandings are different from Rorty's (1982) use of Harold Bloom's conception of "strong misreadings" in which a reader "beats a text into a shape which will serve his own purpose" (p. 151).

[10]Levine utilizes the term "post-Milan" to refer to variety of approaches, including but limited to the following: Andersen's reflecting process, the conversational model of Anderson and Goolishian (1988), the narrative approach of White and Epston (1989), and the solution-focused models of de Shazer (1982), Hudson O'Hanlon and Weiner-Davis (1989), and others.

reviewing a video), neither the clients nor I could ever truly "understand" what was "actually" meant for the meaning can only be known in the transaction, and that meaning is always open for continual reconstruction and interpretation. While encouraging therapists to take a position of "not knowing" and allowing new ideas to emerge in the conversation, I realize that there are still many instances when therapists believe that they know what might be a more useful course of action than another. These ideas should not be ignored but considered as only one of many different directions that can be taken.

Here, again, hermeneutics and social constructionism may offer some added support. Hermeneutics, as described earlier, stresses the value of understanding, not of a true world "out there" but of a socially constructed one in which perceptions fit within some consensual domain. As described in an earlier article (Lax, 1992), understanding is a valued component of the therapeutic interaction. Both the client's and the therapist's perceived experiences of being understood help facilitate the conversation. When there is misunderstanding it does not mean that there is a break in the therapeutic relationship but a state of transition and tension. It is a time when *curiosity* can be present on both the client's and the therapist's parts. It is out of this misunderstanding that a different understanding can arise. For even when we present our version of what we understand of a client's presentation, it is still not an "accurate representation" of his/her world. Even in the most pure Rogerian model, when we are mirroring or reflecting back to clients what they just said, it is different from the original. Again, we are only communicating in metaphors. We cannot know their meanings but only the ones we construct. This is not to imply that all words are up for continual reinterpretation, for as Rorty (1989) has said, "Metaphors are unfamiliar uses of old words, but such uses are possible only against the background of other old words being used in old familiar ways" (p. 41). Misunderstanding can further open the door to a clinician's sense of curiosity (cf. Cecchin, 1987). The creation of a new narrative occurs in the context of this curiosity, match, and mismatch between the participants. Communication researcher and cybernetician Steier (1991) notes that not only is this mismatch frequent but it is exactly what researchers or therapists *should be* looking for and examining in their work.

Thus, it is out of this position of "misunderstanding" that understanding may arise, with understanding always transitional. We are never at a static place as long as we do not reify any particular position and believe that it is the best for all times and contexts. The therapist can try to stay with misunderstandings more intentionally, asking questions, as it is out of the unknown that creativity may arise.

PRACTICAL CONSIDERATIONS

Offering Reflections: Bridging Local Communities

When a psychotherapist and a client "enter into a therapeutic relationship, they become part of a local community (even as small as two) that has implicitly agreed to develop a local reality via the methods, techniques, ideas, and narratives of the psychology of the day and the region as they understand them" (Peterson & Lax, in press). A reflecting team is, as White (1994) has said, "another form of community that offers ideas, opinions, and acknowledges the other community's (the client's) life experiences." Within these newly constructed local communities, we are continually in the process of having interactions with the risk of "changing our minds" (Geertz, 1986, p. 114). The process between client and therapist is then one to "explore the character of the space between them" (Geertz, 1986, p. 119). This is what therapy is about: a co-construction of meaning based on an exchange of each participant's local position with the risk that our narratives will change through the conversation that takes place *between* us. If the narrative of one's life is truly developed in the shared space between individuals, then the reflecting process highlights both the separation and the connection between the two locals worlds.

Within this postmodern perspective, the offering of reflections to clients can be understood in many different ways. Andersen (1991) has described it as an extension of the talking and listening positions, in which the clients can be in each position with their respective benefits. For example, I have talked with many therapists who have been in non-reflecting-style group supervision where they present a case to the others and are in the talking position throughout the conversation. When the other group members offer ideas (at times competitively to see who's ideas are more "on target"), there is an expectation that the presenting therapist will respond to each comment. This process winds up like the trading of baseball cards that some of us did when we were younger: "Got it, got it, need it, got it." When one is not in the talking position but in a listening position, hearing comments–reflections, one feels a decreased pull to respond to each comment and is able to listen to a range of ideas, taking in what is relevant and potentially allowing a gestalt to form. This gestalt may be a compilation of several ideas, arising from a sense of cooperation not competition, multiplicity not reductionism. Sells et al. (1994) describe how clients say that being in the listening position gives "them more confidence and made them feel more comfortable" (p. 260). Clients state: "The pressure is off. I sit back, take a break, and listen to them (the team) dissect it (the earlier interview) . . . you see the problem differently" (p. 261).

With the reflecting therapists in the talking position, a variety of types of reflections can be offered. These may include metaphors, stories, direct suggestions, hypotheses, positive connotations, alternative descriptions, unique outcomes or sparkling moments, personal reminiscences or feelings, restatements of clients words, other questions to be asked, theoretical explorations, pragmatic suggestions, and even wanderings into reverie.

In offering reflections, we need to be aware that this entire process may be foreign to the clients in form, style, and content. Clients will be *talked about* rather than *talked to.* Reflections may be done in a style that is somewhat distant or "intimidating" initially to the clients, as the therapist(s) may not be known to them or maintain eye contact with the clients (Sells et al., 1994). The words they speak, while flowing from the initial conversation, may be different, with new ideas presented. Hence there needs to be a joining phase of reflecting comparable to that of therapy. If clients have not met the reflecting therapists before (perhaps they have been in separate rooms), an introduction is often useful, as well as stating the team members' names and affiliation to the site or setting.[11]

Role of Reflections

Reflections themselves follow a pattern similar to a client's story. There is usually a beginning, a middle, and an end. However, as we see with our clients and our own lives, narratives are not always coherent and do not always move toward closure with any certain continuity. As feminist writers such as Mary Catherine Bateson (1990) and Mary Gergen (1992) have described, narratives may be discontinuous, make abrupt changes or shifts, or even be somehow illogical yet still be viable to the individual. Reflections retain these same characteristics of freedom toward discontinuity, lack of closure, or the offering of radical shifts in content and context. If anything, they should *not* be reductionistic in nature with all reflectors agreeing on one idea, nor should one singular theme be presented.

Andersen (1991) believes that reflecting conversations can be extended to include "interventions" as ideas offered to the client system. These may be in a variety of forms but are not intended to be "given" to the client as the way to be. Rather, these more direct forms of intervention are given as *ideas* of an intervention that the client systems may want to examine for themselves (cf. Hoffman, 1992). This perspective maintains a view of collaboration with the clients but does not move

[11]White (1994) requests that members of a reflecting team begin by telling the clients who they are and identifying their professional affiliation. He asks each person to repeat his/her name before making comments.

to the modernist position of the therapist as an expert who "knows" what might be best for his/her client. It allows therapists to call upon their expertise and experience, making them available to the clients.[12] These ideas of interventions are an addition or expansion to those ideas of the client.

In contrast to Andersen's reflecting process, White (1995; Madigan, 1991; Dickerson, Neal, & Zimmerman, 1995) has developed his own style of reflecting. White (1995) proposes four parts to an interview: the therapists's interview of the clients, the reflections, the clients' responses to the reflections, and a debriefing and "deconstruction of the therapy itself" (p. 182). During reflection he proposes four classes of therapist responses. He encourages reflecting therapists to join with the clients initially, and then to orient themselves to the clients' unique outcomes and connect the sparkling moments that were expressed in the interview. He describes this response as orienting to a "mystery," in which the reflectors are curious and also "respond to those developments that they believe *might* constitute preferred developments to the people seeking consultation" (p. 183). Next, reflectors may engage in conversation about "landscape of action" and "landscape of consciousness" questions (p. 184). This is a zig-zagging process of connecting behaviors and meanings together through time: past, present, and future. Finally, there is deconstruction, in which reflectors ask questions of one another, as described earlier in this chapter.

White's work stresses the role of reflectors as participants *and* witnesses to the therapy process, providing support for the already existing changes that are or may be unfolding in the therapy context. The witnessing process can be extended to diverse areas of therapeutic encounters. One of these is exemplified in the Vancouver Anti-Anorexia/Anti-Bulimia League established by Madigan (1994), which is an expansive network of supporting witnesses.

White dislikes the use of interventions in reflections, as he believes that they continue the power imbalance between therapist and client and maintain the subject–object duality of a modern world. For White (1994), "intervention constructs a one-way account of therapy." He is more concerned with the reflections focusing on individual's personal relations to the conversation and extending one community to another. White sees as the purpose of the reflecting team not to introduce interventions but an opportunity to support clients in an examination of the unique outcomes that they have developed and what these outcomes may have

[12]It would be foolish to believe that these comments do not carry some weight, as they are coming from socially sanctioned "professional." However, a commentary on power differentials also may be proposed by the reflecting therapist(s).

touched in the lives of those watching them. It is also an opportunity for others to support clients' resistance to the dominant narratives of the culture under whose influence they have come and provide some external recognition to their development of alternative narratives in their lives.

Regardless of the style of the reflections, as stated earlier there are occasions when reflecting comments are completely ignored by the client. At these times clients and therapists report various experiences, including not having any connection to the reflections, the team "missing the point completely," or not being able to listen to the reflections, as they were still engrossed in some aspect of the prior conversation. I have had this last experience most frequently with couples who are strongly disagreeing. They are not able to let go of their former positions even to free themselves to listen, despite any elucidation of alternative behaviors or new descriptions, and the reflector(s) do not recognize this until after the reflections are over. It is the role of the therapist to explore this experience. Questions can be asked of the clients such as, "What would you have liked them to have said?" "What parts of our conversation did you understand and what parts did you not?" Again, rather than see the ignored reflections as "mistakes" (or client "resistance") they are better experienced as misunderstandings that require further inquiry as a transition to other understandings. Curiosity on the parts of reflecting therapists can facilitate the transition from ignored comments to new understanding.

There are also no rules about how many reflections may be offered during an interview. When there is a team present and there is a changing of rooms or positions, time becomes more of a factor than anything else. Usually more than two reflections become too time consuming for the length of an interview. A therapist working without a team may offer numerous reflections during the course of the interview, having a "conversation" with him/herself while the clients listen. The therapist can explain to the clients that this is how he/she works and would it be acceptable to the clients if the therapist has these reflecting interludes, sharing his/her thoughts with them while they listen. The therapist can look away from the clients, talk to the wall, or even his/her shoe. Clients are then free to be in the listening position and then comment or ask questions of the therapist after the therapist is done.

At the end of the reflections, the clients are left in the position of being able to take with them what they find useful in the conversation. Often these are underscorings of aspects of the prior conversation and sometimes new ideas. At times a gestalt is formed in which the clients develop a new understanding that was not present during the earlier interview *or* in the reflections. At these times it is even difficult to determine who the "author" of the new idea was, as it appears to emerge from that middle ground between client and reflectors. I am no longer surprised when I hear a client say, "I'm not sure who said this, but . . ." and describe something that no one had specifically said. In their listening to the comments, something new emerges that was authored by neither the clients nor the reflectors. This is a creative jump where the bridge between clients and therapist has been made and something has developed within that space between the two participants or local communities.

Types of Reflections and Rules of Procedure

Griffith and Griffith (1994) summarized Andersen's (1991) rules of procedure very succinctly. They list six categories:

1. Speculations are restricted to the conversations that have taken place in the room;
2. Ideas are presented tentatively, with qualifiers such as "I was wondering," "perhaps," "possibly," or "it's just an idea . . .";
3. Comments are formed as positive or logical connotations as opposed to negative attributions or blaming;
4. Team members maintain eye contact with one another, without being discourteous, maintaining the separation between the listening and talking positions;
5. Perceptions are shared and "consultants' thoughts, images, or imaginings are more emphasized than evaluating, judging, or explaining what was observed" (Griffith & Griffith, 1994, p. 161); and
6. Reflections attempt to present both sides of a dilemma, moving from an "either–or" position to a "both–and" position.

This last rule can be expanded to include a shift to a "neither–nor" position where something quite different from what was discussed is presented as a reframe. In keeping with Andersen's idea about comments following in a similar fashion to those of the therapist during the interview, reflections should not be too usual or unusual from the pacing, style, or wording of the conversation preceding them. Therapists should try to use the language and metaphors of clients, avoiding psychological and diagnostic terms. Here again attention is to the difference that might make a difference in the conversation. The task of the reflecting therapist(s) is to balance the tension between levels of difference. Comments must be connected to what has preceded them but be neither too much the same nor too discrepant.

To move too much in the direction of either side may not be useful to the clients and the emerging joint narrative.

Another type of reflection is new information that while stimulated by the therapeutic conversation, is somewhat tangential to it. Andersen (1991) refers to this type as a "surprise" (p. 67). Surprise comments may seem too unusual to the clients, yet when prefaced by some explanation of how the therapist got to this idea they may make more sense to the participants. When surprise comments are offered, there is the wonderful opportunity for opening up even more conversational space to all and further challenge the dominant discourses of both clients and therapists. Surprises can also be generated by one reflecting therapist asking questions of another, with the intent of deconstructing the reflecting therapist's comments. This is a process of making the unsaid "said" and available to all participants rather than between only the therapist and his/her colleagues in a conversation that may take place afterwards: questions such as, "What in the clients' conversation led you to these ideas? How did you come to that idea? What life experiences of your own led you to these comments?" Again, the discourses that led to these formulations are examined and not left as a priori truths leading to an all-knowing answer to the dilemma. The clients are freer to choose what of these discursive offerings are actually useful to them and not have the therapist make these decisions for them by withholding information about their "underlying thoughts."

At times, all reflecting team members may share the same idea. When one reflector states an idea, even if the next person has the same idea, it is that person's responsibility to come up with something else.[13] If all therapists state only one thought, the clients may be left with the idea that this is the only option. The emphasis here is on a "smorgasbord of ideas" rather than a reductionistic presentation. This is aided by not permitting any private talking among the reflectors watching the interview, thereby not allowing the reflectors to influence one another's thinking prior to the presentation in front of the clients.

Consistent with the above, there is another aspect that has received little attention in the literature: the role of modeling that is inherent in the offering of reflections. We stress how important it is to be respectful of clients and break down the subject–object dualities that exist in the larger culture. By acting in a manner that demonstrates multiplicity of ideas, active agreement *and* disagreement within a conversation, careful listening to one another's views, and respectfulness, we are providing our

[13]Clearly there are exceptions to this idea, particularly when the clients have come to a single resolution that has already shown its benefits. However, the door to alternatives should never be closed.

clients with another experience in the world. For example, reflectors on teams do have different ideas and opinions. One way to avoid an either–or position is to preface a potentially polarizing comment by saying something such as, "That is interesting. I have some other thoughts about that." "Other thoughts" are in *addition to,* not *opposed to,* and make a big difference. It is not up to reflectors to determine what should fit for the client, as that is the client's business. This is also augmented again by encouraging clients to ask questions of both the therapist and the reflectors during and after the interview. This is an experience we would like to foster as it subverts dominant paradigms and ways of being that people have been subjugated to throughout their lives. In addition, by our not being knowing experts who operate from a hierarchical position, we are allowing clients to take greater authority over their lives. This modeling should not be done with a new political correctness of "how life should really be led" but from a genuine sense of appreciation of the interaction with the actual life of the other in this shared work.

Following Andersen's (1987, 1991) guidelines, reflections should be brief, taking no more than 5 or 10 minutes. Recipients of reflections seem to be able to absorb only so much information at any one time, so reflectors need to be aware of not providing too much information, whether it is new or not. If each person on a four-member team made two comments and then there was a conversation, there would already be nine related but possibly different ideas presented. Length of comments ("more is better") is not the significant factor in an interview. Often a few short remarks with a conversation among reflectors examining them leads to the most fruitful reflections.

Regarding size, different formats and settings require different size groups, and no specific limitations have yet been found as a "rule." However, in usual clinical practice, my colleagues and I have found that up to four or five might be the maximum, with three as a good number.

It is also important to include in the reflections comments related to all members taking part in the interview. It is just as powerful to be omitted from commentary as it is to be addressed. This includes the therapists, as often they are left out of the reflecting comments yet are very much a part of the conversing system. Earlier it was mentioned how questions may be posed that were not asked in the interview. Teams of therapists who have worked together for a while also get to "know" one another. There may be interviews in which the reflectors are surprised that a particular therapist *did not* ask about some aspect of the conversation that usually that therapist might have. Reflectors can comment on this surprise, saying something such as the following: "I noticed that Sarah did not ask about [drinking/parenting/gender issues, etc.] during the interview. That is unusual for her and I was wondering if she just did not think about asking about it, or she decided not to. I wonder what would have happened if she had? Maybe she will be willing to tell us and/or the clients her thoughts on this later." In that way the therapist is free to comment or not on the topic, and it is at least introduced in the room.

SUMMARY

Asking questions of reflectors (or even therapists) about their thinking helps to open up other dialogues/topics that perhaps were thought not relevant to the therapeutic conversation (Madigan, 1991). By deconstructing therapists' comments, they are able to further explore their own unsaid discursive practices, helping them become more expansive in their ways of thinking and interacting. By making this unsaid "said" and more available to all participants, rather than between only the therapist and his/her colleagues in a conversation that might take place afterwards or not at all, clients are invited to take greater ownership of the therapy process and determine what narrative threads might be usefully woven together. The process of questioning allows for a mutual meaning-making process to occur between the two or more participants. This further breaks down the subject–object separation that our Western culture supports. Asking questions also serves to "thicken" the narrative that is unfolding, aiding and supporting creative processes and change in therapists and clients.

Obviously, this process makes interviews longer and perhaps "slower" than the usual type of therapeutic conversation. However, the length of therapy often becomes shorter in terms of sessions, as it also brings other conversations to the forefront that had been marginalized (by their not being overtly stated) that all participants can comment upon.

By valuing misunderstanding rather than marginalizing it, pressure is taken off the therapist to be an all-knowing "expert" or even to be "right." Mismatches and misunderstandings are integrated into the therapeutic conversation perhaps leading to sparkling events in the present. These misunderstandings may provide a path to new understandings between therapist and client that neither had considered before.

By emphasizing this process of questioning and valuing misunderstandings, the therapist reintroduces reflexivity into the therapeutic process. The therapist makes his/her own process an object of observation for both him/herself and the client. We can again become participants in the world along with our clients, striving to gain freedom from restrictive patterns of thought and action.

ACKNOWLEDGMENTS

My appreciation to Sydney Crystal, MSW, Steven Friedman, PhD, Roger Peterson, PhD, Joseph Pumilia, EdD, and my colleagues and students at Antioch New England Graduate School and the Brattleboro Family Institute for assistance in developing the ideas in this chapter and for comments on an earlier draft.

REFERENCES

Andersen, T. (1987). The reflecting team: Dialogue and meta-dialogue in clinical work. *Family Process, 26*(4), 415–428.

Andersen, T. (Ed.). (1991). *The reflecting team: Dialogues and dialogues about the dialogues.* New York: Norton.

Andersen, T. (1992). Reflections on reflecting with families. In S. McNamee & K. J. Gergen (Eds.), *Therapy as social construction* (pp. 54–68). London: Sage.

Anderson, H., & Goolishian, H. (1988). Human systems as linguistic systems: Preliminary and evolving ideas about the implications for clinical theory. *Family Process, 27*(4), 371–395.

Bateson, M. C. (1990). *Composing a life.* New York: Dutton.

Cecchin, G. (1987). Hypothesizing, circularity and neutrality revisited: An invitation to curiosity. *Family Process, 26,* 405–413.

Chalsma, W. (1994). *In the chambers of memory.* Unpublished doctoral dissertation.

Davidson, J., & Lussardi, D. J. (1991). Reflecting dialogues in supervision and training. In T. Andersen (Ed.), *The reflecting team: Dialogues and dialogues about the dialogues* (pp. 143–156). New York: Norton.

Derrida, J. (1982). *Margins of philosophy.* Chicago: University of Chicago Press.

de Shazer, S. (1982). *Patterns of brief family therapy: An ecosystemic approach.* New York: Guilford Press.

Dickerson, V., Neal, J., & Zimmerman, J. (1995). *Guidelines for reflections.* Unpublished manuscript, Bay Area Family Therapy Training Associates, Cupertino, CA.

Fish, S. (1989). *Doing what comes naturally.* Durham, NC: Duke University Press.

Gadamer, H.-G. (1975). *Truth and method.* New York: Continuum.

Geertz, C. (1973). *The interpretation of cultures.* New York: Basic Books.

Geertz, C. (1986). The uses of diversity. *Michigan Quarterly Review, 25,* 105–123.

Gergen, K. J. (1985). The social constructionist movement in modern psychology. *American Psychologist, 40*(3), 266–275.

Gergen, K. J. (1994, October). *Therapeutic communication: New challenges.* Paper presented at New Voices in Human Systems, Northampton, MA.

Gergen, K. J., & Kaye, J. (1992). Beyond narrative in the negotiation of therapeutic meaning. In S. McNamee & K. Gergen (Eds.), *Therapy as social construction* (pp. 166–185). London: Sage.

Gergen, M. (1992). Life stories: Pieces of a dream. In G. C. Rosenwald & R. L. Ochberg (Eds.), *Storied lives* (pp. 127–144). New Haven, CT: Yale University Press.

Gianino, A., & Tronick, E. Z. (1988). The mutual regulation model: The infant's self and interactive regulation and coping and defensive capacities. In T. Field, P. McCabe, & N. Schneiderman (Eds.), *Stress and coping across development* (pp. 47–68). Hillsdale, NJ: Erlbaum.

Gottlieb, C., & Gottlieb, D. (1990). The marital cotherapist team as a reflecting team in couple's therapy. *Journal of Couples Therapy, 1*, 67–76.

Griffith, J. L., & Griffith, M. E. (1992). Speaking the unspeakable: Use of the reflecting position in therapies for somatic symptoms. *Family Systems Medicine, 10*, 41–51.

Griffith, J. L., & Griffith, M. E. (1994). *The body speaks: Therapeutic dialogues for mind–body problems.* New York: Basic Books.

Hall, D. L. (1994). *Richard Rorty: Prophet and poet of the new pragmatism.* Albany: State University of New York Press.

Hoffman, L. (1992). A reflexive stance for family therapy. In S. McNamee & K. Gergen (Eds.), *Therapy as social construction.* (pp. 7–24). Newbury Park, CA: Sage.

Hudson O'Hanlon, W., & Weiner-Davis, M. (1989). In search of solutions: A new direction in psychotherapy. New York: Norton.

Katz, A. (1991). Afterwords: Continuing the dialogue. In T. Andersen (Ed.), *The reflecting team: Dialogues and dialogues about the dialogues* (pp. 98–126). New York: Norton.

Kerby, P. (1991). *Narrative and the self.* Bloomington: Indiana University Press.

Lax, W. D. (1989). Systemic family therapy with young children in the family: Use of the reflecting team. In J. J. Zilbach (Ed.), *Children in family therapy* (pp. 55–74). New York: Haworth.

Lax, W. D. (1992). Postmodern thinking in a clinical practice. In S. McNamee & K. Gergen (Eds.), *Therapy as social construction* (pp. 69–85). Newbury Park, CA: Sage.

Levine, W. (1991). Post-Milan therapy and the mutual regulation model. *Dissertation Abstracts International.*

Lussardi, D. J., & Miller, D. (1990). A reflecting team approach to adolescent substance abuse. In T. C. Todd & M. Selekman (Eds.), *Family therapy with adolescent substance abuse* (pp. 227–240). New York: Norton.

Madigan, S. (1991, Fall). Discursive restraints in therapist practice: Situating therapist questions in the presence of the family. *Dulwich Centre Newsletter*, pp. 13–20.

Madigan, S. (1994). Body politics. *Family Therapy Networker, 18*(6), 27.

Miller, D., & Lax, W. D. (1988). Interrupting deadly struggles: A reflecting team model for working with couples. *Journal of Strategic and Systemic Therapies, 7*(3), 16–22.

Penn, P., & Frankfurt, M. (1994). Creating a participant text: Writing, multiple voice, narrative multiplicity. *Family Process, 33*(3), 217–231.

Peterson, R. L., & Lax, W. D. (in press). Toward theoretical and supervisory multiplicity. In W. T. Forbes, K. Edwards, K. Polite, & S.-Y. Tan (Eds.), *Clinical training in professional psychology: Approaching the year 2000.* Washington, DC: American Psychological Association and National Council of Schools and Programs of Professional Psychology.

Prest, L. A., Darden, E. C., & Keller, J. F. (1990). The "fly on the wall" reflecting team supervision. *Journal of Marital and Family Therapy, 16*, 265–273.

Rorty, R. (1982). *Consequences of pragmatism*. Minneapolis, MN: University of Minnesota Press.

Rorty, R. (1989). *Contingency, irony, and solidarity.* Cambridge, England: Cambridge University Press.

Sampson, E.E. (1993). *Celebrating the other.* Boulder, CO: Westview Press.

Sarbin, T. (1986). *Narrative psychology: The storied nature of human conduct.* New York: Praeger.

Sells, S. P., Smith, T. E., Coe, M. J., Yoshioka, M., & Robbins, J. (1994). An ethnography of couples and therapist experiences in reflecting team practice. *Journal of Marital and Family Therapy, 20*(3), 247–266.

Shotter, J. (1989). Social accountability and the social construction of "You." In J. Shotter & K. J. Gergen (Eds.), *Texts of identity* (pp. 133–151). Newbury Park, CA: Sage.

Shotter, J. (1993). *Conversational realities: Constructing life through language.* Newbury Park, CA: Sage.

Steier, F. (1991). Introduction: Research as self–reflexivity, self-reflexivity as social process. In F. Steier (Ed.), *Research and reflexivity* (pp. 1–11). Newbury Park, CA: Sage.

Stern, D. (1985). *The interpersonal world of the infant.* New York: Basic Books.

Sykes Wylie, M. (1994). Panning for gold. *Family Therapy Networker, 18*(6), 40–48.

Taylor, T.J. (1992). *Mutual misunderstanding: Scepticism and the theorizing of language and interpretation.* Durham, NC: Duke University Press.

Weinsheimer, J. (1991). *Philosophical hermeneutics and literary theory.* New Haven, CT: Yale University Press.

White, M. (1989). *Selected papers.* Adelaide, Australia: Dulwich Centre Press.

White, M. (1992). Deconstruction and therapy. In D. Epston & M. White (Eds.), *Experience, contradiction, narrative & imagination: Selected papers of David Epston and Michael White* (pp. 109–152). Adelaide, Australia: Dulwich Centre Press.

White, M. (1993, October). *The narrative approach.* Workshop presented at Ackerman Institute, New York, NY.

White, M. (1994, July). *The narrative approach.* Workshop presented at Family Institute of Cambridge, Cambridge, MA.

White, M., & Epston, D. (1989). *Literate means to therapeutic ends.* Adelaide, Australia: Dulwich Centre Press.

White, M. (1995). Reflecting team as definitional ceremony. In M. White, *Re-authoring lives: Interviews and essays* (pp. 172–198). Adelaide, Australia: Dulwich Centre Publications.

White, M., & Epston, D. (1990). *Narrative means to therapeutic ends.* New York: Norton.

Zimmerman, J., & Dickerson, V. (1994). Using a narrative metaphor: Implications for theory and clinical practice. *Family Process, 33*(4), 233–245.

CHAPTER 8

Through Susan's Eyes:

REFLECTIONS ON A REFLECTING TEAM EXPERIENCE

Zeena M. Janowsky
Victoria C. Dickerson
Jeffrey L. Zimmerman

THIS CHAPTER INVOLVES a unique view of the reflecting team experience through the eyes of a client, who also happened to be a therapist. Upon arriving home from her reflecting team interview with us, she took a seat in her garden where, in the presence of her cats, she spontaneously taped her thoughts about our meeting for the next 20 minutes. Rarely have we been presented with such a specific response to the reflecting team experience, and one articulated so clearly only one hour after the reflecting team meeting. It is especially interesting to hear the perceptions of a therapist who had no previous knowledge of the reflecting team process or the theories informing our work. Susan's voice also stands as a distressing commentary on the subjugating experiences suffered by therapists in training, as they are subjected to some of the mainstream cultural practices indigenous to the "professional" psychotherapy field.

THEORETICAL MUSINGS: NARRATIVE, QUESTIONS, AND REFLEXIVITY

In a narrative therapy (White & Epston, 1990; Zimmerman & Dickerson, 1994), problems are viewed as existing in the meaning people give to their experience. People have their own specific experiences in the world, which they then compare to what their social knowledge tells them is "usual" for others. Based on this comparison, they construct stories to justify their response; these may be stories about themselves and/or others. These stories limit their interpretation of and attention to certain aspects of their ongoing experience. Over time, these stories begin to evolve and continue to develop in a particular direction. Rarely do people reflect on the meaning of those experiences that do not fit into the stories they have constructed; these experiences become trivialized, ignored, and discounted (White, 1988); they are "unstoried." In therapy, asking questions about "unstoried" experiences invites the client to attend to and become curious about them in a new way. These previously unattended-to and unstoried experiences thus become entry points into an alternate story.

Karl Tomm (1987) has theorized that asking questions creates more space for a client to notice possibilities for change than making statements does. In therapies that attempt to be evocative of the client's experience, this creation of space is critical to the work. Nevertheless, the context of a therapy interview, that is, a therapist asking questions of clients and their responding, does not leave much room (or time or space) for the question to "stir up" unattended-to, and thus marginalized, experience. On the other hand, listening to others (two or more) raising questions, without having to *immediately* respond, may put the client in a more reflexive position, one that would allow more possibilities for pondering.

A reflexive position can occur when people find they have some space to consider, think over, examine, and explore their own thinking. In particular, it allows persons to wonder about multifarious possibilities for understanding their experience. There are several ways that we have found to create a reflexive position in the therapy context: One is for the therapist to speak to one person in the room at a time while others listen; another is for the therapist to wonder out loud about what might be occurring in the room; a third is to take a break, so that both therapist and client can have some thinking time; a fourth might be to make specific suggestions to clients asking them to pay attention to or notice some preferred ideas or intentions or activities. We have utilized all these at one time or another; however, what we are currently finding most helpful is the structured creation of a reflecting team. In our use of a reflecting team, the members interview each other, raising questions about what has popped up in the interview as possible preferred outcomes.

When this occurs, a space is created in which clients can call to memory past incidents, make new associations, attend to some, but not all, questions, and generally wonder about what is being asked. When therapists on a team are purposefully raising questions about previously marginalized experience, this reflexive space is created. When, in addition, they offer their own experience as a basis for the origin of their questions (what we call "situating" their questions), clients also have the space to compare their own experience to that of the team members. Whether there is a fit or a difference between the client's experience and that of the team member, we have found that this comparison is helpful to the client. Our belief is that an experience of being in a reflexive position may offer a great deal more to clients than the usual listen-and-respond mode that characterizes most therapies.

THE PARAMETERS FOR REFLECTION

Presently our reflecting team/consultation group is made up of six therapists, three females and three males. Our seventh member is our consultant, also one of the authors of this chapter (JLZ). He helps provide ongoing training with regard to aspects of our work. With this emphasis in mind, team members have utilized the reflecting team for cases in which they are feeling "stuck," or when they think the team's reflections would be helpful to the therapy or to the client. Third, group members have used the team interview to provide an audience for the circulation of a client's difficult dilemma or change or the punctuation of a new accomplishment in the client's life. It is also not unusual for a therapist to bring a case to the team as part of the course of the therapy when no special problem or agenda exists.

The current format we use has a number of parts. Our use of all or some of them depends on the nature of the case and the client's needs along with the client's level of comfort with the interview. Clients are invited to the interview by the therapist and are told the sequence of the five-part process of the interview, which is as follows:

1. The therapist briefs the team about the clients with a minimum of information, usually only names and descriptive data; this precludes discussions of long case histories and thus avoids the risk of providing information about clients without their participation. The clients are then introduced to the team members.

2. The therapist and clients meet and talk together in a session that lasts 20 to 40 minutes, with the time varying according to the pace and needs of the clients. The team observes this session from behind the mirror or through closed-circuit television. Team members often take notes. They do not talk to one another behind the mirror. This practice safeguards the possibility of excluding the clients and the therapist from all the sharings. The avoidance of gossiping about the session also prevents

the risk of lapsing into pathologizing commentary behind the mirror, which has traditionally been interpretive of the clients' experience.

3. After the interview, the team switches places with the therapist and clients. Behind the mirror the clients are offered pad and pen in case they want to take notes. The consultant remains behind the screen to observe the team interview so that he/she can ask questions of the team later in the process. The team reflects on the session for about 10 minutes and then both sides switch places again.

4. The therapist and the clients discuss what they heard for a few minutes. The therapist invites the clients' initial response to what they heard. The clients are asked whether they heard anything useful or not useful or anything that provoked their thinking.

5. After this brief discussion, the therapist and clients are joined by the team and the consultant in the interview room. This final segment of the reflecting team interview brings all participants together to reflect and comment. In our case the consultant extends and develops the themes and "plot lines" that emerged in the interview. This is facilitated by the consultant directing questions to the team members and also to the therapist, specifically asking each of them to "situate" the comments they made. This additional layer of transparency collapses the distance between the team's and the therapist's comments and the origin of their observations. (We will discuss these ideas more later.) The clients are invited to ask the therapist any questions they might have about the therapist's questions. In an attempt to leave room for clients to ponder over the session in private, an effort is made to not pursue them regarding their responses. Because no one is being viewed through mirrors or screens, sitting together in this circle dispenses with the last bit of separation.

GUIDELINES FOR REFLECTING

Our understanding of *what* to share and *what not* to share during the process of reflecting is linked with our ideas of *how* to think and *how not* to think as a reflecting team member. These ideas also inform our approach to therapy. Our use of a reflecting team may, thus, differ from how others think of this process. We focus specifically on "unstoried" experiences that may be "unique outcomes" or aspects of the client's experience that would not be predicted by a telling of the problem story (White, 1988). We also are interested in raising questions about these unique outcomes, wondering whether or not they are preferred and what meaning the client may have put on these events. We are thus interested in inviting clients to an alternate performance of meaning.

Other reflecting team approaches (Andersen, 1991) do not stress the importance of asking questions about unique outcomes and place less emphasis on the client's experience. Our intent, of course, is to help clients be in a reflexive position in which they might be more apt to notice possibilities that could be useful and helpful to them. With these differences in mind, we have formulated the following guidelines for reflection.

Focus, during the interview, on "unique outcomes," thinking of them as entry points to an alternative story. Our interest is in staying with what has been discussed but in a way that allows us to pay attention to contradictions to the problem story and what might be considered preferred developments. We do not introduce new ideas or solutions. If, however, we think of unique outcomes as entry points, we are interested in raising possibilities for new meanings so that clients can consider an alternate meaning-making process. We ask questions about these previously unnoticed aspects of the client's experience and invite others on the team to ask us questions about our questions.

Formulate your curiosity and wonderings into questions. Asking questions has the effect of contributing to an evolving conversation that opens space for the client to ponder future possibilities. It helps the reflecting team not lapse into subjective comments or interpretive remarks that refer to theories of causation. Curiosity becomes privileged on an equal basis with theoretical understanding and expert knowledge. It allows the team members to remain connected to their personal experience and to share that experience through the lens of transparency. Because we work under the assumption that we cannot truly know the client's experience (White & Epston, 1990), we prefer to provide a sequence of possibilities that invite clients to select for themselves what is most useful.

Situate your questions. The process of situating means that we attempt to hold ourselves accountable by engaging in a specific kind of self-disclosure; that is, we say what personal experience, previously held theories, or newly concocted fantasies have led us to the content of our particular question. For example, a team member might say, "I was noticing how Susan had decided to fight her experience of self-doubt and pay attention to her own thoughts and ideas as if they had as much credence as anyone else's. I wondered if there were some specific thoughts she had prior to this decision that spurred her on. I am asking this, because my own personal experience is that I get a burst of confidence or self-certainty—almost like a flash—just before I find the courage to think about and privilege my own thoughts." This process of "situating" prevents our comments from being accepted as "truth" and offers "the information necessary to determine how they (clients) might 'take' the views that are expressed. . . ." (White, 1991, p. 37). When one team member makes an unsituated statement, the next person to comment invites the team member to situate his/her last statement; for example, "Why did you think about that?" The situating of our comments allows us to be "transparent" in a way that highlights our personal biases and viewpoints as well as providing a social, cultural, historical, and political context to our responses.

Use ordinary, not "psychiatric," language. After hearing the team reflect, clients often share feelings of relief that their expectations and fears of being pathologized were not met. There are often responses such as, "You talked just like people." This is sad testimony to the commonly held perception of the therapist as someone other than a helpful person. Due to client-degrading practices in psychotherapy, and many clients' previous experience with therapy, therapists are seen as experts, persons who see themselves as having the corner on the truth about human behavior. Consequently, clients are often wary of the therapist. Positioning the team in the domain of genuine conversation bridges this ill-begotten gap.

Reflections are wholehearted. We do not consider reflections either strategically therapeutic or interpretive. Instead, comments incorporate the experience of the team members as they listened to the interview. This is a conversation that takes place with a frankness between team members that has historically been withheld from the client's gaze. The conversation remains between team members and is not directed to the client. The tone is sometimes thoughtful, sometimes excited, sometimes concerned or contemplative. The team carries on their conversation until a natural stopping place is reached. At times this is when the client and the therapist know they have heard enough. We generally reflect for 10 minutes or less; otherwise our experience tells us there is overload for our clients.

Freire's (Freire & Faundez, 1989) work concerning societal change and power is applicable here to both the therapist's and the clients' relationship to power. "In order for power to be rediscovered, it is essential that we do not know everything that should be done. We must not be too certain of our certainties! We cannot, however, for that reason dispense with proposals as to what to do, suggestions to be tried out. By saying that we must not be too certain of our certainties, I do not mean that the correct course is to wander without direction trying to guess what to do" (p. 83). This posture of the "uncertainty of certainties" creates an ethical dilemma for the therapist with regard to his/her relationship to power and expertise. It introduces an accountability for the therapist's contribution of new ideas that encourages the therapist to self-monitor the coproduction of new knowledge and to be certain that it is firmly rooted in the client's self-knowledge. At this threshold between the worlds of the client's self-knowledge and larger dominant knowledges, an attempt is made for power to rest between the client and the therapist rather than to set one over the other.

SUMMARY OF THE THERAPY

Susan initially entered couples' therapy with her partner, Marty. Susan was finishing her training as a therapist, while Marty worked as a lawyer. Susan was also suffering from chronic fatigue syndrome. The couple came to therapy to discuss the effects of Susan's illness on their relationship. This led to other discussions about areas of their life together during which Susan voiced strong concerns about how the illness affected her ability to work. This eventually led to Susan's requesting some sessions specifically to discuss her career future after her illness prevented her from taking the final oral exam that stood between her and a license to practice therapy as a marriage, family, child counselor in the state of California. In one of these individual sessions, Susan told of a particularly humiliating experience with the licensing board that had recently occurred.

Because of her illness Susan had requested the right to pass on the impending oral exam with the intention of taking it in the next round of exams six months later. The current bureaucracy of the state licensing board would not allow her to pass on the exam without her attending the orals in person, where she was required to present herself to the exam proctor as too ill to function. No amount of medical documentation would suffice. If she decided to not present herself at the exam site, she would have to pay the expensive exam fee again and reapply with the complicated paperwork included. On the day of the exam Susan was driven to the exam site where she lay on the floor of the building hallway (she was too weak to stand) until the exam proctor came down to meet her. The proctor quickly acknowledged the humiliation that the inhumane bureaucratic policies had led to and sent her home. However, to add insult to injury, the board dropped Susan's entire application for the exam. Thus, Susan came to her individual sessions to discuss her ambivalence toward her career choice and the pronounced self-doubt this experience had provoked. At the end of this session, I (ZMJ) invited Susan to meet in our next session with a reflecting team as part of the process.

THE REFLECTING TEAM INTERVIEW

I met with Susan for approximately 30 minutes while the team observed. Susan and I discussed the sense of self-doubt and incompetence that led to confusion about the direction of her life. Previously, Susan had discussed the loudness of critical thinking that played frequently in her head. This "old story" about herself was linked to ambivalence about being a therapist and alienation toward what we had come to call the "hyperprofessionalism" of the psychotherapy field. The term I had originally used was expropriated from Charles Waldegrave (1990), who refers to "the excesses of professionalism" to describe the "excesses and limitations of some professional approaches and Western cultural bias . . . " (p. 10). Susan's coining her own phrase, "hyperprofessionalism" better described her experience. This hyperprofessionalism fed the critical thinking in a way that got her to doubt her own viability as a professional.

When the team entered into conversation they shared a number of questions between themselves about the lines of Susan's "old story" of "self-doubt" and "critical thinking" and began to explore the construction of "new story" possibilities. Susan had previously experienced this narrative text analogy (White, 1990) during our first few individual sessions. It was thus extended through the reflections of the team when they focused on an emerging new story of competence in which Susan was noticing how she could validate her own experience. This new story was further extended by Susan when she engaged in a meaning-making postinterview self-conversation on audiotape, which she subsequently shared with the team.

Included below are some of the team's questions and comments during the reflection that seemed to have prompted Susan's quick response.

- How was Susan able to imagine the experience of her new story?
- Where did that [this ability] come from?
- Who in Susan's past would know this new story about her? Who would not be surprised?
- Susan seems to have a strong connection with people, given her comment on the scariness of the new story and how it will affect her life's work.
- It also seemed so important for her to have that connection of love toward herself. . . .
- How did she get out from under the heaviness of the old story without criticism following her through the door?
- Do you think she's noticing that she has gotten away from the old story without criticism following her?
- I think I saw her leave the old story behind much of the time. . . .

- Susan said that "Marty might not like it" [the new story]. . . . Who will help her construct the new one?
- It seems that the new story is becoming unhidden, or coming forth from the old story, and it can't hide it anymore.
- I really related to Susan speaking about finding her creativity. I know that finding my own creative self has plucked the strings of my soul. . . .

What these questions and comments provide is a circulation of Susan's "newsworthy" experience. This circulation opens space for the process of restorying to occur. The comments and questions follow the trail of information left by the previous segment of the interview, which becomes a conversation that is extended and expanded on by the team. Ideally the conversation will continue beyond the interview space into Susan's life, which in fact is what occurred.

At the conclusion of the third part of the interview, I (JLZ), as the consultant, left Susan with an invitation that sparked her interest. Given Susan's dilemma concerning creativity and the oppressiveness of the specifications she experienced in having a "professional self," I said that I would appreciate hearing from Susan in the future, not just about her personal self but what her professional opinion included, in relation to the reflecting team interview. Susan's response was almost immediate.

SUSAN'S RESPONSE

I am sitting in my garden and I am just reflecting a little bit on the session I had today with Zeena and "the team." I am struck by many things, but right now the thing I am most impressed by, or thinking about, is the question that Jeff asked me: Could he hear from me sometime in the future, not just about my personal, but also my professional, opinion about what happened while I was there.

It is interesting to me that it seems that question was just part and parcel of the whole experience for me. What happened for me with that question was the old story came in really strong and said, "oh-oh, professional opinion? You don't have any professional opinion. You had better get out of here quick. Put it off. You don't know how to answer this. You aren't good enough. You don't know enough to answer it right anyway."

It seems that Susan left the session resonating to a number of the open-ended questions and comments made by the team. In her observation of the team Susan began to self-select those comments and questions that struck some timbre in her that, as Andersen (1991) so skillfully discerned, held the "appropriately unusual" (p. 160).

All the old story line came in strong with that. While I was driving home, the new story started coming in, saying, "Now just wait a minute, wait a minute. Don't assume that you don't know the answer to this question or that you don't have any professional self. See, that's the old story, saying you don't have any professional self, you don't have any professional opinions. You just don't know enough to do that." But the new story was saying, "Just give yourself a little space around this and think about it."

A whole lot of things came to me in terms of my view of what happened from my professional self. Even that was very freeing. I am sitting here thinking, "Wow, maybe I do have a professional self. It's all part of the new story." So, the reflections of my professional self are as follows:

I guess the first one is that it seems like such a refreshing way of working with people. I felt very refreshed, professionally and personally (but I will stay with the professional part), basically because the work is not pathologically oriented. After years and years of being trained and trying to work with people in a very different way, I appreciate the nonpathological view. I also felt that this particular way of working with people is based in the questions that the therapist asked the client and in what I see is a real avoidance of overinterpretation by the therapist, which is something that always made me feel a little nauseated.

When I worked with clients, I was supposed to be interpreting what they thought, so it seems like the questioning really makes it be an incredibly client-oriented work, in the true sense of the word, because the therapist is just asking the questions. It is up to the client to fill in the answers. I really like that.

I think we need to listen to the relevance of Susan's message about her experience of this process and its association with some people's beliefs about how to practice therapy. Unfortunately, hers is a common experience for many therapists in training. Susan was not traditionally trained. In fact, her internships took place in clinical settings where feminist and humanistic theoretical models were embraced. Nonetheless, the dominant indigenous ideas in the field of psychotherapy seem to engulf her preferred views of herself as a therapist. Susan cites the pathological interpretation of a client's thoughts and feelings as a basis for the therapist's "expert" status. Later in this transcript she goes on to acknowledge how frequently these interpretations are often methods of client blaming in disguise.

The intention behind the questions and wonderings of the team were all about how to help the client or what to encourage the client to reflect on, in themselves.

It seems like it is very basic and very simply being with people. I could be wrong about that, but that is the sense that I got in hearing the questions that Jeff asked the team and the way the team answered the questions. There was no psychological jargon. It was very balanced in terms of the team answering the questions, both from a professional viewpoint and from a personal viewpoint.

Susan was clearly impressed and touched by the team's transparency. Being with people in this honest way seems to have been somewhat shuttled to the side in a therapist's training. Susan was almost disbelieving of the team's forthrightness. In fact, during our next face-to-face individual session she asked whether we had gossiped about her after she left, because she could not believe that we had not discussed her behind her back. Susan is not a product of her own paranoia. She is the product of training that encourages the trainee to enter into a sense of being under critical surveillance, which is indeed the case in many training settings. Psychotherapy has inadvertently created a practice of scrutiny that replicates a societal surveillance instead of an experience of support and curiosity.

So the theoretical base just seemed so refreshingly simple and basic. It really seems like it's about being with people, which I feel I have been trained out of through my years at graduate school and through my internships. I am just longing to get that back. I saw a lot of that today.

The other thing that I felt was a great equality. I didn't feel as if the team was sort of a "therapists' club," which I have felt a lot in my experience with internships and all that. (It just seems like there is sort of an elite therapists' club that you have to be a part of. You have to join it and it has a lot to do with what Zeena and I have been calling the "hyperprofessionalism.") It just seems to fit. I felt that we were a bunch of people. I felt like I was gaining some benefit. I felt like the team was gaining some benefit. I felt like we were all people just doing this thing; we were all helping each other.

I did not feel condescended to. From a professional viewpoint, it would seem to me that it would be very freeing to not have to maintain some sense of pretense of being better than or knowing more than the client, or being the expert, and the client being the one who needs to be helped.

Susan's experience of the mutually beneficial nature of the interview is congruent with White's (1994) recently expressed ideas on the mutually beneficial relationship that exists between therapist and client. White's discussion includes a challenge to "the one-way representation of this process (that is) marginalizing of those persons who seek help." He links the production and practices of therapy as a mirroring of the production of the dominant modern culture where "a critical review of the one-way account of therapy exposes the workings of, and reinforcement of, the subject–object dualism that is so pervasive in the structuring of relations in Western culture."

Susan's comments point out that people helping each other in the simplest of terms seems to have gotten lost in the protection of the "hierarchies of knowledge that privilege professional knowledge" (White, 1994). The question is, can we admit to ourselves, our colleagues, and our clients how much this mutually satisfying work does for ourselves as people and as therapists?

The following statements call us into account for the kind of therapy that often engages in and/or mirrors a relentless perpetration of a culture of blame.

As I am reflecting on it, there are some of these things about this form of working with people that resonates with my feminist thinking, too, in terms of the equality between the therapist and client and the sense of the client not being the "sicky" and the therapist being the "expert," but rather the client knowing about him or herself, and also the social–political aspect. I did feel acknowledged in terms of my illness, which was nice, instead of having the feeling of "Ah hah, she's sick because. . . ." I got the feeling that people were really just acknowledging that I am sick and that's part of what's happening for me.

It seems like a nontheoretical theory. I like that and I felt comfortable with that and I think, as a therapist, I could feel comfortable with that because my discomfort with being a therapist has been around feeling separated from the client and feeling like I am supposed to be a certain thing.

I know that's part of my personal stuff, too. It's also part of the training. You are supposed to look a certain way, be a certain way. Many of the discussions I have had throughout my supervision sessions, internships, and graduate school have been very painful to me in terms of, for example, a group of therapists talking about how so-and-so client couldn't come in because they didn't have the money. "Oh right, sure they didn't have the money; if they really wanted to come in they would find the money." That kind of thing was so painful to hear; it was almost like a big gossip group. I really didn't like that. It was very, very uncomfortable to me, and I get the feeling that this does not happen with this particular kind of work.

Given the myriad of theoretical discourses informing this work, Susan's "nontheoretical" supposition is actually somewhat the opposite. Nevertheless, Susan's sense that this is a nontheoretical way of working provides us with confirmation of the acute awareness that most clients bring to therapy. It is an awareness that anticipates a sense of being operated on and analyzed through a lens of pathology. The reflecting team's adherence to a standard of curiosity rather than one of interpretation allowed Susan to reclaim her own lost voice as a professional with her own story to tell.

As the dominant story begins to peel away, Susan's voice strengthens as she begins to relate in detail a body of experience that previously had been kept secret and therefore invalidated. This secret history and knowledge of herself emerged with a painful candidness and sense of relief that exemplifies the process of both liberation from an old story and the constitution of a new, preferred self. The philosopher Odo Marquard's (1991) echoes this as he states:

> It is necessary for human beings to have not only one unique history or story, or a few of them, but many of them. For if they—each individual human being, and all of them together—had only one unique history or story, they would be utterly in the power and at the mercy of this sole history or story. Only when they have many histories or stories are they freed, relatively, from each story by the other ones, and thus able to develop a manifoldness that is, in case, their own . . . by virtue of the separation of powers; by virtue also, ultimately, of the separation of the powers that histories or stories are, and by virtue even of the separation of the powers that the tellings and interpretations of histories and stories are. (p. 67)

I don't need to be grappling over and over again with the convoluted pathological view of myself and feeling like I have to work with my pain and my suffering over and over again and look into my childhood and connect it all up. Perhaps that has been helpful for me in all the years I have been doing that kind of therapy. My professional feeling is also how wonderful not to have to grapple constantly with it getting so convoluted.

On the personal side, I appreciate moving away from that, moving into a more spacious place with all this, feeling acceptance, not having to look at, what did I do, how did I create this, what's wrong with me? Rather, looking at, who am I? It seems like it's the same question we look at in the sitting practice. [Susan practices meditation.] Who am I? . . . the inquiry . . . the old story versus the new story. It just feels freeing, and I feel very grateful to be able to do some of this work.

It feels scary, too. There is that element of the unknown. Today has sort of helped me to see that it is not as unknown as I thought it was. Yes, I think the new story has been with me all along. The feeling is now that I can really find it. I was so struck by Carol when she said that finding her own creative self has "plucked the strings of her soul." That's a beautiful phrase. So, I go away today feeling that it is within me . . . who I am, is within me.

What is so striking here is Susan's seemingly effortless paradigm shift. She goes from being under the influence of a number of currently popular dominant theoretical ideas of psychotherapy to a broader sense of herself as the author of her own thoughts, feelings, and actions. Although Susan articulates these ideas with a certain sophistication, it is not unusual for a client to have this experience after a team reflection. For a client to arrive in the liminal state of uncertainty and report feeling excited about new possibilities is about as good as one could expect. This privileging of the client's experience in direct relation to the theoretical posture of the therapist creates a powerful integrative loop of collaboration. Susan's final comments share the outcome of this.

The way to find who I am is to simply follow my vitality, follow my energy, follow that feeling place inside of me that does become so alive. It feels really hopeful, it feels really exciting. Let the process continue!

SUSAN'S FINAL THOUGHTS

I (ZMJ) recently invited Susan to read a rough draft of this chapter and the original transcript of her audiotaped response to the reflecting team interview. I have included the highlights of what she had to say as she looked back on this experience.

In looking back on the experience I had with the reflecting team, my memory of the experience itself was that there was a great deal of safety, respect, honesty, a sense of equality, a sense that I was involved in a community of people who were working together. So I'm left with a very, very wonderful memory of that experience. That in itself is something that I feel that I carry with me in my daily life. The experience has stayed with me, and I feel has changed me in some ways.

On a personal level, I feel that the pathological view that I had of myself, especially in connection with my long-term illness has greatly decreased. In other words, I am seeing myself from a healthy perspective, much more so than from a pathological perspective. So I can say about myself now: I'm a person, I have a long-term illness, and I can focus more on the things that I can do, rather than the things I can't do. I can say that I'm a person and I have a long-term illness, and it doesn't mean that I'm a bad person, or that I did anything wrong, or that I'm paying some dues, or anything like that. So the level of guilt for being "a sick person" has diminished greatly for me. I feel that is a direct result of the team session. There have been other factors in that change of view, but the team session really helped quite a bit with that.

I'm also, on a personal level, feeling that I'm more in the moment, more current with myself instead of focusing on difficult history. I'm able much more easily to stay with what is happening in the moment; if there's a problem or some kind of conflict, to just stay with the conflict in the moment and to resolve it with the moment, rather than having to delve into some kind of history, dynamic, or something of that nature. I feel that's a result of the team session as well. I'm not sure how that connects up, but it does feel connected. I think partly it's because there was so much emphasis on the new story.

I really found that the new story was something I already knew and believed about myself anyway; it was right there! Whereas the old story was very connected into history and the past stuff and the old dynamics and looking at pathological aspects of myself; so the old story now, as I look back on it, feels very old. The new story feels very current, and alive, and feels that it's a way I'm living my life much more. Certainly the old story comes in, and I recognize it, but I feel that I don't give it as much weight as I used to.

Another area that I experienced change with the team is in the area of my relationship with my partner and my close relationships with my friends. I'm finding that I'm asserting myself more easily. I'm able to say "no" to things that are uncomfortable to me. I feel okay about saying "no." I know my limits. I don't feel bad about myself because I have limits. I'm more genuine. It's as if there's a part of me I'm reaching down to inside of me, and I'm able to access it more easily and get it out and express it more easily. It seems like this has been greatly appreciated by my partner and all the other people in my life. I've gotten a great deal of feedback from people about how direct and honest and real I seem to be, in being with them. It has greatly enriched my life.

In terms of a professional point of view, which I would like to include here, my vision of doing the work with people, how I worked before I got sick, has really expanded. To be specific, I feel the split I had in my professional life was characterized as professional versus personal. With the work I did with the reflecting team, and the work I did with Zeena, I have found that the professional can be personal, and the personal can be professional. There doesn't have to be that split. That is just such a revelation for me, and such an opening. So I can envision the merging of my professional and personal self in the work that I will continue to do someday as I get better. That's very exciting to me.

These "final" thoughts are far from final. They speak for themselves, and they speak to the potential power of the reflecting team experience. What follows is not a conclusion but rather a countercommentary about the culture of therapy, including the reflecting team potential in our current economy.

DISCUSSION ON COST-EFFECTIVENESS

I (ZMJ) wasn't sure I wanted to participate in a discussion on the reflecting team and its questionable cost-effective merit. At the moment I find myself repelled by the conundrum occurring over the future of national health care in the United States. In California the present manifestation of this is taking place in the form of huge insurance conglomerates slurping up providers and small health maintenance organizations faster than we can consume root beer floats on a hot day.

Initially the idea of throwing the reflecting team approach on those waters was unappealing. We appear to be entering a period of intensified widget watching by insurance company watchdogs, and it's hard to know what it will all shake down to in the next five years. I found myself thinking of practical solutions such as the replacement of traditional case consultation with reflecting team interviews. I thought of research projects that would show that reflecting teams can result in a need for fewer sessions. Then I began to wonder what other countries with national health care do? Somehow, they have managed. Somehow those wishing to participate have done so, and I assume they feel that they have gained from it. In my experience the addition of a reflecting team in a clinic setting has always been welcomed. It is a commodity that sells itself.

Most likely it will never be understood by insurance purveyors, who will always value the most "bang for their buck" over intangibles such as increased hope and the renewal of meaning in someone's life. While thinking about this I came across a treatise on Internet entitled "The Economy of Ideas" by John Perry Barlow (1994), executive chair of the Electronic Frontier Foundation and lyricist for the Grateful Dead. This is a 25-page document concerning intellectual property and copyrights in the digital age. This expanded my thinking to include a broader spectrum from which to examine what we are up against when we talk in terms of cost-effectiveness. It occurred to me that cost-effectiveness may be far from the bottom line. Perhaps we need to view insurance companies as the current reigning emperors that have no clothes and are, therefore, of temporary importance. I quote from Barlow (1994), who got me started on this vein when he stated:

> Information Has to Move. Sharks are said to die of suffocation if they stop swimming, and the same is nearly true of information. Information that isn't moving ceases to exist as anything but potential . . . at least until it is allowed to move again. For this reason, the practice of information hoarding, common in bureaucracies, is an especially wrong-headed artifact of physically based value systems. (p. 8)

We can extend this analogy by examining the historical evolution of two-way-mirror work. The mirror has developed from a training mechanism rooted in hierarchical structure, to a collaborative therapeutic conversation. This has taken less than 20 years. Going back to Barlow (1994) again:

> Familiarity Has More Value than Scarcity. With physical goods, there is a direct correlation between scarcity and value. Gold is more valuable than wheat, even though you can't eat it. While this is not always the case, the situation with information is often precisely the reverse. Most soft goods increase in value as they become more common. Familiarity is an important asset in the world of information. It may often be true that the best way to raise demand for your product is to give it away. (p. 12)

What I am saying here is that if we get stuck on how to fit a well-rounded experience into a square hole, we will have stopped moving. We will sink to the bottom of the bureaucratic morass and become shark food. So, my thoughts are that we should get on with it and give away this gold with the wheat.

ACKNOWLEDGMENTS

We would like to gratefully acknowledge Susan, whose "authoring" of her own story and reflections on her experience encouraged the writing of this chapter. We also want to acknowledge the members of the reflecting team, Lucia Gattone, Russ Messing, Bob Poole, Dian Barkan, Michael Reins, and Carol Griff.

REFERENCES

Andersen, T. (Ed.). (1991). *The reflecting team: Dialogues and dialogues about the dialogues.* New York: Norton.

Barlow, J. P. (1994). The economy of ideas [On-line]. Available: URL=http://www.not wired.com/Lib/Wired/2.03/features/economy.id

Freire, P., & Faundez, A. (1989). *Learning to question.* New York: Continuum.

Marquard, O. (1991). Universal history and multiversal history. In *In defense of the accidental.* New York: Oxford University Press.

Tomm, K. (1987). Interventive interviewing. Part II: Reflexive questioning as a means to enable self healing. *Family Process, 26,* 167–183.

Waldegrave, C. (1990). What is just therapy? *Dulwich Centre Newsletter, 1,* 10–16.

White, M. (1988, Winter). The process of questioning: A therapy of literary merit. *Dulwich Centre Newsletter,* pp. 8–14.

White, M. (1991). Deconstruction and therapy. *Dulwich Centre Newsletter, 3,* 21–40.

White, M. (1994). *The politics of therapy: Putting to rest the illusion of neutrality.* Presentation at the Narrative Conference, Vancouver, British Columbia.

White, M., & Epston, D. (1990). *Narrative means to therapeutic ends.* New York: Norton.

Zimmerman, J. L., & Dickerson, V. C. (1994). Using a narrative metaphor: Implications for theory and clinical practice. *Family Process, 33,* 233–246.

CHAPTER 9

Widening the Lens, Sharpening the Focus:

THE REFLECTING PROCESS IN MANAGED CARE

Steven Friedman
Sally Brecher
Cynthia Mittelmeier

> It is like the movie *Rashomon*. It is about an event which is narrated by four people and the event changes depending on who is narrating it. . . . It was true. You have to take all of those pieces together.
>
> —*A father's comment*

THE FIELD OF FAMILY THERAPY has been rapidly evolving from an emphasis on biological or functional metaphors to ones that privilege narrative and story. This change is not simply a linguistic one but reflects a major shift in thinking away from underlying structures or meanings in therapy and toward an understanding of the family's predicament as one piece of a larger tapestry containing a variety of potential stories (e.g., Friedman, 1993a; Gilligan & Price, 1993). Drawing on this metaphor, we view predicaments and problems presented in therapy as threads of stories that have become self-determining, that have come to define for the individual and the family both the present and the future. It becomes the job of the therapist to look for, and access, alternative stories, ones that contradict the problem-dominated one. By so doing, the therapist sets the stage for clients to notice aspects of their lives and relationships that help define new, more empowering life stories. Strengths and resources become woven into the development of new narratives that generate hope and create a context for change.

Working in a managed health care setting requires that we maximize the time we have with our clients and make our therapy time-effective (e.g., Brecher & Friedman, 1993; Friedman, 1992, 1993b, 1994, in press; Mittelmeier & Friedman, 1993). In order to do this we have found it useful to integrate a variety of ideas into our clinical practices. Our work is conceived of as primarily competency-based (Friedman & Fanger, 1991), combining aspects of solution-focused (e.g., Berg, 1994; Berg & Miller, 1992; de Shazer, 1988, 1991) and narrative thinking (e.g., White & Epston, 1990) with the goal of offering clients new perspectives on their dilemmas and predicaments.

We also incorporate the reflecting team as part of this process (Andersen, 1987, 1991, 1993; Hoffman & Davis, 1993). The reflecting team offers both clients and therapists an opportunity to connect and collaborate in ways that remove hierarchical barriers and open avenues for generating new meanings and options for action. When we began seeing families together, using the one-way mirror, one of us would talk with the family while the others would follow the conversation hidden behind the mirror. At various points in the interview, the team would signal the therapist to leave the family and join the team for a brief discussion about what was being observed and what intervention might be given to the family. The family was seen as the object of treatment with the assumption that we had a better idea of how this family should behave than they did. Over the years, our thinking and experiences have led us away from this idea that there is one operating truth or way of understanding the family or that we can ever know what is normative family development (Lax, 1992). With that in mind, we view our goal in therapy as generating collaborative conversations that connect our observations with the ongoing narratives of the client's life (Friedman, 1993a).

In this chapter we explore an integrative, competency-based model that we have found useful as a way to generate new ideas and expand therapeutic possibilities for both the family and the therapist. Our work can be understood as encompassing two mutually interactive processes: a widening of the therapeutic lens to incorporate multiple perspectives and ideas about the client's dilemma and a sharpening of focus that funnels these ideas into workable action plans. The therapist and team shift between widening the lens—opening space for new narratives and ideas—and sharpening the focus—on solutions and action steps. This continuous and fluid process of adjusting lenses allows both the client and the therapist to entertain new ideas and co-construct preferred stories.

This chapter is organized into two sections. In the first section, we offer examples of the variety of ways we have incorporated the reflecting process into our clinical practices. The second section offers the reader an opportunity to listen in to a complete reflecting team conversation and to then observe how the therapist builds on the team's reflections to move the therapy process forward.

THE REFLECTING TEAM

> We are here to deal with their feedback on what we said, and our feedback on what they said we said.
>
> —*An adolescent's comment*

The reflecting team serves as a springboard for new ideas and options for action. Our goal is to maintain a collaborative, nonhierarchical and transparent stance by recognizing the family's expertise of lived experience. The comments of team members arise spontaneously as they connect with what family members are saying. While observing the family and therapist conversation, team members are silent. After about 30 minutes or so, the team trades places with the family and engages in a conversation while the family listens in. The following are some illustrations of ways the reflecting team has operated in our practices:

1. *To generate metaphors and images that activate, intrigue, and alter the client's understanding of the problem*. This includes the idea of "externalizing the problem." (White & Epston, 1990). In the example that follows, the reflecting team consisted of Sally Brecher and Steven Friedman.

SALLY: A question that just got raised for me is whether the family has come under the grip of fear and whether fear has begun to take over their lives in ways they haven't been aware of. . . . I'm wondering whether there are times when the fears aren't as strong and the family doesn't get recruited into worrying so much about Nancy.

STEVEN: I like that idea. I think I can see how the fears have gotten a grip and what it ends up creating are detectives for the fears, trying to study and research and understand them better.

SALLY: Trace their origins.

STEVEN: Trace their origins. And that in a way pulls people into the grip of the fears. That's part of the fears power of pulling them in. . . . In some ways it feels like the fears can take such control that they can just swallow the family up. . . . Yet like you were saying, there have been times where the fears haven't taken over completely and that Nancy has not cooperated with the fears. And again, are there some ways she can continue to do that and other ways her parents can help her not cooperate. Though it is always tempting to be a detective, the fears are really so tricky and sneaky and difficult to understand that it could become a never-ending process that could further envelop them.

SALLY: I got the feeling that maybe the parents and Nancy were becoming exasperated by all the work they were doing on trying to understand the origin of the fears and trying to fight off the grip of the fears. I'm wondering whether it's become intolerable in the sense that they really want to begin to stand up to these fears so they don't take over their lives as you were suggesting and push them in directions that aren't particularly productive. I would be interested to know, and maybe Nancy can tell us, of times when she's been fear-free. . . . Also, I'd be very interested in how the family might have gotten recruited into this view of fears taking over their lives. . . . Maybe the family can enlighten us. I'm also curious about what might be useful in helping them to reclaim their lives fear free and to stop being recruited into this view of the world as dangerous with the fears about to take over at any point. Also, I would be interested to know what sort of ideas Nancy might have about standing up to the fears. I'd love to be a spectator at her life when she was much younger and be able to have a sense of what it is she was able to do that helped her strengthen herself and be strong in the face of difficult problems that come along. . . . It's funny when we hear a story that is so filled with a sense of fear, it doesn't allow room for other stories about Nancy's strengths to come out. That would also be important to learn about.

This conversation, which took place while the family listened behind the one-way mirror, captured the attention of the family, and altered their sense of where they needed to put their energies. The reflecting team's conversation shifted the focus of the work with the family from that of being a detective for the origins of the fears to being a detective for ways the family could experience a fear-free lifestyle.

2. *To notice and comment on "exceptions" to the client's problem-focused view of self or others.* In the example to follow, the 12-year-old daughter was having temper outbursts. This excerpt from the reflecting team's discussion involves a conversation between Sally Brecher and Amy Mayer. A full account is given by Friedman (1994).

SALLY: I was thinking how Rose moved from "temper talk" to "Rose talk" and that more and more the temper isn't having a voice in what she says and what she does. First the temper was stealing her voice and now I get the feeling that she's stealing back her voice from the temper. And I'm wondering if the temper is feeling a little unhappy . . . "I'm losing my place in this family . . . and maybe I want to act up and tempt Rose again . . . because I enjoy bossing her around." When a temper is desperate it tries to pull some dirty tricks and I'm thinking that we can all fall for a tricky temper.

AMY: I was impressed about the times Rose was not letting the temper be in control. But there may be times when she doesn't realize this and that is how the rest of the family can be helpful . . . noticing and pointing out those times when Rose is in charge. The situation with the TV is a good example of how she was in charge, not the temper.

SALLY: The temper wasn't talking, Rose was talking. I wonder if Rose and her parents can sit down and talk about when the temper isn't in control of Rose and her voice, and when the times are going well for her. Because I think the temper really has her saying things she doesn't mean like "I don't care." That doesn't sound like Rose. And Rose's parents have found ways this week to get on top of the situation and they should be commended. They haven't let the temper push them around and Rose's not letting the temper push her around. My feeling is we're seeing real progress . . . real change.

[The reflecting team and family change places. The therapist is Cynthia Mittelmeier and the consultant is Steven Friedman.]

THERAPIST: I wonder what fit for you in what the team said and what didn't fit. Who wants to start?

MOTHER: I will. It's nice to see a different perspective of what you've experienced. It's nice to hear a positive message. One thing I heard was that the real Rose is not the same Rose we see when she's angry. This is important for me to remember because I take it personally.

FATHER: They seemed to be impressed with last night, with Rose cooperating. It was nice and they felt positive about it, which is good. It gives me hope.

CONSULTANT: You mentioned the step the team noticed about the TV situation. The fact that Rose had her own voice in this situation and wasn't being influenced by the temper, what does that tell you about the future?

FATHER: Hope! Maybe we can change this around. It was a nice feeling. I went to bed feeling calm. It wasn't an hour of screaming. . . . It was nice to be able to say "No" and get cooperation.

CONSULTANT: And you saw that that was possible.

FATHER: Yes. Right. It was. It was nice.

MOTHER: (*to Rose*) What do you remember about what they were saying about your voice and the temper's voice?

ROSE: They were saying that they heard my voice and not the temper's.

CONSULTANT: The goal here is really for your voice to get stronger and the temper's voice to get smaller and smaller. One of the benefits you have is that you are growing and getting stronger but the temper stays the same—so really the temper gets smaller and smaller and your voice gets stronger and stronger (*demonstrating with his hands*). . . . I'm wondering if it would be valuable to have a sign. If your parents see the temper sneaking around they can grab the sign, hold it up, post it up—"temper in the area."

ROSE: It would be kinda embarrassing in front of my friends.

CONSULTANT: Yeah. Well, it wouldn't have to be up all the time.

ROSE: (*laughing*) If my friends were over, I could just see my Mother come marching along with a sign. . . .

CONSULTANT: What I think would also be useful is tracking those times when Rose's voice is being heard without it being influenced by the temper.

MOTHER: Yeah. I would like to not listen anymore to the temper. Because I feel I get really hurt when I hear that voice. I think I need to say, at that point, for my own self-respect, for our relationship, I don't want to listen to that voice, because it is not you talking. And I'm going to walk away at that point.

3. *To "authenticate" change by making comments that embody and embed the changes in observed behavior.* In the following reflecting team discussion, team members respond to what the family considers preferred developments and show their interest in learning how these changes were achieved. As they puzzle aloud, their comments are expanded and embodied in an open and nonjudgmental conversation. This excerpt from the reflecting team discussion involves a conversation between Steven Friedman and Cynthia Mittelmeier. A full account is given by Brecher and Friedman (1993).

STEVEN: I'm very curious about the respect that I was observing the children showing to their Mother. . . . how that evolved to that point, because the last time we saw them that respect didn't seem to be there. Something as happened that has created the possibility for the children to show that respect in the way it was happening.

CYNTHIA: I'm curious about that too. In fact, when the family came in today they looked very different from the last time I had seen them . . . but I also thought, like you were saying, that people were acting different toward Mom and treating her with more respect. She came in and said "I'm the Mother of this group" . . . so I was also very curious about that.

STEVEN: How she got to that place . . . in spite of the difficulties, the concrete reality difficulties of her life. . . . I'm puzzled how she can maintain her composure and her consistency in the face of the demands on her time . . . how she's able to maintain that.

CYNTHIA: You said you were puzzled. What made you puzzled?

STEVEN: Because, after seeing the children the last time I could see how hard it would be to maintain your consistency. . . .

CYNTHIA: She really had her work cut out for her.

STEVEN: And so . . . it just threw me to see that. . . .

CYNTHIA: I was interested to hear the Mother talking about her Mother. She sounds like an interesting woman. I was interested in her comment about, that although her relationship has been tense, that she was really thinking about making the trip and maybe seeking her Mother's advice about some things. This is an area where she had a lot of respect for her Mother. And I wonder how she got to that point of opening herself up to that.

STEVEN: Yes . . . So there seemed to be the reaching out to the sister and now to the Mother and that takes a lot of courage.

CYNTHIA: A lot of strength in that reaching out; saying "I'm doing the best I can. . . . I'm doing a good job . . . but I can use some additional input. . . ."

STEVEN: "And if I reached out to my Mother in some way is that going to help my children reach out to me in other ways. . . ."

[The reflecting team and family switch places. The therapist is Sally Brecher.]

THERAPIST: The team was very curious about a lot of new developments. I wondered what you found interesting about their comments. Was there something that fit, that didn't make sense?

CARL [one of the children]: All of it was true.

MOTHER: I enjoyed the observations that they made. The impression I got was that they saw me as a strong person . . . and that I'm trying to be in control of these children that I couldn't get in control a couple of months ago. So that was positive for me. . . . It was nice to hear that the children have changed, from people looking in. That means something is working. They do show a lot more respect now. I have even seen that. I think with Matt, he's much more mature now and I think he's trying really hard. Ellen's changed so much it's been great.

THERAPIST: (*trying to engage the children in a discussion about the team's comments*) The team made so many positive comments about you guys having changed. . . . Do you know what they were talking about? Did it make sense to you? Was it like from outer space? What do they mean you changed? What were they talking about . . . you made changes?

CARL: They were talking about us.

THERAPIST: What is it that you are doing differently now that wasn't happening before?

MATT [another child]: Acting better?

THERAPIST: How is that so?

MATT: Mature.

THERAPIST: That's for sure. You know what I've noticed is your not interrupting each other so much.

MOTHER: They're more courteous to each other.

THERAPIST: There's more respect. This is a very tight-knit family. You've been through a lot of pain and suffering but you've come out on top.

MOTHER: Yeah.

4. *To generate alternative stories (ones different from the client's problem-saturated view) that open space for fresh perspectives.* The reflecting team was made up of Cynthia Mittelmeier, Ethan Kisch, and Sally Brecher.

CYNTHIA: I was really surprised to learn that Phil seems to have tackled alcohol. I was wondering how he went about doing that. I'm curious whether this is something he did on his own or if his family helped him. It's not clear when Phil will make a touchdown, but at least he's made a first down. I guess what his parents would like to see is him run with the ball . . . to take more responsibility. And as he moves forward he's gaining their trust and confidence. I guess I was wondering what would happen if the parents could be on the sidelines and take a break from worry . . . if they could continue to cheer Phil on.

ETHAN: As far as I know, Phil was able to stop drinking pretty much on his own. From what I can tell, he was worried that it was getting out of hand. I think he was able to tackle the problem on his own. Your metaphor of having his parents cheer him on is a good one because I think Phil wants that. Every athlete plays better to an enthusiastic audience.

SALLY: I am intrigued by your metaphor as well. I liked the thoughts the family was generating about how things would look in the future. The playing field you've described is really a future picture of a winning streak where Phil and his parents can be in it together. I was interested also in Phil's wishes to control his own destiny . . . speaking out against medication was a way to say "I can control things on my own" without the use of other help. I was wondering if he took more charge of his life in this way, would his parents have to take as much charge, whether the balance would look very different. I agree with you, if the parents show up at his games, and cheer him on, that would be a very important thing.

ETHAN: I think you're right, Sally, that Phil is making a decision now to do it on his own without medication, to be as independent as possible, to take charge of his life.

SALLY: I was thinking about the future and I was struck by the Father's comments that Phil has the potential in football to be quite excellent. I was seeing a real future there for him if these other things were dealt with. I was feeling quite optimistic because some of these other things have been dealt with and maybe there needs to be more history behind them, to establish that he's on the road to more touchdowns.

Following this conversation, the parents began to shift from a position of feeling they needed to do more to help their son to a position of seeing Phil as capable of "taking the ball and running with it." The Father commented: "Maybe he [Phil] would be more responsible if he thought we were worrying less."

5. *To identify and comment on aspects of self that are hidden, ignored or unnoticed; to take a humble position about the complexities of people's lives.* The following are comments from two different reflecting team discussions:

"I felt somewhat protective of the Father, and I think he was trying to tell us that there is more than meets the eye and that this is a long and complicated relationship, and that perhaps we were not valuing some of the unspoken things, the hidden things; for example, the degree of loyalty that they feel toward one another, and even the degree of connectedness that is there but doesn't emerge during the time of removal from one another. I think that his comment was a signal to us of outrage that we were minimizing in some way the many complex components of this relationship. That we have to stop perhaps at this point and give them time to reassess and absorb some of the things that were said today."

And from another reflecting team conversation:

> ". . . . [This] seems to be a certain transition where the daughter is no longer the Mother's little girl . . . where the Mother isn't sure how much she needs to protect, should protect, and how she can let go and let the process continue. I think it's a very painful time . . . in a way. It's [also] an exciting time because the daughter is becoming her own person. . . . This is very exciting , while at the same time there is a sadness about the Mother losing the little girl that once was more dependent on her. There has been a shift . . . and that is not an easy time to get through. My feelings from my own experience is that, often trying to be open about things, trying to share more of my inner feelings and concentrate less on rules and limitations, sometimes is a way of maintaining the contact or the closeness while the growing is going on. . . . I think the Mother has done an exceptionally good job in bringing Jane to this point. But it's bittersweet. I guess that's what I'm hearing . . . is that it is somewhat bittersweet."

LISTENING IN: A REFLECTING TEAM CONVERSATION AND THE THERAPEUTIC PROCESS

In this section, we listen in on a reflecting team conversation and then watch as the Therapist builds on the team's comments to move the therapy forward. As we will see, the reflecting team contributes a "both–and" perspective that pulls together the clients' differing points of view in ways that builds bridges of understanding and constructs alternative descriptions for the development of preferred stories. The reader will notice that the Therapist is active in raising issues generated by the reflecting team and asking questions that open space for the clients to acknowledge their successes and to become activated in the pursuit of their stated goals.

The couple described here are representative of many clients we see who find themselves immersed in long-standing and complex difficulties. As we will see, the reflecting process becomes a useful forum for moving the "standstill system" (Andersen, 1991) forward. Sam and Agnes, both over age 70, and married for 45 years, came to therapy because they were experiencing ongoing problems in relation to their adult children. But for brief periods, two adult daughters, both in their 30s, continued to live at home with their parents and to support themselves only marginally. Their parents attempts to get them to leave were met with resistance. Both Sam and Agnes were immersed in a view that had them convinced that neither their own actions nor those of their spouse could bring about change in this situation. Yet both parents felt that their lives would be better off if their daughters functioned independently out from under their roof. The reflecting team was introduced to offset the couple's sense of powerlessness by simply directing their energies toward helping them see themselves as agents of change.

We will now listen in on the reflecting team conversation and then observe the therapist (Sally Brecher) in her postsession interview with the couple.

Reflecting Team Discussion: Generating a Both–And Perspective

The members of the reflecting team were Ethan Kisch, Cynthia Mittelmeier, Naami Turk, Steven Friedman, and Madeline Dymsza.

ETHAN: Listening to him talk about his vision for the future with his wife, I was profoundly moved. Hope springs eternal. He's really ready to enjoy the time that the two of them have together, and take a risk doing it. Sam's a man who's not afraid to take risks. Because when you go to an audition for a play, you're taking a risk. You don't know whether you'll get a part or not. When you go to a show or you go to an opera, you don't know if it will be a lemon or if it will be great. Moving to have their children leave the house and spend the rest of their time just the two of them together is a huge risk, but one that I have a feeling neither of them is shrinking from. So I was really moved by their courage and by their optimism.

CYNTHIA: I wanted to thank Sam and Agnes for letting us in, in terms of what's happening in their lives, and to thank Sally for including us in this process. I feel very fortunate to have gotten to know this family. Just a few thoughts regarding Sam and his daughters' criticism of him. I guess my thought was, boy they're lucky to have him around and that not all adult daughters have Fathers at this point. I hope that Sam can rise above it in some ways, and not get too focused on it, not let it wear him down. I also think that these parents, Sam and Agnes, are preparing their daughters for the future when they aren't around. These are the steps that will, in the long run, be best for them. They are doing them more of a favor now than a disservice by taking these steps. Otherwise they're not going to be prepared for the future. So they're continuing to be good parents to their daughters, although it's really shifting into more of an adult/adult relationship which is appropriate at this point.

NAAMI: That makes me think about where they started out, where they're at now, and where they're headed. Agnes and Sam together have taken lots of steps to really move things along. What keeps on coming up in my mind is Sam's sort of skepticism but also sort of mobilizing comment about, I won't believe it until there's a date that's set [for the daughters to leave]. It's two things at the same time is what I was hearing. He's very wary of this. Seeing is believing, but I'm not sure he really believes it yet, even though he wants it to happen. On the other hand, I think it's a really mobilizing comment. They were both really listening to one another talk about what they're trying to do to move this along. But when it came to that particular issue, it was hard for them to connect around it.

STEVEN: Around which?

NAAMI: When Sam would start to say, "I won't believe it until there's a date that's set." They were really together, they were really communicating. Sam knows to sort of check in with Agnes to figure out what the plan is going to be about how they're going to manage their daughters' requests and so forth. But when it gets to the date they get stuck, and I'm wondering what that's about with them.

STEVEN: I was wondering about that too. Are they really just talking about the same things? It reminds me of a couple I saw that were about to get their kitchen remodeled, and the husband wanted to demolish the whole kitchen in three days and get it all done, and the wife wanted to do parts of it slowly, little by little, living with the old while the new was coming in. And the husband had trouble with that. He had built a lot of the original kitchen, and if it was going to go, he wanted it gone. Their goals were the same—to remodel the kitchen. The question was how to go about it—in a quick way or in a slower, more gradual way, where you're living with some of the old even though changes are happening.

CYNTHIA: I see that tension as actually useful and healthy. There really are these different perspectives. I think it does run the risk of being a potential road block, for Agnes and Sam to get locked into their own positions. But I also think, in a couple, that this can be useful—to have both styles represented. As Sally mentioned, these can fall along male–female lines.

MADELINE: They're really acting as a team in a lot of ways, too. She wants them out, and he's prepared to kick them out. Those are the two pieces that need to happen. You need to want them out and you have to possibly ask them to leave. So we have all the components there. It's just a matter of how they're going to put it together, I think.

STEVEN: I was thinking also of the Sam and Agnes boarding house. They're the landlords and they've got these tenants who are just giving them trouble. How do you go about getting them out? Do you evict them quickly or do you try to help them see that it would be better for them to move elsewhere and not live in your place?

MADELINE: And it sounds like they're giving the second approach a try. How long are they going to let that approach go.

STEVEN: They're seeing progress though. Progress is happening. The question is how patient or impatient they will feel with the progress. I was hearing Sally emphasize the progress, that their efforts are paying off already. Although Sam was having some trouble hearing that. He's getting more impatient, which is a very good sign, I think. Because he's letting his wife know he's supporting her in getting the kids out and working together. And he's also saying, as you were saying Ethan, before, he's ready to take that risk of he and Agnes starting a new life together without the kids.

MADELINE: I remember hearing about this couple in the fall, and I can just see how much progress has been made in this family, and all the changes that have happened.

STEVEN: Yeah, I'm impressed with the changes too. They're working together in a nice synchronous kind of way.

NAAMI: But I'm curious why it seemed like Sam had such a hard time seeing some of the changes, what that was about?

CYNTHIA: Well I think he's the healthy skeptic. Again, I think there's some utility in that.

STEVEN: The daughters seem to be becoming more background noise. They're able to lower the intensity, the volume.

NAAMI: Yeah. So how can they give themselves credit for where they are, as Steven was saying before, and not get caught up in this date business becoming a contentious issue. To give themselves credit, to celebrate where they've gotten to, to keep working on this path.

CYNTHIA: I was thinking, maybe they could set aside a time or a date for themselves each month to celebrate, to acknowledge, like the opera, like the symphony, since they have so many interests, to use that as a time to go out to dinner before or after and talk about the progress that they've made, and to take note. Because I think it is important to take note of our successes, to stop and mark them in some way.

NAAMI: It's sort of like birthdays in some ways. You mark developmental occasions with a celebration, and there is a real developmental shift here. Agnes and Sam have really moved in the direction of being a couple by themselves again.

ETHAN: I was thinking that it would be nice if they could see it less as an either–or situation—either the kids are out of the house or they're not—and see it in some ways as both–and. We're moving toward getting the kids out of the house, and while they're here we're setting some limits with them so that they're not really going to interfere with our lives and with the time that the two of us have together for each other. So I think if Sam and Agnes can see it that way, it will be easier for them to be cognizant of the progress that they are making in accomplishing what they want to.

MADELINE: I like that idea. It's sort of like they don't need to think about what they're going to be like as a couple without the kids. In some ways they're already there. They're already getting there. They're already doing a lot of things together. They're communicating like a couple. The kids are background noise, increasingly so. So it's not an either–or.

Sam and Agnes's Response to the Reflecting Team's Comments

[As you read the following dialogue, consider how the experience of seeing and hearing the reflecting team is integrated by each partner into their views about change. In what ways does each partner's reality impact on the other? What story is this husband and wife of 45 years fond of telling? What new story is the therapist working to co-construct based on the team's comments? In what ways has the reflecting team's conversation affected this couple's sense of hope about the future? How does the therapist's questions engage the couple in thinking about their predicament in new ways?]

SALLY: I'm wondering what you felt, what your reactions were to what you saw.

AGNES: They're narrowing in on one particular area, which is okay. I find that their assessment is more or less what I thought. They feel that we're doing well. We're getting along. We're getting them [daughters] out of the corral (*laughs*) and into the field. We'll open the fence, open the gates, and perhaps they'll go out.

SALLY: Was there anything in particular that struck you, Agnes? I mean, anything that one of them said that resonated for you, where you said, "Aha! They're hearing what we're doing."

AGNES: Well, I thought they were all hearing what we were trying to do. We're trying to get the girls to be willing to leave, and leave on their own, without yelling and hollering and saying, "This is it—you gotta go," and dragging them out.

SALLY: What do you think they were hearing in what you and Sam were saying together that got them to appreciate the fact that the two of you are working so hard? What was it that they were picking up?

AGNES: I think that they heard that we're trying to back each other up. I think that was part of the main point. And the more backing you have, the easier it is for you to go ahead and accomplish what you want to do. I think that they were zeroing in on that.

SALLY: Do you think they were picking up this whole business of stick-to-it-iveness?

AGNES: Yeah, well they were encouraging us to keep doing the same thing—to stay together and show the children one face, and one idea. And the idea is that they've got to look for an apartment on their own, one way or another.

SALLY: I had the feeling they were picking up that the two of you aren't defeated by some of the setbacks that have occurred. In fact, you mobilized around them.

AGNES: They seem to feel that we're very positive. If things aren't working out, we continue to go on. We're not becoming too depressed about it.

SALLY: How about you, Sam?

SAM: Well, what was absolutely outstanding in my mind was, they kept saying, "Sam and Agnes." And that's how I see us—as Sam and Agnes. I always have. But I am under the impression, after 45 years, that Agnes sees it as Sam being married but living his life only concerned with Sam. I don't see it that way at all. I think I'm very much concerned with us as a pair. She's never expressed to me that she ever saw that in me.

SALLY: So you were pleased by the team's comment of "Sam and Agnes," and seeing you as a couple really working towards the same goal.

SAM: They said, "Sam and Agnes this," "Sam and Agnes that." And that's how I see it. I can only give you my perspective. I can't give Agnes's. She's a different way.

SALLY: But let's just stick with your perspective about Sam and Agnes. Are you saying that somehow that gives you a sense of: you're in this together, you feel stronger, you're moving forward with more determination?

SAM: I see it as a couple, and sometimes she responds to that. I'll settle for that. What the hell? Life isn't any utopia. I have to take what I can get out of it.

SALLY: You're a realist. But, in some ways, they're suggesting that after the children leave, there's a Sam and Agnes.

SAM: They see it as, "Oh gee, Agnes and Sam—isn't that a great couple? I see they're getting ready to get rid of their daughters, and they're going to have a great life together, and they're going to live happily forever after." The music plays, and it fades out, and it's the end of the movie. However, again, if I'm talking with Agnes, we'll sit down and we'll talk about our life together and things, and I'll say, "I realize that we have our problems, but I think most of the time we get along fine, and we've done so many things, and this and that." Her response will generally be, "Yeah, most of the time we do this or that. But basically we don't get along." It's almost like we're talking about two different couples, when I talk and when she talks.

SALLY: Agnes is laughing on this one.

SAM: Yeah. But what's the real picture? It must be somewhere in between what I'm saying and what Agnes is saying. Which is okay with me too. If it were what Agnes is saying, then I've been cheated. Because somebody's been hoodwinking me. Because that's the way I see our marriage. I was 30 years old when I married this lady, and I started living for the first time.

SALLY: She opened up a life for you?

SAM: Absolutely. . . .

SALLY: So you love her. You're in love with this view of "Agnes and Sam," the view that the team saw.

SAM: Yeah, I see the same thing that they did. I see the same couple.

SALLY: Did the team's discussion of your relationship in any way broaden your understanding of how differences work in your relationship?

AGNES: The main people involved are Sam and me, and we don't do that well with each other, and it just carries on. I feel that what they were talking about is zeroing in on our working together to get the children out and I think that they're observing that we are headed in that direction. So I see that.

SALLY: Was there anything you heard from the reflecting team about your working to benefit your relationship, as opposed to making your relationship more conflictual?

AGNES: Well, they seemed to be homogenizing it—taking everything together and giving it to us as one unit, which was a very good way to present it. But I see a lot of things in back of that. It hasn't really reached that point that they're assuming it has.

SALLY: All right. But you could look at differences. You can look at it as "the cup's half empty" or "the cup's half full." Differences can be a plus or a negative in your relationship. I was wondering whether you picked up any of that in this discussion. Were they seeing these differences as something that could be useful to the two of you?

AGNES: They didn't seem to observe that we both are going at it in a different way. And we are. . . .

SAM: Excuse me. Isn't that interesting? They're neutral observers. They come without any prejudice. They're observing what's going on, and they're reacting to what they saw. And they seem to be saying—*all* of them are saying—"Gee, isn't this wonderful? Here's two wonderful people that live together. They enjoy doing things together. After 45 years, they're still optimistic. There's more good things to come even though right now they have a problem with the kids. They want the kids out, but nevertheless, they're enjoying their life together. They relate to each other." This is what they seem to be saying. I didn't tell them to say that. I didn't tell them to say anything. They're telling from their experience with human relations. They're making their observations, and I'm very optimistic. I see the cup as brimming over. I can only speak for me. I was really listening very carefully. And I feel very optimistic. After all, there are five people. They all seem completely in agreement. They said, "Gee, I wish my Father and Mother were like this." And I feel very good that I'm the guy that seems to be enjoying these things.

SALLY: Right. But maybe Agnes has a more cautious view on this.

AGNES: They're commenting on what was given to them. And what was given to them was our working together to get the children out. From what they saw in terms of that, what they said makes a lot of sense, and we are doing what they said, and then they comment on it in a positive way. But I'm seeing that there's other things, other ramifications, like if we came before this point, and told the problems that we're having between ourselves. . . .

SALLY: Right, Agnes, I don't think this is to say that there aren't problems in your relationship—real problems that need to be worked out. I don't think that they're saying there couldn't be those problems. But if you simply try to get into what they're seeing about your relationship—even if you understand that this is only a partial view—what were they seeing in your relationship that gave them the impression that you were challenging the problems influencing your life?

AGNES: I thought they were very aware that we are making progress in this direction and that's what this is all about.

SALLY: What do you think was jumping out at them, that they were seeing about the two of you. . . .

AGNES: Well, they said, gee, they're over 70, and we still feel that there's other things to do in our lives besides having the children in our home.

SALLY: Was there anything particular in your relationship that they might have noticed that said, gee, you're standing up to these daughters. Your taking back control of your life, basically.

AGNES: Well, by actually both doing the same thing at the same time, we're letting them know that we're acting together.

SAM: One person said, "Gee, this is really something. These people are perfectly willing to get their daughters out. And they're willing to risk a new relationship together, to face their problems together." They did say that. If you want to go back in the tape and you'll see that. They were aware that we're not the ideal two cooing lovebirds. We have our differences.

SALLY: I think they made that pretty clear. I think they know that.

SAM: They feel that if we have the courage to be alone together, to work out our problems, that's pretty good. And that's how I see it.

SALLY: Do you think the team had the impression that you had fallen under the domination of your daughters.

AGNES: I think that they sensed that.

SAM: Not exactly domination, but more that they were interfering.

SALLY: Yes.

SAM: Interfering with whatever we wanted to get on with.

SALLY: You had been recruited into the view that they had so many problems and difficulties that it would be impossible to ask them to leave. Now, somewhere along the line, you refused to have this problem defined in that way. You changed how you were defining the problem.

AGNES: I faced it more.

SALLY: You faced it more. You said, to me that you now wanted time to yourself. You didn't want to be cleaning up after them. You didn't want to be. . . .

AGNES: I didn't want to before, either.

SALLY: Right.

AGNES: Then, I didn't make it a definite issue and face it. And now I have faced it.

SALLY: Right. Something about you and Sam deciding to stand up to a life without this influence of the daughters seemed to be a shift. Do you think that the reflecting team was seeing this?

AGNES: I thought they saw it.

SALLY: They could understand this.

AGNES: Yeah, that was very obvious.

SAM: So what they're saying is, we appear to be willing to work out our problems, whatever they may be. And a lot of people in our position would just as soon have one of the daughters as a buffer, to be there. And we don't. We want them out so that we can work on our own, and I think that's good, regardless of what our problems are or they aren't. The fact that we're willing to face the situation and do it.

By staying present and future-oriented, the reflecting team set the stage for the couple to see a set of emerging possibilities rather than see themselves as immersed in a hopeless situation. The reflecting team also helped the therapist avoid being inducted into the problem-saturated story of the past, which was filled with pessimism and mutual recrimination. The accuracy of what was said by the reflecting team was less important that its power to generate a sense of agency in the couple.

Following this session, Sam and Agnes began to hone in on specific steps they could take together in reaching their mutual goal. The therapist, utilizing the ideas generated by the reflecting team, kept subsequent sessions focused on amplifying the small gains leading to change. However, as we have learned, personal solution fits are seldom predictable and therein lies the excitement and uniqueness of collaborative therapies. By experimenting with practical approaches requiring negotiation, Sam and Agnes discovered a comfort zone within which they could maintain momentum for change. No longer recruited into the old story of doing penance for past parenting mistakes and being fully responsible for their daughters' welfare, Sam and Agnes began to stand up for themselves. In subtle ways they became less involved in assisting their daughters. Agnes believes this was accomplished by "our getting out of the way and doing our own thing." At last contact both daughters were actively looking for jobs with an eye to moving out. One daughter had left home for a one-month job in another state. Sam and Agnes were off on several pleasure trips and attending to matters in their own lives.

In the above clinical example, two mutually interactive processes—a widening of perspectives, and a sharpening of focus—activate the standstill system. Perspectives are broadened by the comments of the reflecting team, and focus is sharpened by the therapist amplifying parts of the conversation that open space for the partners to think about their predicament in new ways. While the reflecting team conversation generates multiple perspectives on the client's predicament (a both–and view), the therapist, by funneling these ideas into the post-reflecting team conversation, opens up hopeful avenues for dissolving the clinical dilemma. In our experience, the reflecting team can be a useful forum for activating and mobilizing the standstill system. It then falls to the therapist to integrate the threads of the reflecting team conversation into the dialogue with the client. As mentioned earlier, our work in a managed care setting puts a premium on doing time-effective therapy. The introduction of the reflecting team, especially with "stuck" systems, has offered us a forum for providing both the client and the therapist a broader set of lenses from which to view the client's dilemma and has opened the door to a world of expanding ideas in a spirit of collaboration. We are not attached to any particular outcome; we view our roles as facilitators of the therapeutic conversation such that the client's goals are heard, acknowledged, and respected and room is made for movement along a path chosen by the client. We see our job as broadening the field of options and understandings while co-constructing, with the client, new possibilities for action. We do this by directing our attention to those aspects of people's lives and relationships that help define new, more empowering life stories.

REFERENCES

Andersen, T. (1987). The reflecting team: Dialogue and meta-dialogue in clinical work. *Family Process, 26*(4), 415–428.

Andersen, T. (Ed.). (1991). *The reflecting team: Dialogues and dialogues about the dialogues.* New York: Norton.

Andersen, T. (1993). See and hear, and be seen and heard. In S. Friedman (Ed.), *The new language of change: Constructive collaboration in psychotherapy* (pp. 303–322). New York: Guilford Press.

Berg, I. K. (1994). *Family based services: A solution-focused approach.* New York: Norton.

Berg, I. K., & Miller, S. D. (1992). *Working with the problem drinker: A solution-focused approach.* New York: Norton.

Brecher, S., & Friedman, S. (1993). In pursuit of a better life: A mother's triumph.

In S. Friedman (Ed.), *The new language of change: Constructive collaboration in psychotherapy* (pp. 278–299). New York: Guilford Press.

de Shazer, S. (1988). *Clues: Investigating solutions in brief therapy.* New York: Norton.

de Shazer, S. (1991). *Putting difference to work.* New York: Norton.

Friedman, S. (1992). Constructing solutions (stories) in brief family therapy. In S. H. Budman, M. F. Hoyt, & S. Friedman (Eds.), *The first session in brief therapy* (pp. 282–305). New York: Guilford Press.

Friedman, S. (Ed.). (1993a). *The new language of change: Constructive collaboration in psychotherapy.* New York: Guilford Press.

Friedman, S. (1993b). Escape from the Furies: A journey from self-pity to self-love. In S. Friedman (Ed.), *The new language of change: Constructive collaboration in psychotherapy* (pp. 251–277). New York: Guilford Press.

Friedman, S. (1994). Staying simple, staying focused: Time-effective consultations with children and families. In M. F. Hoyt (Ed.), *Constructive therapies* (pp. 217–250). New York: Guilford Press.

Friedman, S. (in press). Couples therapy: Changing conversations. In H. Rosen & K. T. Kuehlwein (Eds.), *Constructing realities: Meaning making perspectives for psychotherapists.* San Francisco: Jossey-Bass.

Friedman, S., & Fanger, M. T. (1991). *Expanding therapeutic possibilities: Getting results in brief psychotherapy.* New York: Lexington Books/Macmillan.

Gilligan, S., & Price, R. (Eds.). (1993). *Therapeutic conversations.* New York: Norton.

Hoffman, L., & Davis, J. (1993). Tekka with feathers: Talking about talking (about suicide. In S. Friedman (Ed.), *The new language of change: Constructive collaboration in psychotherapy* (pp. 345–373). New York: Guilford Press.

Lax, W. D. (1992). Postmodern thinking in clinical practice. In S. McNamee & K. J. Gergen (Eds.), *Therapy as social construction* (pp. 69–85). Newbury Park, CA: Sage.

Mittelmeier, C. M., & Friedman, S. (1993). Toward a mutual understanding: Constructing solutions with families. In S. Friedman (Ed.), *The new language of change: Constructive collaboration in psychotherapy* (pp. 158–181). New York: Guilford Press.

White, M., & Epston, D. (1990). *Narrative means to therapeutic ends.* New York: Norton.

CHAPTER 10

Rap Music with Wisdom

PEER REFLECTING TEAMS WITH TOUGH ADOLESCENTS

Matthew D. Selekman

> My method of enlightenment is simple . . .
> Teach one to reach one. Tell every sister
> or brother through my music to walk, talk
> and think profoundly before they speak.
>
> —*Profound*

PROFOUND, AN UP-AND-COMING rapper, writes and sings positive rap music that empowers youth to take charge of their lives, reach out to others who need support, and steer away from gangs and drugs. His music is truly a rap music of wisdom. Over the past 10 years, I have worked with many youth who have been gang-involved, have heavily abused drugs, and have presented with other chronic behavioral difficulties. Despite the serious nature of their individual and family problems, many of these adolescents had at least one or more friends in their lives who were concerned about them and were not in constant or any trouble themselves. Once I started experimenting with utilizing these concerned peers as consultants in family therapy sessions, I observed dramatic changes occurring both in sessions and outside the therapeutic context. Like Profound's words of wisdom, these peers' "rap music" was opening up space for possibilities with stuck and disempowered youth and their families.

In this chapter, I present a very brief overview of my solution-oriented brief family therapy approach (Selekman, 1993). This overview is followed by a discussion of five ways in which I use peers as consultants in family therapy. Finally, I describe the mechanics of how I convene peers and determine the session format. The case example of a 16-year-old gang-involved youth is presented to help illustrate the efficacy of utilizing peers in family therapy.

SOLUTION-ORIENTED BRIEF FAMILY THERAPY

Solution-oriented brief family therapy is a cost-effective family wellness approach that capitalizes on the strengths and resources of the adolescent, family members, the adolescent's concerned peers, and involved helping professionals from larger systems to rapidly resolve the presenting problem. The model is comprehensive and flexible and integrates the best elements of solution-focused brief therapy (de Shazer, 1985, 1988, 1991); therapeutic ideas from Michael White (1984, 1985, 1986, 1987, 1988; White & Epston, 1990); the Mental Research Institute's (MRI) brief problem-focused approach (Fisch, Weakland, & Segal, 1982; Watzlawick, Weakland, & Fisch, 1974); and narrative-based ideas from Tom Andersen (Andersen, 1987, 1991) and the Houston-Galveston group (Anderson, 1993; Anderson & Goolishian, 1988, 1991).

The solution-oriented therapist typically begins family therapy by keeping things simple, by capitalizing on pretreatment changes and assessing what family members' strengths and resources he/she can bring to bear in the presenting problem area. However, some adolescents with more chronic problems describe the presenting problem as oppressive in nature and do not respond well to the solution-focused approach. For these adolescents, it may be more useful to externalize the problem (White & Epston, 1990) or make room for family story telling unedited by the therapist (Anderson, 1993). When there are multiple helping professionals involved, the therapist must actively collaborate with these key members of the problem system in order to maximize opportunities for them to notice changes in the family and hear the problem situation being communicated about differently. As part of these family–multiple helper meetings, I like to include any concerned peers of the adolescent client to serve as helpful consultants in the solution construction process. Once progress has been made in the family's goal area, I will utilize consolidating questions (Selekman, 1993) to help highlight differences and to further amplify family changes.

At times, when at an impasse with more challenging adolescent cases, I use a reflecting team format (Andersen, 1987, 1991). Not only do I have my colleagues serve as reflecting team members, but I utilize my adolescent's peers for this purpose as well. In fact, I tend to get more therapeutic mileage with my adolescent clients when they are serving as reflecting team members than I do when my colleagues play this role in the treatment process. In the next section of the chapter, I will discuss five ways in which I make use of peers in family therapy. For a more detailed overview of the solution-oriented brief family therapy model, readers are referred to *Pathways to Change: Brief Therapy Solutions with Difficult Adolescents* (Selekman, 1993).

RATIONALE FOR UTILIZING PEERS IN FAMILY THERAPY WITH ADOLESCENTS

There are five important ways in which peers of adolescent clients can be utilized in family therapy. It has been my clinical experience that not only can enlisted peers greatly contribute to the change process, but they can empower a stuck treatment system (therapist + family + helpers from larger systems) by the sharing their pragmatic and creative ideas and their collaborative efforts outside family therapy sessions.

Adolescent Developmental Theory and Peer Relationships

Developmental theorists (Elson, 1986; Erikson, 1963, 1968) and family theorists (Fishman, 1993; Minuchin, 1974; Minuchin & Fishman, 1981) have stressed the importance of adolescents' peer relationships for identity formation and consolidation, for social skills development, for the establishment of personal values and ideals, and to help demarcate generational boundaries between the parental subsystem and adolescents' social world. Elson (1986) contends that one of the most important developmental tasks for adolescents to master is to deidealize their parents and idealize their peer group.

Despite all the developmental research and clinical reports (Fishman, 1993; Haber, 1987; Selekman, 1991) that indicate the importance and centrality of peers in adolescents' lives, most family therapists have failed to capitalize on this potentially valuable resource when treating adolescents and their families. One good reason for this is all the national and media attention that Nancy Reagan's "Say No to Drugs" campaign has received. This campaign served to perpetuate the popular belief that peer pressure tends to be of the negative variety and that peers are responsible for causing "straight" adolescents to use drugs. Several studies, however, have demonstrated that adolescents typically are active participants rather than passive respondents to social influences (Glassner & Loughlin, 1987; Meier, Burkett, & Hickman, 1984; Tec, 1974; Weinstein, 1978). Tec (1974) reports that adolescent drug users tend to be less dependent on their friends' expectations than do nonusers. Peers often are *positive* influences who aid in the control and abandoning of drug use. Weinstein (1978) and Meier et al. (1984) found that pressure from peers is provided as a reason for never using drugs, discontinuing use, and abandoning unhealthy peer relationships.

Often, my new adolescent clients are surprised that I take an interest in their social life and recommend the involvement of their close friends in the treatment process. I have had some former adolescent clients tell me they thought I was "cool" because I wanted to bring in their friends as helpful consultants to us both in sessions and outside the office.

Peers as Facilitators of Trust

With adolescent cases in which there is an absence of trust between the identified client and his/her parents, peers can be recruited as expert consultants to assist the therapist, parents, and adolescent client in helping rebuild trust, especially if all members of the treatment system feel that they are at an impasse with the trust issue (Selekman, 1991). Often with these cases, the parents have never met their adolescent's peers and cling to their pretreatment beliefs that the latter are involved with drugs, gangs, or trouble in general. The trust-building process is typically set in motion once the adolescent agrees to introduce his/her friends to their parents, especially if the former has refused to comply with similar parental requests in the past.

Once the peers are engaged for a family session, the parents can explore with the peers and their son/daughter the activities they do together. The therapist can also tap into the peers' wisdom and expertise about how after times of trouble, they won back their parents' trust. Any successful past problem-solving efforts on the peers' behalf can be useful for the parents and adolescent as potential models for present and future successes. For one of my former adolescent clients who was on probation, this peer trust-building interventive strategy proved to be so successful that his mother threw a big barbecue party for her son and his friends because the latter had helped him stay out of trouble. This adolescent client also systematically brought all his close friends and new peers to our family sessions for the mother and me to meet and for them to receive "the Good Housekeeping seal of approval."

Peers as a Natural Support System for Relapse Prevention

Some adolescent clients vehemently oppose the idea of attending therapy groups or self-help groups such as Alcoholics Anonymous or Alateen. Parental and therapist coaxing to attend these groups can lead to needless antagonism and possibly push the adolescent to drop out of treatment. With adolescent cases in which added support outside the therapy context could be beneficial, it can be therapeutically useful to employ some of the adolescent client's concerned peers as an alternative natural support system for them. It has been my experience that more challenging adolescent clients (i.e., chronic substance abusers) are much more likely to cooperate with this therapeutic strategy than with the shotgun approach of immediate abstinence and group therapy or self-help group participation. For example, I once worked with a chronic marijuana-abusing 16-year-old girl who had experienced multiple treatment failures and was on probation. Early in treatment, she had refused to go to Narcotics Anonymous meetings, despite her parents' and probation officer's wishes. After successfully negotiating the idea with the parents, probation officer, and adolescent, we tried an alternative strategy and employed the latter's "straight" friends who had kicked their own drug habits as a natural support group. In this manner, we were better able to pave the way for the identified client to become drug-free. These peers were very resourceful and had a wealth of creative ideas to help the identified client and her parents. One of this peer group's most innovative ideas was to establish their own 24-hour crisis hot line to help the adolescent client in times of trouble. They also shared their helpful wisdom with her parents about what their parents did that further perpetuated their drug-abusing behavior, as well as what they were doing now that was helping them stay drug-free and out of trouble.

Peers as Integral Members of the Solution Developing, Solution-Construction System

Anderson and Goolishian (1988) pioneered the idea that problems occur in language and that once a label has been used to describe a "problem," a system of helping professionals, family members, and significant others will coalesce around the identified problem out of concern and in an effort to resolve the difficulty. In expanding on Anderson and Goolishian's (1988) concept of a "problem organizing, problem dis-solving system," I have found it to be more useful to view the problem system as a solution-developing, solution-construction system. When conducting a macrosystemic assessment (Selekman, 1993) with families, I want to know from each family member who they think is most concerned about the identified problem situation and which of these key individuals should be invited to participate in family–multiple helper collaborative meetings. I particularly want to know from my adolescent clients of their closest peers—those whom they have called upon in the past for support when they were faced with problems—with whom we could collaborate in the family–multiple helper meetings and with the solution-construction process.

Once engaged for family–multiple helper meetings, I will invite peers to share their advice about the current dilemma the adolescent client is faced with, and any stories of successes they have experienced in the past at resolving similar difficulties with their parents and with problem-solving efforts in other social contexts as well (i.e., at school or in the community). The peers' wisdom offered in the context of the family–multiple helper meetings can empower the treatment system when it is stuck. Another interesting phenomenon that has occurred in the context of such meetings is that of peers and helping professionals spontaneously teaming up to help the identified client, for example:

- Probation officers and peers working together in the community to help the identified client stay away from gang members or solo–group delinquent activity.
- Peers working together with counselors in the school context to help curb in-school misbehavior.

Peers as Observers of "Newsworthy" Changes

Peers can be used in second and subsequent sessions to help highlight "newsworthy" changes that have occurred in the parent–adolescent relationship, at school with the identified client's behavior, and with his/her behavior in the community. In the context of family therapy sessions, it can be a newsworthy experience for the parents to hear from their son/daughter's friends that they have noticed changes in how they are interacting with one another or that their adolescent is no longer getting in trouble in the classroom and in the community. As Bateson (1980) has pointed out, *information is a difference* that can lead to "news of a difference" that makes a difference. Through the help of the adolescent client's peers, new constructions of the family situation can help challenge parents' outmoded beliefs about their son/daughter. Thus, the parents' relationship with him/her can be improved and pave the way for the creation of a new solution-determined family story.

THE MECHANICS OF CONVENING PEERS AND SESSION FORMAT

Prior to presenting the idea of incorporating the adolescent's peers in family therapy sessions, there are some preliminary steps the therapist needs to take with the family and the peers. First, the therapist must determine the purpose for enlisting the adolescent's peers as consultants.

Second, the therapist has to explore with the parents and adolescent whether they are receptive to pursuing this interventive strategy. Finally, the peers' parents should be contacted by the adolescent client's parents to explain the rationale for incorporating their son/daughter into the client's family therapy. I also like to have my clients sign consent forms to allow me to release confidential information to the peers and the peers' parents if I need to speak to the latter.

Convening Peers

Typically, I do not explore the idea of involving peers in the treatment process until second and subsequent sessions. When I have my adolescent clients recruit their close peers, I have them take responsibility for explaining to their friends what their current difficulties are and how the friends could be helpful to them, their parents, and the therapist. The adolescent client and his/her parents are responsible for making sure that the peers and their parents understand the importance of respecting their confidentiality. If the adolescent clients' parents have any questions that they plan to ask the peers in their first session together, I will make copies of the parents' list of questions and make sure that the identified client gives a copy of the list to each peer, which will help better prepare them for the first family–peer meeting.

Session Format

Because each adolescent case is unique, the peer-reflecting team format is determined on a case-by-case basis. Often, the adolescent client and his/her parents prefer that the peers sit with us in the therapy room, rather than hidden behind the one-way mirror. Also, many families tend to welcome spontaneous reflections from the peers throughout their family therapy sessions whenever the latter have some pragmatic and creative ideas to share. After the peers share their spontaneous reflections, family members can be invited to reflect on their ideas. However, with some cases, the peer reflecting team will make one reflection approximately 40 minutes into the hour and the family will reflect on their reflections. During the session, I may invite one or a few of the peers to reflect on interactions occurring in the room on both a process and a content level. Finally, the peers can be asked to join the therapist and his/her colleagues in brainstorming a useful therapeutic task or experiment the adolescent and parents could do between sessions. The parents and adolescent determine how often the peers are included in their family sessions.

When it is contraindicated to include the identified client's peers in treatment because of their strong gang affiliation or heavy substance abuse, I may introduce the idea of bringing into a family session some former adolescent clients of mine who are doing well and have experienced similar problems. Some of these "alumni" have been very successful at helping my stuck adolescent clients remain drug-free, secure jobs, and learn how to get along better with their parents.

For example, for 15-year-old "Wendy," who was actively involved with a local street gang and heavily abusing drugs, family treatment had been failing until I brought two female adolescent alumni into our fifth session. "Elizabeth" and "Carol" had also been involved with gangs. The transcription below from that session demonstrates the power of utilizing alumni as reflecting team members. Elizabeth and Carol had the following words of wisdom to offer Wendy in their reflection midway through the session:

ELIZABETH: I used to think that gangs were it . . . but when I saw my boyfriend get shot . . . that's when I said, "I got to get out of this!"

CAROL: When I used to party [get "high" on drugs] I didn't care about nothing . . . I just wanted to get ripped . . . and one night I had totally lost my memory at a party and found out later that I was gang-banged [raped] by some guys that I had never met before . . . that's when I stopped doing drugs!

Wendy was shocked by the girls' horror stories. In response to their reflections, she requested help from them in changing her lifestyle. Both Elizabeth and Carol proved to be instrumental in helping Wendy get a job and stay out of further trouble with the law. Without the help of these two alumni, treatment would have remained at an impasse and Wendy could have possibly lost her life.

The case example that follows illustrates how to employ peers as expert consultants for relapse prevention purposes and to help highlight changes for the family.

CASE EXAMPLE: *MARKED FOR DEATH,* HENRY AARON, AND GOOD-BYE TO GANG LIFE

Case Background

"Steve" and his family were referred to the Juvenile Offender's Program at our social service agency after Steve assaulted a police officer while heavily intoxicated on alcohol. On the evening of Steve's arrest, he and his gang-involved peers were walking home from a party well after their curfew. The local police had been keeping a watchful eye on Steve and his gang-involved friends because of reports by school officials and people in the community that they might be connected to a crack cocaine drug-dealing ring. Steve had been placed on probation for nine months. He was failing most of his major subjects in school due to his cutting classes and not doing homework.

According to the probation officer who made the case referral, Steve's stepfather was "a drunk" and his mother might have a "drinking problem" as well. The probation officer also reported that Steve got along with his biological father but disliked his stepfather. When doing his case study, the probation officer found out that Steve was not a regular abuser of alcohol and marijuana and that he did not seem to be involved in any drug dealing. Steve told the probation officer in the case study interview that it was out of character for him to strike a police officer, or any adult for that matter. The probation officer appeared to be more concerned about the "family alcohol problems" and the "dysfunctional home environment" than Steve as an individual. He stressed the importance of trying to get the parents to "take responsibility for their alcohol problems" in the context of my family therapy with Steve.

Brief Summary of the First Family Interview

Present at the first family interview were Steve, his mother, "Barbara," and the probation officer. The probation officer was invited to share his story of involvement with Steve and Barbara. He also presented his probationary contractual guidelines for Steve, which included no alcohol or drug use, regular classroom attendance and staying on top of his homework assignments, not breaking curfew, following parental rules, and not associating with gang members. These were his treatment outcome goals for Steve as well. The probation officer had also voiced his concerns about the stepfather's failure to attend this session and his drinking problem. Barbara indicated that her husband thought counseling was a "waste of time" and "refused" to participate. Steve had no problem with agreeing to comply with his probationary contract. However, he did disclose his concerns about being able to steer clear of the gang leader, "George."

Prior to the conclusion of this initial family meeting, I asked Steve whether he had any "straight" non-gang-involved peers who could help him outside our sessions and who might be willing to come to the next family session. Steve had two friends, "John" and "Warren," whom he thought could be helpful to him while he was struggling with his confidence around having the inner strength to stay away from George and the street gang. Both Barbara and the probation officer thought that this was a useful therapeutic strategy to pursue. I explained the importance of client confidentiality and had Steve and his mother sign consent forms so that we could include these peers in the next family session and so I could collaborate with the probation officer and concerned school officials. Because Barbara knew John, Warren, and the former's mother, it was not a problem for her to contact John's and Warren's parents to secure permission to include these peers in the next family therapy session. Steve planned to meet with each of his friends over the next week to discuss the whole situation.

The Second Family Interview

In attendance at our second family session were Steve, Barbara, and Steve's closest straight friend, John. Unfortunately, Warren could not attend our session because he had to work that night at a local grocery store. After presenting to the group the various types of reflecting team formats we could utilize, both Steve and Barbara requested that John sit with us and feel free to contribute any helpful ideas he might have during the course of the interview. It was also explained to John that I might call upon his expertise to reflect on interactional exchanges between Steve and his mother in the room, as well as invite him to share strategies he used to stay out of trouble with his parents and school officials and to cope with propositions to join gangs or use drugs. The following is a transcription of portions of the second family interview between Steve, Barbara, John, and me.

THERAPIST: I was wondering, John, if you have any hot ideas about how Steve could stay away from George [the gang leader] and drugs?

STEVE: Stay with you . . . right, man! (*laughing*)

JOHN: (*laughing*) Well, if you see it [drugs] walk away from it . . . tell yourself, "I'm not going to do that stuff!"

THERAPIST: What about with George, what steps could Steve take to avoid the gang?

JOHN: Well, we go to the show a lot and collect baseball cards.

THERAPIST: Guys, give me your Siskel and Ebert movie review . . .

STEVE: Well, we've seen *Marked for Death* and *Child's Play II* . . . (*both smiling*)

THERAPIST: (*looking at Barbara*) Both are five star movies! Right! (*laughter*)

JOHN: Yeah, we have seen all of the Steven Seagal movies together.

BARBARA: You guys are serious baseball card collectors, right?

STEVE: Yeah, he [John] refuses to trade his Henry Aaron card for my Mickey Mantle.

JOHN: No way . . . Henry Aaron is worth $500. That's what the man at the baseball card shop said.

THERAPIST: (*looking at Steve*) What other kinds of things do you, John and Warren do that keep you off the streets?

STEVE: Well, we shoot hoops [basketball], play football, go to the game room at the mall . . . we also like checking out the baseball card shop.

BARBARA: Sometimes when I take the boys over there to the baseball shop, they spend hours there trying to decide what to get.

STEVE: It's going to be hard for me to stay away from George because his girlfriend is real tight with my girlfriend . . . they hang out a lot together. I heard at school that George was looking for me. I still owe him $10 from a dime bag of weed [marijuana] that I had bummed off of him a few months ago.

BARBARA: Look, would it help if I gave you the $10 to pay off George and get him out of your life?

STEVE: That won't matter . . . I can't escape from George; (*turning to John*) remember what George did to Frank when he tried to get out [of the gang] . . . he got his ass kicked!

JOHN: Steve, take the money . . . pay him off and just hang out with Warren and me all of your free time . . . I've never seen George over by my house before.

BARBARA: I think that sounds like a good idea . . . maybe you should spend all of your free time over John's house or Warren's.

STEVE: (*looking angry*) Yeah, but then "Roger" [the step father] will be yelling at me all of the time about not cleaning up the house and doing this and that . . . I really hate him, mom! He's always bitching at me about something . . . that's why I try and stay out of the house when he's around, he's just a drunk . . . he's an asshole!

BARBARA: I've told you many times before, let me handle Roger . . . don't listen to him, he bitches at me about things, too.

STEVE: Why did you marry that guy? All he does is get drunk all of the time. I'm tired of him calling me an idiot!

THERAPIST: John, you have a stepfather, right?

JOHN: Yeah.

THERAPIST: What kinds of things have you done to deal with him when he gives you a hard time or does things that you don't like?

JOHN: Well, I go to my mother when I need help in dealing with him . . . or I listen to music in my room to cut him out of my mind.

BARBARA: (*turning to Steve*) That's not what you do . . . you usually start yelling back at him and slam doors, right?

STEVE: Well, but he's such an asshole . . . he makes me mad . . . sometimes I wish I would come home from school and he would be gone.

JOHN: You know, I think like that sometimes, too, but your mother's married to him and we can't change that.

BARBARA: Look, Steve, come to me if Roger is being unreasonable . . . you know that usually happens when he drinks too much.

STEVE: (*turns to his mother*) Yeah, why isn't he here, he's the one with the real problem?

BARBARA: I know, I've asked him to get help and come here, but he said that counseling was a waste of time and he hates shrinks!

JOHN: Steve, you can always give me a call if Roger is getting on your case.

STEVE: Thanks, dude.

Throughout the first part of the interview, I utilized John as an expert consultant by having him reflect on my questions regarding useful steps that Steve could take to avoid the gang leader George, remain drug-free, and cope with a stepfather's troubling behaviors. In total, John contributed nine useful problem-solving and coping strategies during the interview. Prior to ending the family session, I tapped into John's expertise again regarding any changes he had observed in the relationship between Barbara and Steve.

THERAPIST: I'm curious, John, have you noticed any changes in how Steve and his mother are getting along now, versus two months ago?

JOHN: Yeah, they don't argue as much.

BARBARA: You've noticed that we get along better now?

STEVE: (*looking at his mother*) Yeah, I've been able to talk to you more lately, you know, about tough things and you don't blow up.

THERAPIST: As an outside observer, describe how Steve and his mother used to communicate with each other two months ago.

JOHN: Well . . . I'd come in the door and they'd be yelling at each other . . . sometimes Steve would be swearing at his mother.

THERAPIST: What did she used to do when Steve would swear at her?

JOHN: She would get real red in her face, yell at him more loudly, and tell him not to come back home if he walked out the door.

THERAPIST: What is Steve doing differently with his mother that seems to work?

JOHN: Well, I haven't seen him swear at her or yell much.

BARBARA: Yeah, I think we are getting along much better now.

Before concluding the session, I explored with the family which of John's ideas they found to be most helpful and whether they were willing to have him participate in a future family session. The family planned to implement all of John's recommended strategies for dealing with George and Steve's stepfather. Barbara particularly liked John's idea about Steve spending his afterschool and remaining free time in John's neighborhood away from "gang territory." Steve found John's support and helpful ideas offered in the session to be empowering to him. The family unequivocally voted that John be included in a future session if he was willing to participate. I thanked John for his help and asked him what his consultation fee was. Everyone laughed. When asked when they wished to come back for another family session, Steve and his mother confidently asked to come back in "three weeks." When asked if they wanted a task to work on over the three-week vacation period between visits, both Steve and his mother indicated that they had gotten enough to work on for now through John's help.

Case Summary and Outcome

I ended up seeing Steve and Barbara eight times over the nine-month period that Steve was on probation. John and Warren participated in the third, fifth, and seventh family sessions. John's proposed strategy of Steve's spending all of his free time at either his or Warren's house proved effective in keeping Steve away from gang involvement. In the fifth family session, the probation officer and school social worker were present. I used the peers' services in the session to highlight differences and changes in Steve's behavior, which proved to be newsworthy for the probation officer and school social worker.

Between the fifth and seventh family sessions, Steve got into a fistfight with his stepfather and it was decided that he would live at his biological father's house. My seventh and eighth family sessions were with the mother, father, stepmother, and Steve. Despite some minor confrontations between Steve and his stepmother, the new living arrangement seemed to be the final step necessary to help him pioneer a new direction in his life. Follow-up telephone calls to the mother and father were made one year after our last session together. Both parents reported that Steve successfully terminated his probation, was alcohol and drug-free and no longer involved with gangs, and had improved his academic performance.

CONCLUSION

In this chapter, I presented five ways to utilize peers in family therapy with adolescents. These peer therapeutic strategies have helped create possibilities with some very tough adolescent cases; they have also helped reduce lengths of stay in treatment. When following up with families that had agreed to utilize peers in their treatment, both parents and adolescents cited the peers as being very instrumental in the solution-construction process. All the peer therapeutic strategies can be used with other family therapy approaches. For example, Fishman (1993) makes use of peers in his structural therapy approach with adolescents.

With the help of my adolescent clients' peers, I have learned some very creative and pragmatic coping and problem-solving strategies, the names and effects of new drugs on the street, and other important aspects of the constantly evolving youth culture. Thanks to the peers with whom I have collaborated, their "rap music" has helped make a difference with many of my most challenging adolescent cases.

ACKNOWLEDGMENTS

I would like to thank Karen Foran for her helpful editorial comments and willingness to type the manuscript. I would also like to thank LaWanda Pope for introducing me to the rap music of Profound.

REFERENCES

Andersen, T. (1987). The reflecting team: Dialogue and meta-dialogue in clinical work. *Family Process, 26*(4), 415–428.

Andersen, T. (Ed.).(1991). *The reflecting team: Dialogues and dialogues about the dialogues.* New York: Norton.

Anderson, H. (1993). On a roller coaster: A collaborative language systems approach. In S. Friedman (Ed.), *The new language of change: Constructive collaboration in psychotherapy* (pp. 323–344). New York: Guilford Press.

Anderson, H., & Goolishian, H. (1988). Human systems as linguistic systems: Evolving ideas about the implications for theory and practice. *Family Process, 27,* 371–393.

Anderson, H., & Goolishian, H. (1991). Thinking about multi-agency work with substance abusers and their families: A language systems approach. *Journal of Strategic and Systemic Therapies, 10*(1), 20–36.

Bateson, G. (1980). *Mind and nature: A necessary unity.* New York: Ballantine Books.
de Shazer, S. (1985). *Keys to solution in brief therapy.* New York: Norton.
de Shazer, S. (1988). *Clues: Investigating solutions in brief therapy.* New York: Norton.
de Shazer, S. (1991). *Putting difference to work.* New York: Norton.
Elson, M. (1986). *Self psychology in clinical social work.* New York: Norton.
Erikson, E. (1963). *Childhood and society.* New York: Norton.
Erikson, E. (1968). *Identity: Youth and crisis.* New York: Norton.
Fisch, R., Weakland, J., & Segal, L. (1982). *The tactics of change.* San Francisco: Jossey-Bass.
Fishman, H. C. (1993). *Intensive structural therapy: Treating families in their social context.* New York: Basic Books.
Glassner, B., & Loughlin, J. (1987). *Drugs in adolescent worlds: Burnouts to straights.* New York: St. Martin's Press.
Haber, R. (1987). Friends in family therapy: Use of a neglected resource. *Family Process, 26*(2), 269–283.
Meier, R. F., Burkett, S. R., & Hickman, C. A. (1984). Sanctions, peers and deviance. *Sociological Quarterly, 25,* 67–82.
Minuchin, S. (1974). *Families and family therapy.* Cambridge, MA: Harvard University Press.
Minuchin, S., & Fishman, H. C. (1981). *Family therapy techniques.* Cambridge, MA: Harvard University Press.
Selekman, M. D. (1991). "With a little help from my friends": The use of peers in the family therapy of adolescent substance abusers. *Family Dynamics of Addiction Quarterly, 1*(1), 69–77.
Selekman, M. D. (1993). *Pathways to change: Brief therapy solutions with difficult adolescents.* New York: Guilford Press.
Tec, N. (1974). *Grass is green in suburbia: A sociological study of adolescent usage of illicit drugs.* Roslyn Heights, NY: Libra.
Watzlawick, P., Weakland, J., & Fisch, R. (1974). *Change: Principles of problem formation and problem resolution.* New York: Norton.
Weinstein, R. M. (1978). The avowal of motives for marijuana behavior. *International Journal of Addictions, 13,* 887–910.
White, M. (1984). Pseudo-encopresis: From avalanche to victory, from vicious to virtuous cycles. *Family Systems Medicine, 2*(2), 150–160.
White, M. (1985). Fear-busting and monster taming: An approach to the fears of young children. *Dulwich Centre Review,* pp. 29–33.
White, M. (1986). Negative explanation, restraint and double description: A template for family therapy. *Family Process, 25*(2), 169–184.
White, M. (1987). Family therapy and schizophrenia: Addressing the in-the-corner lifestyle. *Dulwich Centre Newsletter,* pp. 14–21.
White, M. (1988). Anorexia nervosa: A cybernetic perspective. In J. E. Harkaway (Ed.), *Eating disorders* (pp. 117–129). Rockville, MD: Aspen.
White, M., & Epston, D. (1990). *Narrative means to therapeutic ends.* New York: Norton.

PART III

THE COMMUNITY AS AUDIENCE
Reauthoring Stories

A social network has within it the resources to develop creative solutions to the human predicaments of its members.

—*Ross Speck and Carolyn Attneave*

By the crowd they have been broken; by the crowd shall they be healed.

—*Cody Marsh*

CHAPTER 11

Public Practices

AN ETHIC OF CIRCULATION

Dean H. Lobovits
Richard L. Maisel
Jennifer C. Freeman

> The foundation of morality should not be made dependent on myth nor tied to any authority lest doubt about the myth or about the legitimacy of the authority imperil the foundation of sound judgment and action.
> —*Albert Einstein*

THE PROCESS OF MAKING meaning is woven from the fabric of language and articulated in a participatory social context (Gergen & Gergen, 1991). It follows that the shaping of liberative meanings requires not only a "storyteller" but an audience. Such an audience is an active and collaborative participant in the process of making meaning, rather than a passive recipient of information (Bruner, 1986). Recent years have seen a flourishing of innovative practices incorporating audiences in the process of therapy. In addition to the use of reflecting teams, these therapies have taken the step of circulating alternative narratives to various kinds of audiences, both within and beyond the therapy session (e.g., through verbal messages, letters, tapes, leagues, clubs, handbooks and libraries).

Our focus is on ideas that have emerged from narrative therapy, "just therapy," and similar approaches of recent years that have made psychotherapy more public through circulation practices. These therapies have opened the way for such practices due to their emphasis on collaboration and their focus on competency, empowerment, and preferred stories, rather than on pathology (Waldegrave, 1990, 1991; White & Epston, 1990a, 1990b). Rather than to instruct or provide expert knowledge for clients, the role of the therapist is to enter the social space where meaning is shaped and support the development of alternative meanings to oppressive stories. Audiences can be engaged to develop clients' preferred stories and to increase the diversity of available viewpoints regarding a client's situation. These stories are advanced by a process of collaborative and recursive commentary among those who are involved in the shaping of meaning.

Circulation practices challenge our traditional notions about the need for absolute privacy in psychotherapy. Ethical and effective psychotherapy is commonly thought to depend on a unique relationship that unfolds in a private and protected sphere. Our thesis is that the need for privacy increases when people who experience problems are viewed in terms of illness/pathology or other problem-saturated descriptions.

Externalizing the problem, wherein "the problem is problem, the person is not the problem," creates a separation of persons from problems and relieves feelings of shame and failure (White, 1989; White & Epston, 1990a). When we explore a person's evolving relationship with a problem, we evoke their competence and strength in relation to it, promote a value-congruent and preferred view of self, and identify virtuous rather than vicious cycles (White & Epston, 1990b). It is these virtuous cycles and preferred accounts of self that primarily are circulated to wider audiences. This approach tends to produce documents or descriptions that have less of a need to be protected from exposure to others. Because the narratives that are recorded usually reflect well on people and further their goals, they are often eager to share this material. This enables the expansion of the boundaries of therapy and offers alternatives to diminish the negative effects of a climate of secrecy and privacy in the therapeutic arena. Such effects include stigmatization, increased risk of exploitation by the therapist, and a lack of therapist accountability (Goffman, 1959, 1961; Lobovits & Freeman, 1993).

TYPES OF AUDIENCES

We make a distinction between two types of audiences. There is the "known audience," which "consists of those in a person's life who interact with and influence his or her unfolding story" (Freeman & Lobovits, 1993, p. 205). These people may be drawn upon to witness a person's changes or preferred story and also to participate in shaping its evolution. They may include relatives, friends, teachers, other professionals, or significant persons either living or deceased. Some known audiences are sympathetic and already shaping positive meaning with clients, whereas others may be skeptical and need to be recruited actively in the renegotiation of meaning.

The second kind of audience is an "introduced audience." This audience is drawn from a wider community of those who have struggled with a problem, who understand its social context, and who are dealing with the problem successfully. An example of this is the Anti-Anorexia/Bulimia League (Epston, Morris, & Maisel, 1995; Madigan & Epston, Chapter 12, this volume). These communities have "the power to appreciate alternative stories in the making, and to offer locally based knowledge and techniques for changing dominant, problem saturated stories that equate a person with a problem" (Freeman & Lobovits, 1993, p. 222). Families may be invited to receive or contribute information to others about problems and solutions (Epston, 1989; White & Epston, 1990a). For example, clients may be asked whether they would like to have their methods passed along to other clients, as in a case that follows, where a father's methodology for improved communication between parent and teenager is gathered to share with other clients. Audiences may be interacted with or invoked in therapy. For example, in another case that follows, a client facing anorexia interacts with the Anti-Anorexia/Bulimia League by way of video and mail, and in yet another instance, the therapist invokes a hypothetical audience of admirable women.

BENEFITS OF CIRCULATION PRACTICES

If we are to change therapy from a private to a selectively public practice, what are some of the effects on our clients and their audiences? We begin here with some of the benefits; later we take up some of the risks and thorny ethical issues and outline some ideas that guide us.

Clients report that their stories of hope and pain are validated by the reflections of a team, applying to a club, contacting a league, or having news of change circulated to others. When their ideas are gathered for circulation to others through tapes, letters, or verbally by the therapist, people have the added satisfaction of making a contribution to others in need. Whereas they might previously have felt degraded by the problem, the opportunity to contribute to others allows people to claim a preferred status (e.g., from patient to consultant or from victim to survivor, from drowning person to lifeguard). Audience participants appreciate being respected for their contributions and like the opportunity to participate in a positive way in another person's or family's life. Below we provide several illustrations of ways in which we have involved audiences in our work.

HANDBOOKS

The idea of involving different audiences to enrich the therapeutic environment has inspired our experimentation. One such adventure has been the development of handbooks in which children and families may read about how others approached a similar problem and offer their own story of success or advice to future readers (Freeman & Lobovits, 1993). Jennifer (Jenny) began in 1990 to record children's stories in relation to problems in a series of "handbooks." Children are invited either to write in an unlined book or to dictate to the therapist and to illustrate their story if they wish. The notebooks have collage images on their covers, and Jenny has added pictures and cartoons to the pages. When children enter therapy, they are offered the chance to see and hear the stories of those who have passed that way before. The handbooks are beginning to be circulated among other therapists working with children who then add their own entries.

Handbooks have several aims: to empower and respect children by inviting them to consult with other children facing a similar problem, to validate their accounts of struggle and success, to provide a way to have fun in showing off success and reaching beyond themselves, and to keep these accounts for inspiration and reference in case the authors themselves experience a setback.

Some examples of handbooks include *The Temper Tamer's Handbook: How to Cool Off and Be Cool; The Fear Facers' Handbook; Rest Well: Sleeping and Such; The Freedom from Habits Handbook;* and *The Different School Book,* including an entry by the Anti-Anti-Math Club.

The latter club deserves some note. It was formed with two nine-year-old girls who had been struggling with math. One girl, a client in therapy, decided to invite her friend in for a couple of sessions after the friend mentioned that she shared the same problem. They quickly grasped the idea of looking at their problem in the social context of attitudes regarding girls and math. Both girls realized that in the careers they were dreaming of, they would need math skills. They decided on a gender revolution in which they made revolutionary art, told stories, and developed a puppet play called "People That Dis Girls and Math and the Girls That Dis Them." Next they hired a math tutor to catch up. They became available as consultants to other girls through their story in this handbook. Here are some comments written by the girls: "The problem of Math: You see, some girls think that just because you get tricked [by the idea that] you don't like math. I mean you say you do not like it and soon enough you don't like it. So don't be tricked like I was" [Shawna, age 9]; "Don't listen to people who tell you some subjects don't count, cause they just want someone to be dumb with" [Alice, age 9].

The following are a few sample entries from *The Temper Tamer's Handbook*: "I think it's better to play instead of staying mad. If your temper comes up when you're playing, just go away and do something else . . . until it goes away and calms down" [Risa, age 6]. Another child, inspired by the invitation to contribute, dictated:

> "I figured some ways to get rid of the temper. I can do it all the time now! I spied on it. It used to creep up behind in a straight line, but since I spied on it, it creeps up in a spiral. I wait till it's close, cause I like to trick it, then I blow the whistle and it jumps up and runs in the air. Then it goes away and falls down. Or, sometimes, I call it names. 'Stop you big bag of clattering screwdrivers, you poophead!' Then it stops and goes away. Like mommy and daddy were going out at night but mommy mixed up the schedule. We were going to have a different baby-sitter than I thought, and I could have been really upset, but I used my ideas and calmed down. Daddy and mommy didn't even know about this, I was so calm." [Maria, age 8]

When Maria and her parents were told that reading her entry was useful to another child, it made them all proud and confirmed her status as a temper tamer.

A PUBLIC AUDIENCE

During a community event featuring visits to artist's studios, Jenny's office was offered as an example of an expressive arts therapy studio. The studio setup was shown, including sand tray, puppet theater, drama dress-ups, art, sculpture, and puppet and mask making, along with clients' work in most of these media. Both the general public and clients were invited to attend. The artwork was accompanied by descriptive captions, poetry, or stories, some of which were written in collaboration with the artists/clients. Most of the work was by children, who were especially excited to show it. Expressions of therapy thus became available to the public as well as to other clients. These therapeutic productions seemed to enter another realm once they were considered something to show and share.

Expressive artwork intrinsically lends itself to externalization. In the context of an externalizing conversation, clients consider their artwork something to be proud of and potentially helpful to others. For example, one child wanted to share a picture and a poem showing how her relationship with fear of loss was evolving, because she felt it was something that might help other kids who had suffered a loss, and because she felt good about the confidence she was regaining to face surprises in her life.

This event, which was experimental, raised boundary issues such as clients meeting each other and meeting the therapist in a different context. Each client was carefully interviewed before the event about any negative consequences that could be anticipated and debriefed after the event. Feedback from clients was positive, which demonstrated to us that they were capable of dealing with the shift in context when such an endeavor was guided by a process of informed consent and collaboration. They felt that they had learned from and enjoyed the work of others. One unexpected benefit was that public visitors also were informed and inspired by the work. Several visitors who read the illustrated stories of children in therapy said they got ideas for working with their own children. One visiting child was inspired to take on a problem with which he had quietly suffered, after seeing the cartoon illustrated story of another child who had faced and overcome a similar problem.

Soon after this show, we were invited to a similar public showing of expressive art by women members of an incest survivors self-help group in New Hampshire.

Denise

In the following section, Richard's (Rick's) work with a woman struggling with anorexia[1] will be presented in order to illustrate some other uses of audiences in the course of an ongoing therapy.

Denise was a 17-year-old woman and a senior in high school. During the previous year she became convinced that she was fat and became determined to lose weight. She thought of almost nothing else and put herself on a starvation diet of 400 calories a day. She was an accomplished dancer and practiced for several hours each day in addition to other forms of exercise. She eventually became so fatigued and malnourished that her pediatrician prohibited her from dancing. He also told her that if she did not gain weight during the following week he would hospitalize her and commence tube feeding. Denise was so determined to keep dancing that she forced herself to eat during the next week. However, she soon began vomiting, and after a few months was doing so approximately eight times per day. After approximately 15 sessions of therapy at a hospital, she was referred to Rick. At the time of

[1]For a more comprehensive presentation of a narrative approach to anorexia/bulimia, see Epston, Morris, and Maisel (1995), and Madigan and Epston (Chapter 12, this volume).

the referral, the frequency of her vomiting was greatly reduced and she was able to eat some food each day. However, her mind was still dominated by anorexia, whose voice she could hear from her first waking moments, ordering her not to eat and calling her "fat, ugly, stupid, and a failure" throughout the day. She also struggled with intense feelings of worthlessness and a lack of entitlement.

Evoking Hypothetical Audiences to Positive Developments

Anorexia often moves in on people at times when they are feeling weak and vulnerable. When Denise was 15 her father died unexpectedly. He had taken an active interest in her academic and extracurricular pursuits and tried to smooth her path in myriad ways. After his death she felt lost, alone, and devastated. Shortly thereafter anorexia held out the promise of attaining a sense of competence and self-control. Anorexia also told her she would win the love, approval, and respect of other people if she followed its dictates: conforming to the demand for extraordinary thinness, striving for perfection in all of her endeavors, adhering to an ethic of self-denial, putting another's needs above her own, and confining herself to subservient and submissive relationships with men.

During one of Rick's meetings with Denise, she described times when she had failed to comply with anorexia's requirement to defer and subordinate herself. Unfortunately, feelings of guilt and self-hatred were evoked when Denise's acts of self-assertion and resistance to anorexia's dictates were attacked by others as selfish, bitchy, and mean-spirited. Rick's questions helped Denise to perceive the wider sociopolitical (i.e., gendered) context of drawing such negative conclusions about herself (White, 1991). Denise decided that she preferred to view her behavior through the lens of a sense of entitlement and worthiness, and that she preferred descriptions such as "self-assertion and protest" to characterizations such as "selfish" or "bitchy." Below is an excerpt from a letter to Denise providing Rick's summary of their meeting:

> *You talked about how often you have been called "a bitch" by so-called friends. This had the effect of convincing you that you were a mean and selfish person. You told me that people have used these words to describe you at times when you have put your needs ahead of theirs, or have protested against some form of injustice. When I asked if you thought these words were used to disqualify and silence women's protest, you said you didn't know. However, you thought any strong woman who stands by her convictions and takes herself seriously probably would be*

subjected to these labels, but could not afford to accept them as valid descriptions.

What you told me next was very illuminating, and I must admit, although I have always admired you greatly, the story you told doubled my respect for you. You told that one of your friends had shown up really drunk to a party that you had taken pains to organize, one in which both your friends and adults would be in attendance. Since he was behaving obnoxiously, you told him off. What do you think I might find to respect in this? Do you think other people at the party appreciated you doing this? You later felt guilty about it and began to wonder if maybe you were a "bitch." If this is being a "bitch" then I think we have to ask what it means to be a "bitch"? What men (and women who identify with them) need to put down women in this way? I mean "put down" not only in the sense of an insult but also in the sense of quashing a rebellion. You said, "so many people have called me a "bitch"; does this mean that there have been many instances in which you have stood up for what you believe to be right? What do you think the women you admire would appreciate about you if they could see you at those times when those you have challenged or confronted or resisted called you a bitch? What descriptions might these women give for what you were up to? What qualities would they recognize? Do you think some boys and men are also capable of recognizing and appreciating these qualities?

A hypothetical audience of "women you admire" was called on to offer a consensus that supported Denise's anti-anorexic behavior and to develop alternatives to the description of her as a bitch. This was designed to open space for Denise to legitimate her behavior according to her preferred interpretations of her conduct as assertive and just.

Consulting the Anti-Anorexia/Bulimia League

In his first session with Denise, Rick had described a videotape he had seen of David Epston's interview with a woman who was the same age as Denise, who was battling anorexia. He described how the woman had continued to claim that she felt energetic despite the fact that her doctor said she could die at any moment and her roommate reported that she was too fatigued even to walk to the mailbox. In response, Denise reflected on how anorexia had been able to "pull the wool over her eyes" and get her to take pride in excelling at her own self-destruction. At the end of this session, Denise asked whether she could see the video, as it would help her see through anorexia's lies and to see it for what it was—a killer.

At one point Denise reached an impasse in her struggle against anorexia. She and Rick decided to write a letter to the Anti-Anorexia/Bulimia League of New Zealand seeking consultation. They hoped that the league's knowledge about the tactics of anorexia as well as any anti-anorexic discoveries could help Denise gain some ground. They also sent the league copies of session summaries, documenting some of Denise's discoveries about anorexia and some of her developing anti-anorexic understandings.

Dear David Epston and fellow members
of the Anti-Anorexia/Bulimia League,

I am writing to you, with the help of my therapist, Rick Maisel, for some input. I am 18 years old and live in California. I first encountered anorexia shortly after my father died of a heart attack when I was 15. I was really depressed and didn't want to deal with anything and anorexia offered me a way out. It gave me something to occupy my mind so I wouldn't have to face my emotions surrounding my dad's death. For about two weeks it had me dieting, and throwing up when I did eat. Finally I blew up at my mom and told her how much I hated her and my life—my mom didn't seem to be as affected by my dad's death as I was and I felt pretty alone.

After expressing these feelings, anorexia took leave of my life for about a year. During that year I was sad about my father's death and somewhat critical towards myself. Anorexia eventually caught up to me again and pretty soon it had me back on a starvation diet. I lost so much weight the doctor told me I wouldn't be able to continue my dancing. I've been dancing most of my life and it is one of the things I really love. I was not about to let anorexia take this from me, so I forced myself to eat again.

Currently I see myself as basically over anorexia insofar as my eating habits are back to normal. Anorexia still tries to put me on diets, and the urge is especially strong when I am around friends who themselves have been captured by anorexia. But I know from experience that what anorexia promises and what it delivers are two different things. However, I still feel there are parts of me that I have not been able to retrieve. I am still struggling to reclaim my sense of self-esteem and self-worth. Anorexia tells me I'm worthless because I'm fat, that I'm mean, and that I am an awful person. Whenever I break anorexia's rules it comes back at me with these kinds of punishments. I have to say that I find myself believing what it tells me. Have any of you been through this? If so, how have you gotten past this? How were you able to see through anorexia's lies to your own worth as a person? Have any of you managed to overcome the desire to be thin, to experience your worth only as a function of your weight? If so, how have you done this? Did anorexia also deprive you of a sense of happiness with your life and pride in your accomplishments? How did you get these back? What role, if any, did friends and family play in this? Any responses you might provide would be greatly appreciated. I will try to respond to any questions you might have for me.

Soon after, Rick and Denise received mail from David Epston, who, serving as archivist for the league, had compiled excerpts from the writings of league members and his own letters. He included a complete transcript of a meeting he had held with a woman, Rebecca (age 22), in which they explored a breakthrough in her struggle to overcome anorexia/bulimia. Rebecca had attributed her breakthrough, in part, to reading the anti-anorexic journal of a 14-year-old girl. Remarkably, it was Rick himself who had worked with this young woman, and they had passed the journal along to the league for circulation.

Denise read the transcript of this session with great interest. The account of Rebecca's breakthrough reminded her of a significant anti-anorexic turning point in her own life. The following letter from Rick to Denise documented the recollection of this turning point and its associated anti-anorexic understandings:

During our past meeting you gave me some of your thoughts about the transcription of David Epston's session with Rebecca. You recognized many of the same messages anorexia/bulimia had been giving to Rebecca. What was amazing is that you also had a similar turning point in your fight back against anorexia/bulimia. It seemed as if this was something you had forgotten about until our session. This turning point came in relation to your boyfriend at that time, a young man in his first year at college. In a flash, you saw this person for who he was, a selfish, uncaring person, who you no longer wanted to be with. Almost immediately after this realization, you went back home and began to eat. You said that at the time you realized, "I don't need to put myself through this. This is pointless and its not getting me anywhere." From this day on anorexia was never fully able to control you and get you to starve yourself. What do you think enabled you to see the injustice of the relationship at this moment? Did this depend upon you getting back in touch with your own worth? If so, how did you see past anorexia's lies and condemnations?

Accessing the Experience of Appreciative Others

Toward the end of Rick's work with Denise, he took a five-week vacation. Upon returning, he learned of a new relationship with a young man named Dustin, which Denise felt had helped her gain ground from anorexia. She spoke highly of Dustin and described his positive qualities. However, when Rick asked what she thought, or even guessed, Dustin appreciated about her, she was unable to answer. While Denise had so readily internalized the experience of critical, demanding, and disqualifying others, she was at a complete loss when it came to looking at herself through the eyes of an appreciative (presumably) person. Rick suggested they write to Dustin who had just moved to Europe to attend university. Soon after, on the telephone, Denise asked him to write to Rick detailing what he appreciated in Denise. The following is an excerpt from a fax that arrived a few weeks later:

> *1. What attracted me to Denise?*[2] *First off, I resent the use of the past tense in the question because I am still very attracted to Denise. But, if you were referring to when I first started to see her, then the answer is as follows. Because I did not know Denise as a friend before I started to see her, I relied on the information that a good friend told me; that Denise was a very "cool" person. But I must admit that Denise's beauty was the major attraction.*
>
> *2. What positive qualities do you see in her? I see many positive qualities in Denise, such as: beauty; realistic attitude and down to earth (a "cool" person); very loving; smart (good conversations that delved below surface level); she is very fun to be around; she is easy to talk to and relate to and therefore well liked; and the best reason yet . . . she likes me (good taste).*
>
> *I hope that my responses are along the lines of what you intended and help you explore the yet uncharted regions of Denise's perilous mind.*

Denise's response to the letter was positive. Some things in the letter surprised her. She hadn't realized that Dustin experienced her as a loving person. This contradicted the prior story of herself as "bitchy" and "selfish." Likewise, she had never thought of herself as fun to be around.

Rick was aware of the possibility that Dustin's compliment about her beauty could become subjugating. In our recruitment of audiences, we need to consider the extent to which we may be complicit in the reproduction of the very same cultural knowledges that generate or support the problems our clients are struggling against. Despite Denise's positive response, Rick began to wonder about some possible unintended

[2]Rick thought he had asked Denise to ask Dustin the question, "What do you appreciate about Denise?" The use of the word "attracted" has dominant cultural associations that emphasize physical appearance.

implications and consequences of recruiting Dustin as an appreciative audience. Did asking her to look at herself through Dustin's eyes inadvertently imply that Dustin's perceptions of her carry more validity than her own perceptions or those of other women? Did this question imply an expectation that she should submit herself to the evaluation of others, and of men in particular? Did Dustin's reference to beauty (even if it contradicted anorexia's view of Denise as being fat and ugly) reinforce anorexia's (and the dominant culture's) emphasis on physical beauty as the most important criterion by which the worth of a woman is judged?

In order to practice accountability in his own process, Rick discussed these questions with some feminist women colleagues and raised them with Denise during his final consulting-your-consultants (White & Epston, 1990a) meeting. To engage Denise's own authority in relation to Dustin's comment, Rick asked her about her reaction to Dustin's emphasis on beauty. Did she feel this was pro-anorexic in any way? Denise said she felt it was helpful to hear him say this because it defied anorexia's insistence that she could only be "beautiful" and "attractive" if she lost weight. She also interpreted his use of the word "beauty" to refer to more than just physical appearance because Dustin had made it clear to her previously that he did not care about her weight and believed that she placed much too great an emphasis on it.

ETHICAL CONSIDERATIONS FOR THE USE OF AUDIENCES

The examples above reveal not only some of the benefits of recruiting or evoking audiences in therapeutic work but also some of the potential risks. Audiences may have the capacity to appreciate and validate the new and preferred narratives of our clients, contribute to the development of positive identities, and introduce alternative and liberating knowledges. On the other hand, could they also have the capacity to support, promote, or impose narratives and prescriptions that impoverish and oppress? In our roles as therapists, teachers, and consultants we have been applying and reflecting on circulation practices with each other, our clients, students, and trainees. What are some ethical challenges arising with these practices? We have been struggling with the question of how to apply these practices in a liberative rather than an oppressive manner. In the remainder of this chapter, we articulate some of the ethics that, at present, guide our practices of reflection and circulation. We then present two examples to illustrate how these ethics actually affect both the content and process of our work with clients.

Focus on Existing Strengths and Competencies

We strive to establish a relationship with our clients that engages their views and experiences. We invite people to let us into their worlds, to tell us their stories. We allow ourselves to be led through the narrative landscape as our clients describe to us its familiar and defining features. We enter this landscape with the eyes and ears of an alert and appreciative newcomer, noticing and inquiring about aspects of our clients' experience which they have hitherto overlooked, dismissed, or forgotten.

We assume that our clients possess knowledges and competencies that can free them from the grip of the problem. Our emphasis is on the identification of evolving processes of change, wherein competence is already to be found. We find it is better to back an existing or historic trend of strength and competence rather than insert a new task or prescription that may diverge from the family's style or imply there is a deficit to be corrected. We may, however, cocreate rituals, tests, or tasks with the family in order to add momentum to positive developments. These developing knowledges and competencies, once identified, can be documented and shared with significant others or those experiencing similar problems.

Informed Consent

We should not let our enthusiasm for circulating client discoveries to wider audiences prevent us from fully exploring any potential reservations our clients may have. In spite of our efforts to be collaborative and obtain informed consent, clients may comply rather than agree. They may wish to please, they may feel grateful and want to give something back to us, or they may be uncomfortable with dissent or conflict.

For newly developed practices such as those we have been describing, our obligation to obtain informed consent increases. The therapist may need to go beyond a readily given consent to engage clients with specific questions in a careful consideration of the possible effects, both positive and negative, now and in the future, of circulation. In order for consent to be truly informed, a person needs to comprehend the implications of the action and must offer the consent voluntarily, without even subtle pressure or coercion. The meta-question is: "If you didn't really want to circulate this information, is there anything that would prevent you from letting me know that?" The focus of attention is on restraints to communicating reservations as well as on the reservations themselves. Once an individual can speak clearly about his/her reservations, the creativity of both the client and therapist can be engaged in problem solving to the satisfaction of the client.

It is our hope that this chapter will inspire the reader to join us in defining existing practices and creating new practices that provide for a truly informed consent.

Private Pain and Social Policy: An Ethical Obligation to Go Public

Because we are privy to stories of pain and injustice, as well as of hope and strength, therapists are in a position to circulate more than client discoveries and competencies. The revisioning of the boundaries of the therapeutic relationship is intertwined with an ethic of social justice. Waldegrave (1992) questions whether traditional clinical boundaries "ensure that [the social] causes of physical and psychological problems never get addressed. . . . In modern industrial societies . . . the helping professions are the barometers of pain in their communities" (p. 18). Therefore, therapists have a moral and ethical responsibility to be "better informed about the broader economic, political, cultural and gender determinants of well-being and ill health" (p. 18) and to make public the social and economic issues that cause their clients pain. This information can then be used to influence social policy.

Transparency of Values

We are not advocating a relativistic ethic in which we accept and work with whatever our clients present without engaging in a critical evaluation of our clients' ideas and practices. Externalization allows us to discuss ideas and practices that we perceive as morally problematic in terms of influences rather than as inherent individual or family traits.

Rather than pretend that we come to our work value-free, we prefer to identify our values and be open about them. We now engage clients more fully in candid discussions of the values that inform our discourse. We are exploring the balance between neither imposing our values nor compromising them. The sensitive process of negotiating meaning occurs within the space between these poles. These encounters, where we struggle with values, can be among the most moving and transformative. We find it useful in this process to carefully consider the negative effects of power and hierarchy and to facilitate a diversity of accounts.

Diminishing Hierarchy and Its Effects

The existence of multiple hierarchies and the operations of power associated with these hierarchies profoundly influence our lives. As Pinderhughes (1989) points out, "The assignment of people to dominant and subordinate groups, in part based on culture, is erected and maintained by social structures that help determine how people are viewed, how they view themselves, their access to resources, and their response to these conditions" (p. 9). People with relatively little or no power may interpret their experience through the lens of the dominant discourse and accept meanings that either obscure or legitimate their own oppression. When people begin to challenge these personalized or psychologized meanings and reexamine their experience in the context of race, culture, class, gender, and the operations of power, they often move from a position of self-detesting to one of attesting and protesting.

We are attempting to develop therapeutic practices that diminish the toxic effects of social and cultural hierarchies. When working with families, we are alerted by Waldegrave (1991) to the possibility that those with the most power will dominate or subordinate those with less power, and we monitor our own complicity in this domination. When we observe tactics of domination in operation, we point them out and invite family members to reflect on the effects of these tactics and the ethical questions they raise (Maisel, 1994). We also try to ensure that each family member has an opportunity to speak, comment, and be heard, and we explore any constraints that might interfere with the full participation of all family members. By valuing what each participant and the audience has to say, we increase the diversity of viewpoints and positions. This tends to promote "both/and" solutions (Lipchik, 1993) instead of reinforcing the accounts of those who are able to wield power from their sociocultural positioning.

When addressing power differentials between therapist and clients, we attempt to diminish the extent to which we might exert undue influence by virtue of our status as professionals. We do this by situating more openly our ideas in our personal experience, our understanding of the experience of those whom we have known or worked with, or as stemming from a theoretical model. When working with reflecting teams, Madigan (1991) and White (1991) suggest that questions be addressed to the therapist (and reflecting team members), in the presence of clients, about the therapist's direction, comments, questions, and so on, in order to reveal their foundations. Such questions can be asked by a cotherapist, members of the reflecting team, or the clients themselves.[3] In therapies without teams, clients can be invited to ask similar questions of their therapist throughout the course of therapy.

In addition to consideration of the therapist–client hierarchy, we must consider the experience of hierarchical domination outside the

[3]For a more complete discussion of therapy practices that assist in the "deconstruction" of therapist knowledge, see White (1991).

therapeutic situation. For example, Archie Smith Jr. (personal communication, October 1994) observes that if an African American client chooses to value a white therapist's nondominant ways of behaving, he/she must then live simultaneously in two worlds. He uses W. E. B. Dubois's (1976) idea of "double consciousness" to clarify this experience. According to Smith, the African American client "may exhibit a double consciousness towards a non-subjugating therapist which is a mixture of genuine gratitude on the one hand and suspicion (a hermeneutic of suspicion) on the other." Both sides of this consciousness need to be developed and expressed in therapy, not one side at the expense of the other. Should the African American client disregard the evidence of history and trust that the same nondominant ways of behaving would occur outside therapy? If the therapist fails to allow for the expression of this suspicion, he/she ignores the reality of racism and may imply that the client can and should expect nondominant behavior from other whites in positions of power outside the context of therapy. Thus, we attempt to cocreate meanings that expose rather than obscure the sociocultural contribution to problems and the operations of power.

Accountability

If we place value on social justice, we must also concern ourselves with the issue of accountability. No matter how sincere our intentions and how disciplined our efforts, we will occasionally (and probably more often than we like to believe) respond in ways that are insensitive. This is inevitable given the ways in which our understanding has been constrained by our own life experiences, our placement in the social fields of class, race, religion, gender, and so on, and our own professional socialization.

When misunderstandings arise, it is necessary that we be willing to stand corrected. Otherwise, our "one-up" position creates a potential for these therapist misunderstandings to shape a therapy that may be colonizing and ultimately destructive for the client (Lobovits & Freeman, 1993; Tapping, 1993). Because misunderstandings are inevitable, we find it easier to admit to and learn from them without the attendant guilt and defensiveness. To occupy this position entails a relaxing of the therapist's need to "be in the know" and an acceptance of the necessity of not only guiding our clients but being guided by them.

At a minimum, making our work accountable to the people we work with requires the constant solicitation of their experience of therapy and an acknowledgment of the extent to which we depend on their feedback for guidance (White, 1991). However, if our minority clients are our only source of feedback about cultural differences, we may place an undue burden on them and deny them the option of not responding. For example, when one of the authors (DL) used an outside consultant to give him feedback about diversity issues in the classroom, students from nondominant groups expressed gratitude for not being placed in the bind of being forced to respond about issues of difference. This bind existed because, if they did not respond, the issues would not likely be raised and if they did respond, the risks of exposure would be borne by them (Lobovits & Prowell, 1995).

The Family Centre of Lower Hutt, New Zealand, has been developing accountability structures to address culture, class, and gender inequities in its therapy and administrative work. The staff assume that the best judges of injustice are members of groups that have been systematically mistreated. These nondominant groups have the right to caucus amongst themselves when a concern arises about the functioning of the dominant group, and members of the dominant group have the responsibility to hear the concern of the nondominant group and to work toward finding a mutually acceptable solution (Tamasese & Waldegrave, 1994).

Although most of us have a long way to go in establishing this kind of structural accountability, some options can be immediately considered. One option is to review our clinical work with colleagues of the same race, culture, class, gender, religious, or sexual orientation as our clients. Another option is to seek the help of "cultural consultants" from the community as audiences to our therapies, who can review tapes or be present at clinical conferences. They can also be invited to be audiences for teams and in other ways have direct input into the therapy.

We also need to find ways of making accountable to the community those clients who have been abusive. Audiences such as other men who have overcome abusive behavior or groups of women may be assembled for the purpose of building a structure of accountability into the lives of people who have caused serious harm to others as well as the therapists who work with them (cf. Jenkins, 1990; Lobovits & Freeman, 1993; McLean, 1994; Waldegrave, 1990).

Diversity of Accounts

Information in therapy is typically limited to the client's narrative, which is often problem-saturated, and the therapist's narrative, which usually includes an expert diagnosis and opinion informed by theoretical approach. Clients can be exposed to a diversity of accounts through audiences, which provide a rich resource of different stories, viewpoints, values, and ideas for approaching problems.

As team members, we no longer attempt to speak with one voice, a "voice of authority." We try to establish a space in which persons feel free to evaluate multiple options and reflect on their own personal preferences.

MAX, JANET, AND JACK

One of the author's (DL's) work with a team and family illustrates several principles. We begin with a discussion of one of our formats for reflecting team interviews.[4] We hope this discussion will reveal some of the considerations that help shape the framework of our conversations with clients. We are indebted to Michael White and David Epston for this format.

The following case illustrates the process of interviewing all those who are involved in the therapeutic system and introduces the idea of *recursiveness.* We adopt a reflexive model for our collaborations with clients, trainees, or students (Lobovits & Seidel, 1994; Steier, 1991). Reflexivity may be accomplished by introducing multiple recursions into an interview.

In this typical case, there were seven recursions:

1. Consultant interviews therapist.
2. Each family member is interviewed separately and asked to comment on each other's comments.
3. The team reflects.
4. The family comments on the reflections.
5. Later, the team writes a letter to the family and/or an audience.
6. The family responds to the letter.
7. After reviewing the videotape, several months later, the family responds in writing to an invitation to reflect on the entire experience.

The interview process begins when the family enters the room. The family is carefully introduced to the team members, who wear name tags. The team is kept small enough that the family can begin to develop individual perceptions about each member's strengths and biases.

The family presented here originally sought help from the agency as Max, age 11, was having school problems. They returned four years later for additional help when Max was suspended for being abusive to

[4]This recursive interviewing process is based on a reflexive research model (Steier, 1991) that utilizes ethnographic interviewing (cf. Sells, Smith, Coe, Yoshioka, & Robinson, 1994).

teachers, then ran away to his grandmother. Jack (step father) and Janet (mother) felt Max was uncontrollable and uncooperative and that Max and his grandmother would undermine the limits they set for him. Max felt picked on for everything he did. He could not talk to his stepfather without getting into an argument. Jack and Max fought especially over chores, sometimes to the point of getting physical. Janet would try to mediate between them but the fighting was so bad that she was considering whether it would be better for Max to live elsewhere.

After the introduction of the interview format, Dean interviewed the therapist (Sarah). When the consultant begins by interviewing the therapist, the family is placed in the role of an audience and often reports feeling taken off the spot. It also provides a demonstration for the family that the consultant will interview everyone in a collaborative and facilitative manner.

DEAN: If you could grant a wish to each member of the family for their therapy what would it be?

THERAPIST: I wish for Jack that he could see the success that he's been as a stepfather in influencing who Max is. For Max, my wish would be that he would continue to grow on his own path and be able to utilize the love and support that he has from his parents and use his parents as advisers. For Janet, I wish that she would have some peace, and wouldn't have to referee the fight between Jack and Max.

DEAN: What do you imagine Max's wish would be?

THERAPIST: His wish would be to have everybody stop yelling and screaming all the time. To do things his way and have it work for the family. He'd like to be able to do his own thinking and act from that thinking and not have it cause a big ruckus.

DEAN: What would Janet's wish be?

THERAPIST: I think her wish would be for peace and agreement. To have Jack and Max get along.

DEAN: What would Jack's wish be?

THERAPIST: I think his wish would be for Max to understand the logic behind his request and the love behind his request and to do what he asks with joy because he understands. Jack wants Max to have the good life for himself.

We evaluated this interview by gathering feedback from the family two months later by mail. Jack felt that Sarah's wishes "opened new doors for hope and optimism." Max felt Sarah's wish helped show Jack's commitment to the family for him in a meaningful way.

After the session, a team member made this comment to the consultant: "By interviewing the therapist, you reinforced that there's something important between her and the family. This showed you were respectful of the family's relationship with the therapist. You demonstrated that you were going to learn something from their therapist and you were going to learn it in front of them. The usual professional way of doing this would be talking behind their back."

The therapist made these comments: "I thought you picked up on my concern that they were not experiencing what they had accomplished so far in therapy. By showing them what I see them wanting, it grounded me in my work with them. It had the effect of grounding them in their work with me. I had not had the opportunity to reflect on who I perceived them to be in front of them and I think it was powerful."

The following section was pivotal in clarifying a liberative theme that was circulated to an outside audience. Janet appeared to have a gendered role as the sole family mediator in the fights between Max and Jack. The bind for her was that when she attempted to set limits on this role for herself, she was seen as a rejecting mother. This interview segment, which focused on gender issues, explored the role of mother in the family in such a way that honored Janet's limits and released her from the bind.

Consequently, she was able to voice the preexisting priority that her home become a place of peace instead of conflict without being labeled "rejecting," even if it meant Max had to move to his grandmother's house.

JANET: The day-in-and-day-out bickering is constantly weighing on me. I don't even want to go home. Jack said to me the other day: "You're the one who wants to send Max away." I said: "But I have a big saturation point, I've just hit it, I just can't think anymore" and that's when I said "he has to leave."

DEAN: Would it be fair to say that if Jack and Max got the better of the bickering that your preference would be to have the family together?

JANET: Of course.

DEAN: But if the bickering is dominating family life then it's better to have peace at home and Max with his grandmother?

JANET: Yeah, honestly yes. Part of me admits that there's times when I don't enjoy being Max's mother. It's hard with all the bickering and the school troubles. It can be a struggle being a parent because there is also a part of me that wants him to be with me.

DEAN: Can I ask you something that would be for the benefit of our conversations about parenting? How did you come by the idea that you are allowed a saturation point? We've experienced mothers who don't feel they're allowed a saturation point. Is there something that you've experienced in your current or past life that convinced you that mothers can have a point where they can say enough is enough?

JANET: Well, I don't know if it's as much being a mother as being a human being and what's thrown at you and what you've gone through. I had a difficult first marriage and I took a lot in then. It's part of my personality that I take a lot in and then, when I get to that point, I talk to myself and cleanse it out.

DEAN: You would locate that ability from your experience in life, your first marriage being an example where you hit the wall? Since you have that experience in your life you know not to go past that?

JANET: Yeah.

DEAN: Would it be a leap to say that you don't let the role of mother block your personhood?

JANET: No, I'm individual too, I've never defined myself as just Max's mother. That's how I preserve a little serenity. We all have our stresses and they're very important to each of us. But when we come home and can't feel quiet at home, it's hard. *(crying)*

DEAN: Would it be okay to say that the tears are not only for not having your peace at home but for your dream of having it?

JANET: Yes! It's a great relief to cry. To let your guard down.

Gathering a Solution Ethnography for Future Audiences

In the beginning of the session, the stepfather, Jack, proposed some changes in his parenting and partnering style that would reduce conflict with Max over chores. Dean realized that Jack had some ideas that might help other families face this common issue of arguments over chores. Dean asked permission from Jack and the family to circulate these ideas to other families who seek help from the agency.

JACK: There has to be a more positive end to the conversation. There has to be clear reasons for the chores. Like raking around the water spigots in the field below the house. In case there was a fire there, we would have to have the outlets for water. My wish would be that I would have more time to explain myself. I've gotten in the habit of giving orders rather than explaining myself. I've been thinking this is why it always escalates between us. If I put a time frame on my requests along with a reason for it, if I put a reward for completing it.

DEAN: Let me see if I've got this. During the week you've been thinking how to strike a more positive note with Max?

JACK: I've been a problem. Trouble has been escalating into violent behavior on Max's and on my part.

DEAN: Would it be okay to say you're taking up your part of the problem?

JACK: Yeah.

DEAN: So, first you've taken steps to accept your part in the problem. You observed that the conversations ended in a negative, violent, or escalated note. Then you came up with a method to change the way your message was delivered. Instead of giving orders and not explaining yourself, you are going to employ three components. The first component of the method is that there is a time frame to a task, second, there is a reason for the task. The third is a reward for the task. . . .

JACK: There's a fourth part to this. I need to find out what Max considers a reward instead of imposing what I think it ought to be.

DEAN: (*writing and saying out loud*) "Consult with Max and find out what he thinks a reward is." Jack, what would you recommend to another family member who came to this agency caught up in escalating arguments like you described? How did you turn yourself around toward solving the problem rather than being a part of it?

JACK: I started by doing the task myself that I was asking Max to do. First, I wanted to show Max I could do it and second I wanted to have a realistic idea of how much work it was. My frustration was that I work a lot differently than Max does. Second, you should depend on your wife. I spent hours and hours talking to her and observing her moderating behavior. I have some very high expectations of myself and I put them on Max. I'm a very emotional person.

JANET: He's a worry wart! (*All laugh.*)

DEAN: In terms of how you do a turnaround, the first thing I heard was that you do the task yourself that you are going to ask the teen to do. That gave you a reference for how much work was involved in the task and that the teen would know that the job you assigned was a job that you could do. The second idea was about knowing your own work style and taking account of differing work styles between you and the teen. The third idea was to consult your partner, observe your partner's moderating techniques and how they reduce blaming.

JACK: Actually this morning I just asked her, "What am I doing wrong?" You have to ask for a critique, not just deny anything is wrong. I think about things a lot. I'm willing to change.

DEAN: I'd guess we'd have to put that number one; be willing to change. In terms of being emotional, were you saying that you put a lot into your love and that was turned into high expectations for others?

JACK: Yeah, I have a lot high expectations for myself too.

Both Janet and Max made comments on Jack's ideas. Janet especially liked Jack's idea of paying careful attention to differences in work rates, and urged Jack to tune his expectations to where Max was developmentally. Max felt that if he was going to listen to Jack's explanations and reasons about a task, Jack would also have to listen to Max's reasons as well. Here is an excerpt of Dean's interview with Max about Jack's ideas:

DEAN: Do you think that explanations like the example Jack gave about the fire danger and the spigots, would these reduce the amount of bickering between you? Is that a bickering-reducing strategy for you?

MAX: Not really because down in that field, if there was a fire, we wouldn't be able to save that field, we'd have to back up and save the house. Around the house I can see doing the raking. There's not enough water pressure down in the field. Stay up at the house and protect the house!

DEAN: So you would carefully clear the spigots around the house because that makes sense to you?

MAX: Yeah, but not down in the field.

DEAN: If Jack comes up with an explanation for a job, for the explanation to reduce bickering it's going to have to make sense to you.

MAX: I guess so.

During the reflection, a team member made the following comment:

> "I was thinking about how Max said you can't put out a big fire with a little hose, and that the anger the family struggles with is like the brush fires they have to contend with and prepare for. In a way, there's a parallel between what Max was saying about needing more water to put out a fire and how the whole family was speaking to

> the idea of collaborating to resolve some of these issues. Instead of each person taking a little hose to put out a big fire, they can each pool together their little hoses, to create one big hose, which would be better at cooling the flames of anger which sometimes get out of control and become violent."

On follow-up two months later, we found that this reflection had continued to make an impact on all members of the family.

During the session Jack and Max continued to disagree on the issue of the fire line. In spite of this diversity of opinion, the metaphor led to a both/and idea: arguing, bickering, and stressful baggage from work or school should not be brought into the house. Janet raised the issue that stressful baggage was often waiting for her on the phone machine as a result of the school calling about Max. The family jokingly referred to these messages as incoming missiles. Dean was inspired by this conversation to propose that a letter be written to the school.

Recruiting a Skeptical Audience

Individual efforts to reduce the fighting by leaving stresses in the field, away from the house, were important. However, this would not protect the family from "incoming missiles" from the school via the telephone. The idea of this letter was to engage school personnel as an audience to the family's aspirations for peace and recruit them to support the commitment to preserve peace within the protected confines of the home. The letter was composed by the team and strove to use the language and metaphors of the family. It invites the audience, the teenager's school, into the latest developments in his relationship with the problem and catches them up with the family's preferred story and goals. The letter was sent to the family for review and approval, and after integration of the changes proposed by family members, it was sent to the school.

An important conversation that has not been excerpted here shaped the letter to the school. Max was interviewed about the fighting between he and Jack over chores and was asked to rate the intensity of the fights. He felt that the intensity level of the fights was as low as 5 on a scale of 10 during summer vacation, but during the school year it would not be lower than a 9. He was then interviewed about his contribution to reducing the fighting to a 5 level. He described avoiding a "click" that would go off in his head, after which he would lose control and "not think." Dean was familiar with clicks from his work with other teens and questioned Max about his click and his methods of controlling it. Max felt that he now had the ability to see a click coming and that clicks and conflicts came together. In fact, he had tried "walking away" from a conflictual situation and had been able to avoid a click.

After gathering this information, Dean reviewed Max's ideas with Jack and Janet as he had reviewed Jack's ideas on conflict reduction with Max and Janet. As we stated earlier, we feel it is important to attend to the hierarchy and its effects within the family. One technique for doing this is to make family members accountable to each other's opinions. The idea is not to achieve a consensus but to make sure that each opinion is validated. Janet's opinion was that Max's idea of walking away from conflicts was only a temporary solution. She felt that conflicts must be returned to and faced to achieve resolution.

Letter to the School

We are writing to you to share our work together with the . . . family. This letter is an invitation to you to see Max and his family differently than you may have seen them before. In the past temper, arguing, and bickering have been dominant features of Max's life. Now, he has joined together with his family to set off on a determined course toward their preferred peaceful modes of family communication.

Max is determined to free himself of being controlled by temper and the negative effects it has had on his home and school lives. He has taken the step of developing "Click Control." A "click" is what precedes "blowing up" or "doing without thinking." These are the things that have caused Max the biggest difficulties in the past, as you may remember.

Max's first step in "Click Control" is to "walk away" from situations in order to avoid a blow up. Janet, Max's mother, feels this is a good step for Max to take. However she feels that it is only the first step. When Max walks away from a problem that may blow up, he then needs to take the second step of coming back to face the problem in a calm and collected manner.

School problems are a major source of stress, argument and bickering for the whole family. Max rates arguments in the family during the school year to be no lower than 9 or 10 on a scale of 10. During the summer, when school is out, arguments and bickering can come down to the 5 level.

Now, it is important for you to know that this family is determined to live in peace together. If they can't, then Max will live and go to school where his grandmother resides. So as you can imagine, it is essential for Max to have a peaceful, low stress year at school in 94–95.

Janet has made the significant point that calls from school about Max and his troubles often await her and Jack at the end of long and stressful workdays. It is our observation that the family is very responsive to the school's concerns about Max's behavior. In order to allow for Max and his family to reduce escalating stress levels, they need to first take a step back from these problems and then, to turnaround and face them. What we feel is that in order to deal with school problems effectively without blowing their family apart, they need some turnaround time.

The adjustment we are suggesting is that if Max experiences a slip in his new course of life using his two-step "click control" method and the school calls home about trouble, the school should not expect an immediate response from the family except in cases of medical emergency. The family will respond to the school no sooner than 24 hours and no later than 72 hours. This should allow for a one- to two-day cooling-off period for the entire family. Time enough we hope, for everyone to take a step away from the problem and reduce arguing and bickering down to a 5 level. When that is achieved then they will step back to face the problem and contact the school with the appropriate response. Of course, we hope it is not necessary to implement this turnaround time plan, but even though we expect the best, it is wise, as you know, to prepare for the worst.

It is important information for you to have that in addition to this effort with your school, the parents have made similar commitments to limit the effects of work related stress on their family life. We hope that this strategy, of creating and protecting a "center of peace" in their family life, from which they gain the equanimity to then cope with outside stresses, is an enterprise that you can join with wholeheartedly!

Yours for peace in the . . . family home,

In the family's response to the school letter Janet said: "We found the letter to be wonderfully written and you have been able to express our family's determination to have a positive 1994–1995 school year. . . . Your agency has been such a shoulder of support for our family. We commend you for the support you give to families and to the individual kids and parents that need to be heard."

On follow-up, the family felt they had continued to articulate their aspirations—"a striving for self reliance, a warm sense of wholeness . . . and a credibility amongst themselves and extended family members." They emphasized the value of having a copy of the videotape of the session because it summarized their counseling experience and could be used as a reminder of their aspirations and a "benchmark" of their progress in the future.

CULTURAL CONSIDERATIONS

Our discussion continues by taking up the crucial issue of cross-cultural contact. In such contact, we are interested in avoiding colonization and its effects. Colonization involves a power-over relationship that does not respect existing ecologies within nondominant cultures—for example the way in which a culture conceives of the ecologies between individuals and families, between men and women, between the personal and the communal, between the people and their land, between the sacred and profane (Lobovits & Freeman, 1993). The ethic of noncolonization encourages respect, curiosity, an assumption of degrees of ignorance and bias, and a willingness to learn and be corrected.

NICOLE, RAY, AND KEVIN

What follows is an excerpt from a meeting between a couple, their therapist, a reflecting team, and a consultant (RM). During this meeting, one of the clients found it necessary to correct a misunderstanding on the part of a reflecting team member. An African American couple, Nicole and Ray, initially sought help for their six-year-old son, Kevin, after he was nearly smothered to death by three white boys at day care. The parents felt the after-school program treated the incident lightly by merely suspending the three boys for one day and withdrew Kevin from the program. Both parents believed that had their child been white and the attackers black, the response of the day-care program would have been stronger. Their sincere efforts to establish accountability and rebuild a sense of security sufficient for them to consider having Kevin remain in the program had been misconstrued by some parents as an attempt to "grind" a racial ax. This placed the couple in a difficult bind: If they challenged these attributions about their motives, it would only serve to reinforce perceptions that they were militant or antiwhite.

Following the attack, Kevin developed symptoms of posttraumatic stress for which he received individual play therapy. Although Kevin's symptoms had almost entirely resolved at the time of the team consultation, Nicole was still preoccupied with protecting her son. Ray felt that Nicole had become obsessed with the boy's well-being to such an extent that she was unable to focus on or enjoy her life and that she was unreasonably restricting the range of Kevin's activities. During the interview, the team learned that Nicole's preoccupation with her son was a self-imposed penance, fueled by the guilt she felt for arriving late to pick up Kevin on the day he was assaulted. She believed that if she had been on time it might not have happened. A majority of the reflecting team comments and questions focused on the effects that this guilt had been having on the family.

TEAM MEMBER (TM) 1: These kind of people are potentially around in all our kids' lives. I was wondering if Kevin could learn better how to deal with these not very nice guys who did this. Perhaps if he learns the discipline of the martial arts, he can get a sense that he can take care of himself. I've seen kids who have this training emanate a kind of quality, a sureness, that kids don't mess with them in the same way. Nicole's fear is that if she lets him go, something bad will happen. What if she says: "I'm going to help you learn how to take care of yourself, honey, so I don't have to feel guilty all of the time because then I really know it's going to be all right"?

Does this comment overlook the context of race and racism which is so salient to this couples' experience of their child's victimization? By suggesting that all kids are equally vulnerable to this kind of aggression, are distinctions based on race made to appear moot? Does the definition of the problem become overly psychologized as the focus shifts from the social context to the boy's vulnerability and the mother's fear? We reviewed these questions with a cultural consultant while writing this chapter. Archie Smith Jr. felt Nicole's fear about her son's safety might reflect the historical concern of African American mothers for their sons' survival. "Mothers want their sons to be men, i.e., aggressive and able to defend themselves, but not too aggressive so as to offend the white world and bring down punishment or death" (A. Smith, Jr., personal communication, October 1994). Considerations of this nature led some team members to respond with reflections that attempted to reintroduce race as an important context.

TM2: I wonder if that would really work because no matter how good at martial arts he becomes he still might get victimized, and guilt could come in and Nicole could say, "Oh, I didn't make sure he learned enough." Is she still going to have square off with guilt?

TM3: I wanted to mention that they are black parents, and being a minority [Asian American] parent myself, it's hard sometimes not to take on that guilt, to listen to that guilt in a different way. I feel that I really have to protect my kid because this isn't a safe world for minorities sometimes. So that can get juggled in there—Am I doing a good enough job if I'm going to be teaching my black child to become a good, loving, kind man, given this hostile world?

TM4: (*to TM3*) Do you feel that by going to the school and trying to get the school to take responsibility, Ray and Nicole are standing against guilt?

TM3: I think that was a way of dealing with guilt. But it would be difficult for me because I need other people to help me to fight the guilt because it's so easy to take it in.

TM1: And the guilt can come doubly in minority situations.

TM5: And when you try putting the responsibility back where it belongs and they don't take it, you're left holding the bag.

The reflections presented above represent a 2-minute slice from a 20-minute reflecting team segment. Even during this brief exchange, we can see the manifestation of several of the ethical considerations we outlined earlier. Due to our concern for social justice, we think that even if this couple had not introduced race and racism as a factor in the problem they were struggling with, we would have raised the issue. The school, according to these parents, had refused to accept meaningful responsibility for the problem. Nicole blamed herself for not preventing these events. This led to a story about herself as an ineffectual and neglectful mother, and obscured the operations of power and racism and their effects.

Presenting our clients with a diversity of perspectives, especially when these are in some ways contradictory, helps insure against the potentially dominating effects of any one reflection. Team member 1 offered a reflection that might have inadvertently mirrored and even reinforced the mother's sense of responsibility for her child's victimization. By presenting this idea and affording other reflecting team members the opportunity to reflect on and debate its implications, Nicole was exposed to alternative and perhaps novel ideas. It is not necessary to censor comments that might inadvertently uphold problem-saturated descriptions, provided that reflectors are mindful of potential effects of reflections and experience the freedom to question or disagree about reflections made by other team members. If it were not for the diversity of views expressed around this issue, we think it is unlikely that Ray would have felt safe enough to eventually share his reaction to the idea that his son could attain security by learning a martial art.

The therapist then invited the couple to evaluate the reflections for what was helpful and unhelpful. Both Nicole and Ray responded only with positives. The team was reluctant to accept this one-sided reaction as the full story. During the interview, Nicole and Ray told the team how their son had been outnumbered, overpowered, and nearly suffocated by a group of white boys and how this account had fallen on deaf ears at the school. In no way did the team wish to replicate the dynamic, and so the team persisted with an invitation to them to engage in a critique of these comments:

PHONE-IN FROM TEAM: The team would like to again ask whether there is anything you feel didn't fit for you, because we really like to learn from people what's helpful and not helpful. So if you have any constructive or even nonconstructive criticism or feedback we are very interested in hearing it.

RAY: Let me just say that, try not take this the wrong way, as a minority family trying to raise a minority son and then having this thing happen to us—my point being that there is not one African American on the panel that's listening. So even though everyone in this room may be educated and really know what they are talking about, and I believe they do, there was still nobody that is from our culture and that really understands our point of view. People are just different. I just think that on a certain level there may have been something missed by the fact that there wasn't enough minority representation listening to us today. Which is fine. It's neither here nor there. One woman who said putting him into a martial arts might help him find some type of discipline, which is true, but the same situation could happen again where it is three people against one and Karate's not going to do anything. Having self-discipline, knowing how to kick somebody in the chin isn't going to do anything if three boys—three *white* boys—jump on you and try to smother you. At six years old to be learning racism outright is scary.

NICOLE: He doesn't know racism . . .

RAY: Maybe you think he doesn't but we really don't know whether or not he does. The way I see it, I think he does.

THERAPIST: So you felt that people might have understood better if there had been African American representation?

RAY: Yeah, it's just how I feel in a very general sense.

Because there was no African American member of the team to provide an outside source of accountability, Ray may have been put in the bind of being the sole source of feedback about cultural differences (see discussion on pp. 238–239). Thus, the choice to not respond was constrained and Ray bore the sole risk of exposure. It may have been the team's encouragement to evaluate which reflections might have been unhelpful, that helped Ray experience this exposure as a bit less risky. When racism and underrepresentation became permitted discourse, Ray and Nicole did not reexperience the exclusionary effect of the school's anemic response to their raising the issue of racism.

PHONE-IN FROM TEAM [delivered by therapist]: The team wants to let you know that they agree with you, Ray. It is unfortunate that there is not any African American representation on the team and that they feel honored that you would feel comfortable enough to share that with us. We also wanted to express our condolences to you for your loss [Ray had mentioned, during his response to the reflecting team, that his grandmother had recently died] and they also want to encourage you both to continue to be in conversation with each other and with me about the many issues which were raised today.

RAY: Yeah, I think the meetings we have are important, so that you can confer with us about just . . . stuff.

THERAPIST: So let's be in touch in the future.

After this message was delivered by the therapist, the team realized that they had not expressed their intention as an agency to address the issue Ray had raised. The issue of staff diversity had in fact been an ongoing subject of discussion and one this agency had been attempting to address. In light of the fact that the afterschool teacher had initially sympathized with this couples' concern but had subsequently not supported the school's taking concrete action, the team felt a need to emphasize its intention to redress the lack of African American representation.

PHONE-IN FROM TEAM [delivered by therapist]: The team wanted to let you know, Ray, that they really are working towards addressing this issue of having more minority and particularly African American representation at the Center, that we not just paying lip service to that because we are aware that it is a problem.

RAY: That's fine . . .

NICOLE: Well, he feels differently than me. He's a little more on the militant side.

RAY: (*irritated by Nicole's characterization*) See, that's why I don't want you to misunderstand me. It has nothing to do with being militant or being pro-black; it has to do with being rational. People are different, you know, most black folks rear their kids different than most white folks. It's just how it is. It's not good or bad, right, or wrong. It's just how it is. So for a room full of eight white folks to sit around and tell us . . .

THERAPIST: Mm hmm.

RAY: I mean, it's like I say, it's all people who I totally respect. I totally respect their points of view, I totally respect them as intellects. But at the same time, all the book reading in the world's not going to give you more insight into our culture. You have to grow up there, you know, you have to grow up walking down the street being pulled over by a cop saying . . . I got pulled over by a cop walking near my home and they said, "Well, we had a description of someone in the area that fits you who just robbed a house." I'm walking home at age 13!

NICOLE: (*obviously uncomfortable with Ray's expression of his experience of racism*) All right!

RAY: I mean, I'm just saying, it's not a militant thing, it's just reality. (*pausing*) I really think that today was really good. It was good to hear all these opinions.

Although at first there could appear to be a conflict between the couple, the conversation may reflect the realities of the "double consciousness" referred to earlier. Ray articulated the realities of his everyday experience outside of therapy, whereas Nicole may have articulated her current experience of trust inside the therapy. Smith (personal communication, October 1994) observes that these positions may be complementary rather than conflictual: "In effect, Ray tells more than Nicole about the cultural dilemma, and Nicole keeps him from telling too much. Between the two of them, a balance is found." Smith's reading of these interactions as complementary rather than conflicting may be an example of the "positive regard and recognition of the Black families coping skills" recommended by Nancy Boyd-Franklin (1989). She points out that such coping skills are often misinterpreted by therapists as "resistance" (p. 66). This discussion surfaced only after Ray persisted in trying to make the therapy accountable to his experience as an African American male. We believe that Ray's persistence required trust that the therapist and team were open to being corrected and informed and would not respond to him in a defensive and disqualifying manner. He visibly relaxed at the conclusion of his comments and his parting remark suggests that he felt a good-faith attempt to listen to and honor his experience was made by all.

CONCLUSION

On reflection, we find that the use of audiences has sharpened our focus on social interdependency. Unexpected solutions to problems may be found as we access a wider range of input and social support for change. We are no longer burdened by feeling as if we are the sole source of support and knowledge for clients. We have become more conscious of how privileged we are to interact with clients and witness their journeys of change. We gain from a greatly enriched fund of creative ideas, as well as stories of pain and hope, to inform us and to share with other clients.

According to an African proverb, it takes a village to raise a child. Similarly, it may take an audience to solve a problem. A community of those who have experience with a problem will contain just what is needed. So let us sow the seeds of belonging with stories of pain and hope and harvest liberation.

ACKNOWLEDGMENTS

We would like to acknowledge the contributions of Victoria Dickerson, David Epston, Ann Epston, Michael Searle, Archie Smith Jr., Susan Sterling, Charles Waldegrave, the Xanthos therapist and reflecting team: Sarah Fisk, Priscilla Caputo, John Karr, Karen Moore, Barbara Easterlin, Mimi Naish, Steven Kruszynski, Emily Seidel, Vanessa Anderson; and the Redwood Center therapist and reflecting team: Andrew Smith, Fran Dayan, Ann Yabusaki, Michael Murtz, and Susan Bressee.

REFERENCES

Boyd-Franklin, N. (1989). *Black families in therapy: A multisystems approach.* New York: Guilford Press.

Bruner, J. (1986). *Actual minds, possible worlds.* Cambridge, MA: Harvard University Press.

Dubois, W. E. B. (1976). *Souls of black folk.* Mattituk, NY: Ameron.

Epston, D. (1989). *Collected papers.* Adelaide, Australia: Dulwich Centre Publications.

Epston, D., Morris, F., & Maisel, R. (1995). A narrative approach to so-called anorexia/bulimia. *Journal of Feminist Family Therapy,* 7(1/2), 69–95.

Freeman, J. C., & Lobovits, D. (1993). The turtle with wings. In S. Friedman (Ed.), *The new language of change: Constructive collaboration in psychotherapy.* New York: Guilford Press.

Gergen, K. J., & Gergen, M. M. (1991). Toward reflexive methodologies. In F. Steier (Ed.), *Research and reflexivity.* London: Sage.

Goffman, E. (1959). *The presentation of self in everyday life.* New York: Doubleday/Anchor Books.

Goffman, E. (1961). *Asylums.* Garden City, NY: Anchor Books.

Jenkins, A. (1990). *Invitations to responsibility: The therapeutic engagement of men who are violent and abusive.* Adelaide, Australia: Dulwich Centre Publications.

Lipchik, E. (1993). "Both/and" solutions. In S. Friedman (Ed.), *The new language of change: Constructive collaboration in psychotherapy.* New York: Guilford Press.

Lobovits, D., & Freeman, J. C. (1993). Toward collaboration and accountability: Alternatives to the dominant discourse for understanding sexual exploitation by professionals. *Dulwich Centre Newsletter,* pp. 33–44.

Lobovits, D., & Prowell, J. (1995, March 3). *Unexpected journey: Invitations to diversity.* Paper presented at the Narrative Ideas and Therapeutic Practice Conference. Vancouver, British Columbia.

Lobovits, D., & Seidel, E. (1994, April 1). *Relational co-research in narrative training and supervision.* Paper presented at the Narrative Ideas and Therapeutic Practice Conference. Vancouver, British Columbia.

Madigan, S. (1991). Discursive restraints in therapist practice: Situating therapist questions in the presence of the family. *Dulwich Centre Newsletter,* pp. 13–20.

Maisel, R. (1994, April 2). *Engaging men in a reevaluation of practices and definitions of masculinity.* Paper presented at the Narrative Ideas and Therapeutic Practice Conference. Vancouver, British Columbia.

McLean, C. (1994). A conversation about accountability with Michael White. *Dulwich Centre Newsletter,* pp. 68–79.

McLean, C., White, C., & Hall, R. (Eds). (1994). Accountability: New directions for working in partnership [Special issue]. *Dulwich Centre Newsletter.*

Pinderhughes, E. (1989). *Understanding race, ethnicity, and power: The key to efficacy in clinical practice.* New York: Free Press.

Sells, S. P., Smith, T. E., Coe, M. J., Yoshioka, M., & Robbins, J. (1994). An ethnography of couple and therapist experiences in reflecting practice. *Journal of Marital and Family Therapy, 20*(3), 247–266.

Steier, F. (1991). *Research and reflexivity.* London: Sage.

Tamasese, K., & Waldegrave, C. (1994). Cultural and gender accountability in the "just therapy" approach. *Journal of Feminist Family Therapy, 5*(2), 29–45.

Tapping, C. (1993). Other wisdoms, other worlds: Colonisation & family therapy. *Dulwich Centre Newsletter,* pp. 3–37.

Waldegrave, C. (1990). Just therapy. *Dulwich Centre Newsletter,* pp. 6–46.

Waldegrave, C. (1991). *Weaving threads of meaning and distinguishing preferable patterns.* Lower Hutt, New Zealand: Author.

Waldegrave, C. (1992, October). Psychology, politics and the loss of the welfare state. *New Zealand Psychological Society Bulletin, 74,* 14–21.

White, M. (1989). The externalizing of the problem and the re-authoring of lives and relationships. In M. White (Ed.), *Selected papers.* Adelaide, Australia: Dulwich Centre Publications.

White, M. (1991). Deconstruction and therapy. *Dulwich Centre Newsletter,* pp. 21–40.

White, M., & Epston, D. (1990a). Consulting your consultants: The documentation of alternative knowledges. *Dulwich Centre Newsletter,* pp. 25–35.

White, M. & Epston, D. (1990b). *Narrative means to therapeutic ends.* New York: Norton.

CHAPTER 12

From "Spy-chiatric Gaze" to Communities of Concern

FROM PROFESSIONAL MONOLOGUE TO DIALOGUE

Stephen Madigan
David Epston

> Neutral dictionary definitions of the words of a language ensure their common features and guarantee that all speakers of a given language will understand one another, but the use of words in live speech communication is always individual and contextual.
>
> —*Bakhtin (1986, p. 88)*

THERAPY, LIKE POLITICS, has always rested on the construction and maintenance of social reality. Until recently, therapists practiced in accordance with a set of enduring or given "truths." Unfortunately, these "truths" acted to conceal and support our monopolistic ambitions to control information on what constitutes right and wrong, normal and abnormal. The purpose of this chapter is to argue for "alternative knowledges" (Foucault, 1980) that derive from those populations most excluded from power (e.g., clients, inmates, and residents). Our intent is to widen the frame of certain therapeutic traditions regarding the utilization of client knowledges and to increase the possibilities of utilizing these knowledges.

Our chapter proposes "communities of concern" as a means of revisioning our relationships with people who seek our help. We substitute such communities for the exclusionary professional–other and the degrading practices that seem associated. From our point of view, reflecting team practice (Andersen, 1987; Lax, 1991; Madigan, 1992a; White, 1995) exemplifies such communities of concern. Our hope in this chapter is to extend the reflecting team idea into areas of (co)research and political action.

Specifically, the chapter illustrates the practice of circulating clients' local knowledges through the establishment of leagues, letter-writing campaigns, and coresearching practices.

A LOOKING-GLASS HISTORY

Since the early 1700s, the deep problems of human concern have been assumed to be the monopoly of a range of health professionals. Therapeutic practice was managed through agreed-on structural, temporal, and ideological tenets. Therapeutic tenets dictated how therapy would be carried out, who would be involved, what information was relevant, how long therapy would take, what constituted a "cure," and so forth. Tenets of therapy were secured through hard-fought struggles at academic, professional, and governmental levels. Tenets were mediated through policy guidelines that dictated appropriate practice procedure. Since the 1700s, not much has changed. What gets to be said, and with what authority, is not viewed within the landscape of the excluded others' story-telling rights (Law & Madigan, 1994). How the problem is defined, who will be involved in the solution of the problem, and how much time is necessary to create change are considered the prerogative of the professional person.

Traditionally, the ideology of professional practice viewed clients/patients as not having expertise in their own lives (Foucault, 1982). Often the existence of a problem is used as prime facie evidence to support such a claim. Health professionals viewed themselves as having "expert knowledge" and spoke openly of this knowledge with colleagues but not with clients. This expert knowledge marked the health professional off as the "observer" and distinguished him/her from the "other." In fact, the positivist methodologies that undergirded expert knowledge required separation of the observer from the "observed other," in what Joan Campbell refers to as "the watchers and the watched" (personal communication, Auckland, July 1994).

Client observation has long been a practice of psychiatry, psychology, and family therapy. From behind one-way mirrors, the family therapy "eye" expanded to a four-by-six-foot gaze. This provided family therapists with a new eminence which they hoped would make them preeminent among their mental health colleagues as looking-glass heroes/heroines. Concealed and quite often anonymous, the behind-the-scenes team offered up ingenious hypotheses and interventions by telephone or in written summaries. Their comments were usually interpretive and strategic in origin as demonstrated by the work of the Mental Research Institute (MRI) and Milan-style "teams."

The negative reactions of many families to these "gazing" practices often went unheeded because negative reactions were often interpreted as signs of perturbation, something that was unequivocally viewed as heralding change. However, both preceding and in the wake of reflecting team practices, questions were being asked as to whose benefit the therapeutic gazing ritual was structured for (Madigan, 1991b, in press) and concern was expressed for "some of the clinical, political, and ethical dilemmas of different ways of reviewing and using one-way screens" (Young, 1989, p. 5).

Postmodernism, feminism, and social constructionism called for a reconsideration of our structuralist and functionalist traditions, as was the case in the social sciences at large. Alongside this discussion, the "other" began to talk back. Anna Yeatman (1994) suggests:

> Many and maybe most commentators agree that [postmodernism] represents a crisis of authority for the western knowing subject, posed by the refusal to stay silenced on the part of those whom this subject had cast as other: natives, colonials, women and all who are placed in a client relationship to expert, professional authority. By insisting on their own voice and status as subjects, these erstwhile objects of modern western knowledge, have disrupted the epistemological order of domination inscribed within modern, western knowledge. (p. 27)

The professional field of family therapy has begun to review the tenets that long dictated the course of what we understood to be family therapy. Therapeutic ideas and therapy practice have begun the painful shift from being viewed as entitled truths to social constructions (Shotter & Gergen, 1989). Who constitutes the self, the status of therapeutic objectivity, structures, and discourse came under revision and have been replaced by coauthoring (Epston & White, 1990), the decentering of the subject (Elliott, 1994; Madigan, 1991a; Sampson, 1989), the cultural effects on problem maintenance (White, 1995; Waldegrave, 1990), and therapist transparency (Epston & White, 1990).

It was through the introduction of reflecting teams that therapists began to oblige themselves to make their opinions visible and audible and, by the same token, accountable and contestable. Liberated from the distant security of the one-way screen, reflecting team members joined with families they observed and sat in observation of their own comments. Having foresaken any allegiance to grand traditions of "truth," they felt entitled to offer up a "smorgasbord" of ideas and not correct interpretations.

They suggested points of view, "not as rigid explanations but as tentative thoughts" (Lax, 1991 p. 133). Clients were offered a chance to talk back, interrogate, question, and reflect back to therapists their thoughts about the therapist's thoughts. Within this recursive conversation, clients were intended a different status; one of inclusion and equity.

It is here that the professional monologue that Foucault has referred to, is substituted for communities of dialogue—a process of talking with, rather than talking to. Foucault (1984) writes:

> In the serene world of mental illness, modern man [*sic*] no longer communicates with the madman [*sic*]: on the one hand, the man [*sic*] of reason delegates the physician to madness, thereby authorizing a relation through the abstract universality of disease; on the other hand, a man [*sic*] of madness communicates with society only by intermediary of an equally abstract reason which is order, physical or moral restraint, the anonymous pressure of the group, the requirements of conformity. As for a common language, there is no such thing any longer: the constitution of madness as mental illness, at the end of the eighteenth century, affords the evidence of a broken dialogue, posits the separation of the already effected and thrusts into the oblivion all those stammered, imperfected words without fixed syntax in which the exchange between madness and reason was made. The language of psychiatry, which is monologue of reason about madness, has been established on the basis of such silence. (pp. xii–xiii)

Through reflecting teams, clients participated as partners to the dialogue, co-constructing the very terms and language of the therapy, thereby receiving a chance to be directly involved in co-constructing the language of their own change. Epston and White (1990), found Myerhoff's (1982) "definitional ceremonies" as apt descriptions of these communities of concern in the manner in which they performed their knowledges and their redescriptions of themselves as persons and families and therapists. They view the performance of reflecting teams as "celebrations of redefinition" which highlight and bring forth previously restrained solution knowledges.

The purpose for the establishment of ideas such as leagues, letter-writing campaigns, and coresearch projects involve the further circulation of "local knowledges" around problems to those not in attendance and can considerably widen the scale of operation. These communities of concern might be considered "virtual communities."

The voices of the client and their family are privileged in these communities of concern as the means to therapeutic ends. These communities may very well extend their activities from concern to more organized coresearch, or in the case of the Anti-Anorexia/Anti-Bulimia League to frank political activism on behalf of its membership and others.

NARRATIVE IDEOLOGY AND PRACTICE

Leagues, letter-writing campaigns, and coresearch are situated in a narrative ideology that acts "as if" it were true that the problem is the problem rather than the person is the problem (Epston & White, 1990; Madigan, 1992b; Roth & Epston, in press; White, 1995). These practices challenge both therapist and client to revise their relative positioning to, and beliefs about, knowing and not knowing about problems. Briefly, narrative ideas are situated in a therapeutic context that does the following:

1. Privileges the person's lived experience.
2. Encourages a perception that change is always possible and occurring through linking lived experience across the temporal dimension.
3. Encourages multiple perspectives and acts to deconstruct claims of "expert knowledge."
4. Encourages the carnival of possible futures through the reconstruction and reremembering of alternative stories.
5. Invites a reflexive posture and demands that therapists be accountable for their therapeutic stance.
6. Acknowledges that stories are coproduced and endeavors to make the clients the privileged authors of their own experiences.
7. Believes that persons are multistoried.

LEAGUES

During the early 1980s my coauthor (DE) began to circulate his client's knowledges to others who were still trapped within the confines of particular problem lifestyles. He collected his client wisdom in what he called an archive. The archive contained an assortment of audiotapes, letter writings, and artwork that represented a rich supply of solutions to an assortment of long-standing problems such as temper taming, night fears, school refusing, asthma, and, of course, anorexia and bulimia. He came to redefine his clients' knowledge as expert knowledge.

He was able to patch together a network of clients with the purpose of consultation, information, and mutual support. He called these client networks leagues. As the leagues grew, he realized that he had ready access to a wealth of consultants. His clients became his colleagues. The archive is now a vast offertory shared by David around the world.

Leagues are a gathering of persons who have a desire to protest the effects of a particular problem on people's lives. The membership constituency usually involves a majority of clients, mixed with an assortment of therapists, family members, friends, teachers, journalists, and community activists. They are structured in similar ways to many other grassroots political organizations, such as Youth against Violence Committee, or a Doctors for Peace Group. A league's focus is directed toward combating a particular identified problem (e.g., anxiety and depression) and the structures that support the problem.

Leagues allow for the distribution of client knowledge from one client to another. In addition, they often voice strong opposition to those cultural and professional institutions that are problem supporting. A league's mandate acts to undo the knotted dichotomy of difference, distance, and status presently wedged between therapists and clients. Leagues can be seen as another step in stretching the ideas of transparency and reflecting teams into the community.

THE ANTI-ANOREXIA/ANTI-BULIMIA LEAGUE

The Anti-Anorexia/Anti-Bulimia League encourages a different kind of self-directed healing and encourages persons to retrieve, and reflect upon, what lies hidden in the wings of their imaginations. Members of the league realize that their ideas represent the tip of an untapped therapeutic iceberg. To assist the readers of this chapter, David compiled a series of written questions about the league's history and membership involvement. Vancouver league members, Jennifer and Lisa, volunteered to coresearch and present the idea of their Anti-Anorexia/Anti-Bulimia League.

Lisa's Coresearch

DAVID: How did you think professionals regarded the problem of anorexia/bulimia?

LISA: I think that, generally, "professionals" regard the problem of anorexia/bulimia as a part of those afflicted.

DAVID: Who do you think they thought had the problem?

LISA: It was the person, not the "eating disorder," that was the problem!

DAVID: Where was the problem located?

LISA: Before hearing about the league, I was strongly indoctrinated with the belief that anorexia was a deeply rooted and integral part of me, and that without it I would in fact lose parts of my own self.

DAVID: How do you recall first becoming aware of the league in the context of your "treatment"?

LISA: Oh God! When I first heard about the league I was involved in a transition group through a hospital youth clinic. Let's just say that, at that point, having been given a rather biased opinion of the league by the staff, I was not exactly in favor of its principles.

DAVID: Did your impressions change over time?

LISA: Yeah, my impressions have changed and continue to change over time. I think most often my impressions change according to how I feel about myself—when I am feeling strong my impressions of the league's activities in anti-anorexia are very strong and that everything is going to work out. When I am feeling fragile the voice of anorexia says "it sounds good in theory but in practice it is wrong." I think people supporting one another is a great idea, and living by the principles of the Anti-Anorexia League is much easier doing it alongside other people than doing it on your own. Being part of the league, and seeing it begin to get together has been a great help to me and has the potential to help a lot of other people.

DAVID: Did the league offer you anything different from the other forms of "treatment" you had undergone in the past or were undergoing?

LISA: Definitely! The league offers a reality that is not offered in therapy. Most often in therapy you are viewed as the problem—that something has to be fixed, that there is a wrong in your past, that you have to overcome this or that. The league has a different view of the problem—that it is something that has visited upon you, that you don't need it to live. In the past, and especially at the youth clinic groups, I would be asked to "check in with my problem," but there was no action taken or offered to relieve anorexia. The league is different; it says okay, this is the way that it was, and this is what anorexia has taken away from you, and these are the pro-anorexic parts of our society. We don't dwell on the horror stories, we just go from here by taking action against anorexia. I think for me that the only way to get free is by taking action against the problem of anorexia and those things that support its life. I think action is the only way to combat eating disorders and the league does this in a variety of ways.

DAVID: Did you sense that this was somehow different than a conventional, run-of-the-mill support group?

LISA: The difference between the league and your run-of-the-mill support groups and 12-step programs is that in these other groups there tends to be a lot of comparison, and story telling, and it is like these worst of the worst stories keep people there—and keep people feeling hopeless and horrible. The person who lost the most weight is the one to be most pitied and most envied! The support groups often just fed into anorexia by supporting ideas of specialness and perfection. However, the Anti-Anorexia/Anti-Bulimia League is supportive of the nonanorexic, nonbulimic steps the person has taken. This is really important and very different. The League's way of thinking needs more attention by other "professionals" and support groups. Also, the League moves within the realm of political activism and does something about it, not only in ourselves but in the realm of the society—changing society. When our anti-anorexia media campaign really gets off the ground I think there will be potential for an anti-anorexic/anti-bulimic revolution—I really do!

DAVID: When did you feel that you started to have a "voice" in matters of your life and death?

LISA: Recently I have come in contact with my own voice and not the voice of anorexia. For so long I believed that anorexia's voice was just who I was, and anorexia just told me what to do—other people believed this as well and helped anorexia along. Now I am able to stop and say *no* to the anorexia. I feel that I have the power and the real desire to say no—this voice is not who I am, I want to have a life and I am going to!

DAVID: When did you feel you were being attended to and taken seriously?

LISA: I think only when a person begins to take anti-anorexic steps will they begin to be taken seriously. I mean a person in a support group can tell you that they are doing fine, but you can see they are not. It is only when they begin to fight back can they be taken seriously, because all of us who have suffered through anorexia and bulimia are experts at saying one anti-anorexic thing and doing another anorexic thing. When you really begin to take back your voice everything changes.

DAVID: In your experience of human associations is there anything about the league that is unique in your experience?

LISA: I think what is exciting about the league in Vancouver, and that which makes it different to a team or club or a family, is that there are so many aspects of support to the league. There is the community-building aspect of it, there is the goal that we are doing something for the community aspect of it, and there is the not blaming the person aspect of it. What I like most about the league though, is that it has the potential to not only help people break free of anorexia and bulimia, but to be able to change the society little bit, by little bit. The league helps women claim back their voice to say, "No this is not acceptable." The advertising, the standards we are made to live up to in the media, what the media considers "normal" is not acceptable by the league. Our society that supports anorexic activity commits violence against women and their bodies and we in the league will not accept this. When people begin noticing our league banners, newsletters, T-shirts and stickers, there will be change and we will make a difference.

Jennifer's Coresearch

DAVID: How did you think professionals regarded the problem of anorexia/bulimia?

JENNIFER: I believe professionals have viewed anorexia and bulimia as a disease.

DAVID: Where was the problem located?

JENNIFER: I believe that if a professional was to point his or her finger at a spot where anorexia and bulimia is located in me they would point to my brain . . . they would say that the problem is located in the way I think. I, of course, would respond that the problem can not be removed from the context of history, society, and politics.

DAVID: How do you recall first becoming aware of the league in the context of your "treatment"?

JENNIFER: My impression of the league began somewhat negatively.

DAVID: Did your impressions change over time?

JENNIFER: Gradually, I began to look forward to league meetings where I felt I had a voice and I was listened to. I also began to feel an immense relief from "guilt" which I had been carrying around with me. I began to recognize bulimia was not only what the medical model suggested [e.g., distorted body image, relentless drive toward thinness]. I became aware that bulimia and anorexia had convinced me that I could not fight back.

DAVID: Did the league offer you anything different from the other forms of "treatment" you had undergone in the past or were undergoing?

JENNIFER: The league differs from the normative support group in that it calls on the so-called patient to be the *expert.* Family members are taught ways to fight anorexia and bulimia from league members themselves. The individual is empowered and encouraged not to be passive, victim or patient. Furthermore through externalizing the problem the league calls on *all* members to consider their values and to critically examine the society in which they are embedded.

DAVID: What would you say to a person who asked, "Isn't this just another kind of Alcoholics Anonymous?" "Another kind of 12-step recovery movement?"

JENNIFER: An Anti-Anorexia/Anti-Bulimia League is entirely different from a 12-step recovery program. While I want to fully recognize and respect those individuals who have attained a sense of "well-being" via the 12-step program it doesn't fit for me. To me the 12-step process is about "letting go"—giving up control and finding peace. Philosophically different, the Anti-Anorexia/Anti-Bulimia League empowers the individual through externalizing the problem. Anorexia and bulimia are proposed as a separate entity in themselves which the nonpatient, nonvictim is fighting back against. The league's perspective also demands responsibility not only from society, community, and the immediate context, but from the individuals own resources. The league acknowledges and respects the power of the individual. It fights back against the problem.

Leagues utilize an "anti-language" for explaining their philosophy and ideological position (e.g., the Anti-Depression and Anti-Anxiety leagues). In doing so league members act to externalize previously internalized problem discourse. For example, the Anti-Anorexia/Anti-Bulimia League utilizes an anti-language to:

1. Establish a context in which women taken by anorexia/bulimia experience themselves as separate to the problem.
2. View the person's body and relationships to others not as the problem; the problem is the problem (counters the effect of labeling, pathologizing, and totalizing descriptions.)
3. Enable people to work together to defeat the effects of the problem.
4. Consider the cultural practices of objectification used to objectify anorexia/bulimia instead of objectifying the woman as being anorexic/bulimic.
5. Externalize and objectify the problem, which challenges the individualizing techniques of scientific classification and looks at the broader context for a more complete problem description.
6. Achieve externalization by introducing questions that encourage the individuals taken by anorexia/bulimia to map the influence of the problem's devastating effects in their lives and relationships.

7. Externalize by deconstructing the pathologizing "thingification" and objectification of women through challenging accepted social norms.
8. Externalize, thereby allowing for the possibility of multiple descriptions and restorying by bringing forth alternative versions of a persons past, present, and future.

Currently the Vancouver Anti-Anorexia/Anti-Bulimia League works in conjunction with the league in New Zealand in establishing numerous anti-anorexic/anti-bulimic networks of activity, through consultations with clients, families, and therapists residing in Australia, the United States, and Canada. Prior to joining the league, members have usually taken part in a variety of anti-anorexic/anti-bulimic therapeutic activities such as individual, group, and multiple family group therapy from a narrative perspective.

The purpose of the league is to traverse the questionable ideological and fiscal gaps that lay within the traditional treatment terrain of mental health. The league promotes the idea of independence and self-sufficiency. Its playing field is twofold: (1) preventive education through a call for professional and community responsibility and (2) an alternative and unconventional support system for those women caught between hospitals and community psychiatry.

Through regular meetings, league members, families, lovers, and friends often take a direct-action approach to the problems of anorexia and bulimia. For example, through the development of a media watch committee it can act to publicly denounce "pro-anorexic/bulimic" activities against women's bodies through letters written to a wide variety of magazines, newspapers, and company presidents. This enables the league to possibly return the gaze through anti-anorexic/anti-bulimic surveillance directed toward professional, educational, and consumer systems.

The school action committee has developed an anti-anorexic/anti-bulimic program for primary and secondary school students; however, they are finding out that diets and concerns with body specification is now the talk of toddlers as young as four.

League T-shirts have the words "you are more than a body" emblazoned across the back of them with the league name and logo printed on the front. They were a hot selling item throughout this last year.

Radical in its philosophy, the Vancouver Anti-Anorexia/Anti-Bulimia League's mandate is to hold accountable those professional and consumer systems that knowingly render women with "eating disorders" dependent and marginalized. Dependency and marginalization can occur through practices of pathological classification; long-term hospitalization; medication; funding shortages; and messages of hopelessness, dysfunction, and blame.

The league's battle is to win the war being waged on women's bodies on both the professional and the consumer front. Through the process of reclaiming their lives from anorexia and bulimia, league members refuse to accept the popular misconception that they alone are responsible for their so called eating disorders. League members are beginning to make a crucial shift in their identities—from group therapy patients to community activists and consultants. In helping at the level of community they are assisting other women and families and, in turn, are helping themselves.

Given the choice of utilizing a league member or another therapist for an anti-anorexic reflecting team, I (SM) would prefer, whenever possible, to access a league member. Clients are always struck by the members' compassionate and direct reflections. It is now common practice for us to pay ex-clients and league members to act as consultants to therapists in training and as reflecting team members.

Below is an excerpt from a videotape that was made by a league member for the explicit purpose of circulating her ideas in the training of therapists on what they might need to know when working with the problem of anorexia and bulimia.

SM: What do therapists need to know when working with persons taken by anorexia and bulimia?

LORRAINE: There are points in the healing process when the words and actions of a support person/therapist can be very helpful and instrumental in the fight against anorexia and bulimia. Anorexia/bulimia relies on anti-logical tactics to keep a person in its grips. I'll give you a more concrete example: A person has just enjoyed a three-day camping trip with friends and for the duration of the trip she felt relatively free from the abusive and controlling voice of anorexia, but upon returning, she is launched into a drastic campaign against her health and towards anorexia's plots and plans for her destruction. At this point, she is feeling like a failure, like the freedom of the past three days is erased and as if she could never turn this destructive path around. The most critical thing for a supporter/therapist to do, at this point, is to hear the panic as a reaction to the vicious messages that anorexia/bulimia is relaying and identify them as such. Once anorexia is heard out and the panic is shared and validated—because it is scary and lonely when one is feeling swallowed by anorexia—then the conversation can turn to how it was that she made a three-day escape and how she might do it again. The most dangerous and unhelpful thing that can occur is that the panic is ignored and unheard because this can fuel anorexia to prove just how ferocious it can be, thus driving a person further into its grips.

SM: When might a therapist be considered pro-anorexic?

LORRAINE: There are many times, but I will give you just two examples that therapists and hospitals might consider. Something that can be very unhelpful in a relationship between client and therapist is the perpetuation and maintenance of a power differential. Traditionally, there has been the assumption and acceptance of a power differential between therapist and client, but if the intent of a therapist is to be helpful and supportive then it is to both parties' benefit if the fight against anorexia is waged on equal ground. Because doctors and patients have often been segregated by the gap in power, perspective, and background, it is challenging to enter into this unfamiliar territory of equality—even more frightening still to recognize that perhaps the real expert is he/she who has lived the experience rather than he/she who has spectated. Anorexia/bulimia acts as a power over a person, and if the therapist takes on this power-over position even the best intentions to help may act in collusion with anorexia instead of against it.

I am wary of the current practice of weight and body-fat focus that is occurring through weekly weigh-ins and skinfolds in many recovery programs. In my experience, this type of surveillance acts as a double-edged sword, and the negative effects seem to far outweigh the positive ones. If anything, the focus on weight and skinfolds acts as a medium through which the ideas of perfection, comparison, and not measuring up are reinforced and fueled.

SM: When might a therapist be considered anti-anorexic?

LORRAINE: Something that is helpful is to focus on moments of freedom from anorexia/bulimia and to celebrate health and wellness. A very dangerous message to be relaying to people suffering the effects of anorexia/bulimia is the idea that he/she is not sick enough for help—this too can drive anorexia to prove itself. It is important to recognize anorexia and bulimia as operating on a continuum that begins with body surveillance and weight preoccupation.

Because anorexia/bulimia relies on convincing its victims that they are powerless, that the future is hopeless, that they are unworthy of a compassionate relationship with themselves and others, a great amount of work needs to be done to recognize and to counter these lies that anorexia and bulimia tell and to create new versions of possibility. At the times when anorexia/bulimia is challenged by an anti-anorexic/anti-bulimic action or thought, there is a strong tendency for anorexia/bulimia to wage an assault on the person in order to try and convince them against attempting any future moments of freedom and enjoyment. This is a sort of anti-logic that occurs on the path to freedom, and it is something that I feel helping professionals and other support persons need to be aware of so that they can help in the fight.

Focusing on issues of power, voice, individuality, and uniqueness have been very helpful for me in my battle against anorexia/bulimia and I believe that these issues are common to the struggle of many persons living in our Western culture.

The element of the sociocultural manufacturing and perpetuation of anorexia/bulimia is a piece that is often ignored in therapy and research on anorexia/bulimia. Taking the focus off of the person/self as the problem and returning the gaze back to the place where the problem originates has been incredibly empowering and relieving for me. Once the blame is relieved, there is so much energy available to use in the construction of a new storyline for one's life. Anorexia/bulimia predicts a mundane story with an ending in death and disappointment. I, as the author of my story, have the freedom to create one of endless possibilities, full of interesting characters and exciting conclusions. A therapist can assist in the authoring of either of these stories with a client—clearly the latter is desirable, yet it presents a large challenge, both to the client and the therapist. The client must take back his/her power and the therapist must relinquish some of their power. In my experience it has been the most helpful thing that a therapist/helping professional/supporter can do.

SM: Would you like to say a few words about the League?

LORRAINE: Definitely! The League is a wonderful thing because it takes these ideas and puts them into practice. Because this has never been done before, it has been a constantly evolving concept and group. Presently, the focus of the group is to bring together people suffering the effects of anorexia/bulimia, their families, friends, and all other supporters and to implement the power of collectivity against anorexia and bulimia. The focus of our work is on addressing the perpetuating elements in our culture by offering conversation, education, and action.

Another aim of the League is to experience the benefits of health, power, and voice and to combat the glamorization of anorexia/bulimia. A medium like the League's publication, "The Undead," which is free from the constraints of advertising regulations, et cetera, offers a chance for voices that are often unheard to be heard and will work to promote these ideas and spread them further.

Is it any wonder that upon viewing the league's "What every therapist needs to know about anorexia and bulimia, but were afraid to ask" videos, the room thunders with applause, interest, and tears? I (SM) asked psychiatrist Dr. Elliot Goldner, director of St. Paul's Hospital eating disorder program in Vancouver, to offer his reflections after reading excerpts of the league's ongoing coresearch project. Dr. Goldner writes:

> *The writings of Lisa, Jennifer, and Lorraine underscore a potent fact—people struggling against anorexia and bulimia possess a wisdom and expertise that must not be marginalized. Their research is pulled from the pores of experience and has not been limited to eight hours a day, academic blinders, and political or financial motivations. To ignore their insight would be folly. Yet, psychiatry and therapy practices have too often disregarded such careful and painstaking research, and have preferred promises of quick fixes, and electrifying solutions from technology and scientism.*
>
> *When I listen, instead, to the words of Lisa, Jennifer, and Lorraine, these are some of the things I hear:*
>
> 1. *Collaboration is helpful in fighting anorexia and bulimia; leagues such as the Anti-Anorexia/Anti-Bulimia League can offer such collaboration.*
> 2. *Anti-anorexic/bulimic actions help to combat eating disorders for individuals and societies; in contrast, nonaction (which characterizes some "therapy" or "support efforts") is not helpful.*
> 3. *Empowerment of those persons fighting anorexia and bulimia is helpful in combating eating disorders; such empowerment is supported by respect and by separation of the person and the problem.*
> 4. *Anorexia and bulimia can hold a person with the vice grip of an abusive partner; secrecy and shame can form the glue that adheres these problems.*
> 5. *Others (including those in "helping professions") may worsen the problem; this often occurs when people confer certain knowledges about a person and constrain that person's identity and selfhood.*

When presenting the league ideas in a public forum, we are continually reminded of their social impact on therapeutic possibilities. It is from within the wisdom of these coresearch projects that therapists can be moved (shoved) toward a reflexive accountability. We would argue that the weight of therapeutic accountability should privilege and be mediated through the knowledges of the once marginalized; not through a professionalized discourse.

Letter-Writing Campaigns

Letter-writing campaigns assist in the re-remembering of unique aspects of a client's life, now restrained by problem saturation. The campaigns are likened to a eulogy or an obituary made on behalf of the client while the client is still living. Members of the family and friends are asked to assist in a re-remembering process through written accounts that outline their memories of their relationship with the client separate from the problem's relationship with the client. The letters, by documenting alternative versions, counteract the infirming effects of the problem story. These accounts hold a tremendous potential for the restorying of persons' lives.

Nigel's Story

The psychiatry department of a local teaching hospital asked if I (SM) would "see" Nigel, a 60-year-old man. Nigel was described as "very suicidal and depressed," and as a consequence had undergone over 40 electro-convulsive therapy "treatments" over the previous year. I was informed that Nigel was at great risk of taking his own life, was unresponsive to "talk" therapy, and they had done everything they could for him.

Nigel and his wife Rose had eight visits with me over the course of four months (on three of those meetings we were joined by a reflecting team). I learned from Nigel that he was having great difficulty remembering much of his life. The problem, which he referred to as "depression," had taken over his daily life from waking to retiring at night. Rose was of the opinion that the effects of the ECT had eroded Nigel's capacity for believing that he had accomplished anything in his lifetime. However, she was quick to inform me that Nigel was well respected by his five children and his community, which was located 300 miles north of Vancouver.

My thinking here was to reinvolve Nigel with the relationship context of his community from which "depression" and "suicidal thoughts" had separated him. It was out of this concern that Nigel, Rose, and I reached an agreement that "depression was a strong foe" and that we needed to recruit an "anti-depression team." We collaborated on writing a letter to possible recruits, which Rose said she would be only too happy to distribute.

Dear friends of Nigel and Rose:

My name is Stephen Madigan and I am a Family Therapist working alongside Nigel and Rose. Nigel, as you may be aware of, has unfortunately been taken over by depression, so much so that the depression has tried to convince Nigel to take his own life on several occasions. The depression tells Nigel that he is "a worthless person," that he "never accomplished anything of value," and that "no one ever liked him." The depression is trying hard to make Nigel blind and deaf to all of his qualities, and wants him to turn away from all of the people who love and care about him. We are writing to ask you to draft a letter in support of Nigel and against the depression's version of him. Thank you for your help in this matter.

Yours in anti-depression,
Nigel, Rose, and Stephen

Within two weeks, Nigel was inundated with mail. One of the hospital staff on Nigel's ward said she thought he might have to get his own special mail delivery person. More than 100 letters and cards poured in. At first, Nigel modestly tucked the anti-depression notes away in his hospital night table, but before long, he felt able to put them on display all around his room. He then began to give "anti-depression" consultations to interested staff and patients on the ward, by reading them his letters and lecturing on ideas of anti-depression.

Nigel is now free of depression and has on occasion offered consultation to therapists training with us in narrative ideas on "how I went free of depression."

Oscar's Story

A colleague referred 70-year-old Oscar and his wife, Maxine, to me (SM). Oscar informed me that he had been struck down by a truck a year before. He was not supposed to live, but he did; he was not supposed to come out of his three-month-long coma, but he did; it was predicted that he would never walk again, but he did, and so on. It didn't take me long to realize I was sitting before quite a remarkable man. However, it seemed that Oscar had paid dearly for his comeback, for now he had lost all confidence in himself and would panic if Maxine was not in attendance "24 hours a day." Maxine had spent the year before organizing the complicated task of Oscar's medical care and was at this time looking forward to getting back to her own business pursuits. Unfortunately, her interests were being pushed aside and taken over by the anxiety.

The anxiety that had been the legacy of Oscar's accident had him believing that "I am only half a man," and furthermore "Maxine will leave me for another man . . . she is planning to put me in an old-age home." And there was an odd twist in that it had him also believe "I did not deserve a good life" and furthermore "I should kill myself." The anxiety was making him forget the life that he had lived prior to the accident and, like Nigel, he was becoming more and more isolated and depressed.

Oscar and Maxine had moved from England to Canada 10 years earlier. We all agreed that the anxiety was gaining on Oscar and that the situation was desperate. With this in mind we agreed to design an international anti-anxiety letter-writing campaign. Below is the letter we coauthored in five minutes near the end of the third session. As Oscar was concerned that his friends might consider the letter "a crazy idea," he insisted that I include my credentials to give it credence.

Dear Friends of Oscar:

My name is Stephen Madigan and I have a PhD in family therapy. Your friends Oscar and Maxine have asked me to write to you so that we might solicit your support. As you are probably aware Oscar suffered a terrible accident 14 months ago, and has instituted a remarkable comeback. What you may not know is that the after-effects of the accident have left Oscar a captive of anxiety, and that it is currently bossing him around. We think you can help Oscar win back his life from this terrible anxiety. You may not believe this but one of the messages anxiety gives to Oscar is that "he is a good for nothing," that "he is a useless human being," and that "sooner rather than later all of his friends will come to know Oscar the way anxiety knows him." Through anxiety's influence, Oscar is beginning to give up on himself, and we ask your support in bringing Oscar back from anxiety's grip. We hope that your letters of support are not too much to ask, and we want you to know that they will be greatly appreciated. Oscar would like you all to know that he will respond to all of your replies.

Warm regards,
Stephen Madigan, PhD,
Oscar's anti-anxiety consultant

During the weeks that followed, Oscar would bring the campaign letters to my (SM) office, requesting that I read them out loud to him. I happily did so and my recitations were accompanied by Oscar's crying, laughing, and telling me "of his good fortune." You see, Oscar had affected the lives of many, many people and, not surprisingly, they welcomed the opportunity to reciprocate by writing to him. His anti-anxiety support team wrote from around the globe—Europe, the United Kingdom, and North America.

Oscar recently wrote to me (SM) from his long-awaited anti-anxiety trip to France with Maxine, which would mark "my arrival at health." He told me that he was sitting alone, drinking espresso, while Maxine had gone shopping for the day. He wrote, "I am thanking my lucky stars that I am no longer a prisoner of anxiety." His only problem now was keeping up with all of his return correspondence, but this was a problem for which he was willing to take full responsibility.

Without the recruitment of their community of concern, Nigel and Oscar might never have rebounded to re-remember all their personal qualities and the contributions they had made during their lifetimes, which their problems were "insisting" they overlook and dis-remember.

Letter-writing campaigns are viewed as attempts to counter this dis-information and to inform both the client/family and their community of "stories" of the person that are at odds with the problem-saturated story. Campaigns are viewed not only as ceremonies of redefinition (White, 1995) but as protest and counterstruggles that undermine a problem-context-dominant story.

In the circumstances involving Nigel's life, there was a dominant professional story to overthrow, which inadvertently supported the "life" of depression. Upon returning to his home community, the psychiatrist responsible for all of the ECT treatments contacted Nigel to resume treatment. Shortly thereafter, Nigel called to tell me (SM) "that I have just given my psychiatrist his walking papers." A short letter followed announcing he was depression-free.

REFERENCES

Andersen, T. (1987). The reflecting team: Dialogue and meta-dialogue in clinical work. *Family Process, 26*(4), 415–428.

Bakhtin, M. M. (1986). *Speech genres and other late essays* (V. McGee, Trans.). Austin: University of Texas Press.

Elliott, H. (1994). *Decentering the subject.* Paper presented at the 2nd annual Narrative Ideas and Therapeutic Practice Conference, Vancouver, British Columbia.

Epston, D., & White, M. (1990, Winter). Consulting your consultants: The documentation of alternative knowledges. *Dulwich Centre Newsletter,* p. 4.

Foucault, M. (1979). *Discipline and punish: The birth of the prison.* Middlesex, England: Peregrine Books.

Foucault, M. (1980). *Power/knowledge: Selected interviews and other writings.* New York: Pantheon.

Foucault, M. (1982). The subject and power. In H. Dreyfus & P. Rabinow (Eds.), *Michel Foucault: Beyond.* Chicago: University of Chicago Press.

Foucault, M. (1984). *The history of sexuality.* New York: Pantheon.

Law, I., & S. Madigan. (1994, Winter). Power and politics in practice. *Dulwich Centre Newsletter,* pp. 3–7.

Lax, W. (1991). The reflecting team and initial consultation. In T. Andersen (Ed.),

The reflecting team: Dialogues and dialogues about the dialogues. (pp. 127–142). New York: Norton.

Madigan, S. (1991a). *Voices of demystification: Questions as performative texts in therapeutic discourse and practice; a post-structural analysis.* Unpublished dissertation.

Madigan, S. (1991b, Fall). Discursive restraints in therapist practice [Special issue]. *Dulwich Centre Newsletter.*

Madigan, S. (1992a). Questions about questions: Situating the therapist's curiosity in front of the family. In S. Gilligan & P. Reese (Eds.), *Therapeutic conversations.* New York: Norton.

Madigan, S. (1992b). The application of Michel Foucault's philosophy in the problem externalizing discourse of Michael White. *Journal of Family Therapy, 14*(3), 265–279.

Madigan, S. (in press). Undermining the problem in the privatization of problems in persons: Considering the socio-political and cultural context in the externalizing of internalized problem conversations. *Journal of Systemic Therapies.*

Myerhoff, B. (1982). Life history among the elderly; performance, visibility and remembering. In J. Ruby (Ed.), *A crack in the mirror: Reflexive perspectives in anthropology.* Philadelphia: University of Pennsylvania Press.

Roth, S., & Epston, D. (in press). Developing externalizing conversations: An introductory exercise. *Journal of Systemic Therapies.*

Sampson, E. (1989). The deconstruction of the self. In J. Shotter & K. Gergen, (Eds.), *Texts of identity* (pp. 3–11). Newbury Park, CA: Sage.

Shotter, J., & Gergen, K. (1989). *Texts of identity.* Newbury Park, CA: Sage.

Shotter, J. (1990). The social construction of remembering and forgetting. In D. Middleton & D. Edwards (Eds.), *Collective remembering.* London: Sage.

Waldegrave, C. (1990, Winter). Just therapy. *Dulwich Centre Newsletter,* pp. 6–46.

White, M. (1995). *Re-authoring lives: Interviews and essays.* Adelaide: Dulwich.

White, M., & Epston, D. (1990). *Narrative means to therapeutic ends.* New York: Norton.

Yeatman, A. (1994). *Postmodern revisionings of the political.* New York: Routledge.

Young, J. (1989, Summer). A critical look at the one way screen. *Dulwich Centre Newsletter,* pp. 5–11.

CHAPTER 13

Consulting Your Consultants

A MEANS TO THE CO-CONSTRUCTION OF ALTERNATIVE KNOWLEDGES

David Epston
Michael White
"Ben"

TRADITIONAL MODELS and metaphors for psychotherapy suffer from many limitations. One of these is the emphasis on "termination as loss," the position that the discontinuation of therapy inevitably is experienced as the painful relinquishment of a therapeutic relationship on which the "patient has become dependent." While we acknowledge that the transition from "patienthood" to full-fledged "personhood" is indeed an important one, we believe that the preoccupation of therapists with the loss metaphor subtly reinforces the dependency of the person seeking assistance on the "expert knowledge" of the therapist. More important, we believe that this dominant metaphor fails to legitimize the person's own role in freeing him/herself from the problem-saturated identity that brought the person to therapy in the first place. In contrast to the practices informed by the termination-as-loss metaphor, we will outline a model of the final stage of therapy as a "rite of passage" from one identity status to another. Importantly, this passage centers around a joining of the person with others in a familiar social world and encourages the recruitment of others in the celebration and acknowledgment of the person's arrival at a preferred destination or status in life. We refer to those therapies that are informed by these practices as therapies of inclusion.[1]

[1] In *Confession: Studies in Deviance in Religion*, Turner and Hepworth (1982) distinguish between two major classes of ritual: those that *include* persons in social groups and those that *exclude* persons from them.

In this chapter we describe a therapeutic practice that encourages persons to document the ways in which they have resisted and surmounted the "dominant stories" of their lives, stories organized around their problems, symptoms, and socially ascribed "pathologies" (White & Epston, 1990). In describing our therapeutic practices, we have found it helpful to view the concept of knowledge as a plural noun and to formulate questioning strategies that elicit from the persons we work with the "solution knowledges" and the "alternative knowledges" about their lives and relationships that have been resurrected and/or generated in therapy. These knowledges then become more available for persons to redeploy when necessary and for others to consult as aids to their own self-development.

We begin by reviewing some of the limitations of the dominant termination-as-loss metaphor and then suggest an alternative rite-of-passage analogy that provides an organizing conceptual frame for our own work. Placing this transition in the broader systemic context of the person's world, we then outline a protocol for establishing persons as consultants to themselves and to others. In doing so, we present, via a clinical interview, an array of questions that assist persons to engage in an archaeology of their alternative knowledges in a way that makes them more available for future use.

THE TERMINATION-AS-LOSS METAPHOR

Of all aspects of the transformative process called therapy, the concluding stage has been among the most inadequately understood. We believe that this has to do with the fact that the termination-as-loss metaphor has dominated the literature on this stage of therapy, blinding therapists to more fruitful ways of viewing and facilitating the termination process.

The dominance of the termination-as-loss metaphor is premised on a particular orientation to therapy. This is an orientation that privileges the therapeutic microworld above all others.[2] It represents the final stage of therapy as one that is dominated by the loss of this microworld and its central and supposedly all-important relationship, and by the requirement for an adjustment to "going it on your own."

[2]In challenging this privileging of the the therapeutic microworld we are not proposing that all aspects of therapy be undertaken in some public domain. We believe that persons should have access to a private place in which they can feel safe and secure and have their desire for confidentiality honored. However, we consider it inappropriate to place this world above all other worlds, and we believe that all knowledges that arise in therapy that are preferred knowledges for persons should have space made available for their circulation to larger communities. We prefer to construe the concluding stages of therapy as being about new beginnings.

We believe that this orientation to therapy—one that constructs an entirely separate and private stage for persons' lives—is in turn premised on certain cultural conceptions and practices. These include the dominant individualizing conception of personhood in Western culture, the idea that the person is the source of all meaning, and the modern practices of the objectification of persons and their bodies which are common to the "disciplines" (Foucault, 1973). Commenting on this individualizing conception of personhood, Geertz (1976) observed that "the Western conception of the person as a bounded, unique cognitive universe, a dynamic center of awareness, emotion, judgment and action organized into a distinctive whole is, however incorrigible it may seem to us, a rather peculiar idea within the concept of the world's cultures" (p. 225). Because they separate the self from social context, we refer to those therapies that are informed by these cultural conceptions and practices as therapies of isolation. Within this highly individualized conception, it follows that the termination of the therapeutic relationship deepens the person's sense of isolation and in so doing accentuates his/her sense of loss.

AN ALTERNATIVE METAPHOR: TERMINATION AS "RITE OF PASSAGE"

We believe that the class of rituals referred to by van Gennep (1960) as rites of passage has a great deal to offer as a metaphor for the process of therapy. Essentially, van Gennep asserted that the rite of passage is a universal phenomenon for facilitating transitions in social life from one status and/or identity to another. He proposed a processual model of this rite, consisting of the stages of *separation, liminality,* and *reincorporation.* In traditional cultures, the initiation of each of these stages is marked by ceremony.

At the *separation* stage persons are detached from familiar roles, statuses, and locations and enter an unfamiliar social world in which most of the taken-for-granted ways of going about life are suspended—a *liminal* space, This liminal space, which constitutes the second stage of a rite of passage, is "betwixt and between" known worlds and is characterized by experiences of disorganization and confusion, by a spirit of exploration, and by a heightened sense of possibility. The third stage of *reincorporation* brings closure to the ritual passage and assists persons to relocate themselves in the social order of their familiar world, but at a different position. This different position is characteristically accompanied by new roles, responsibilities, and freedoms. Traditionally, the arrival at this point is augmented by claims and declarations that the person has successfully negotiated a transition, and this is then legitimated by communal acknowledgment.

Rite of Passage and Therapy

We have found that this rite-of-passage metaphor provides a useful map for orienting therapists to the process of therapy and for assisting those persons who seek therapy in transiting from problematic statuses to unproblematic ones (Epston, 1985, 1987).

Our interpretation of this metaphor structures a therapy that encourages persons to negotiate the passage from novice to veteran, from client to consultant. Rather than instituting a dependency on the "expert knowledge" presented by the therapist and other authorities, this therapy enables persons to arrive at a point where they can take recourse to liberating alternative and "special" knowledges that they have resurrected and/or generated during the therapy.

In therapy, the "separation" stage can be invoked through a range of interventions, including those that encourage persons to distinguish themselves from their problems by engaging in *externalizing discourses* in relation to these problems (White & Epston, 1990). That is, therapy enables them to see their problem (e.g., depression, bedwetting, or, anorexia) as something outside themselves that can be resisted, rather than as essential features of themselves. This dislodges persons from certain familiar and taken-for-granted notions about problems and from the dominant internalizing (and self-blaming) discourses that guide their lives. This initiates the experience of liminality.

It is in this liminal space that new possibilities emerge and that alternative knowledges can be resurrected and/or generated. It is in this liminal space that person's experiential worlds is "subjunctivized," that is, treated as hypothetical and malleable rather than as real and fixed. Thus, Turner (1986) speaks of "the liminal phase being dominantly in the subjunctive mood of culture, the mood of maybe, might be, as if, hypothesis, fantasy, conjecture, desire—depending on which of the trinity of cognition, affect, and conation is situationally dominant" (p. 42). It is the "as if" nature of the therapeutic reconceptualization of their problems that enables people to begin to envision an alternative self-identity or alternative life story.

Therapists can best gauge the extent of their participation in the stage by the degree to which they lose track of time and are unable to estimate the length of the session, and by the degree to which they experience a sense of "communitas" with the persons who seek therapy. Individual, family, and group therapists and clients operating in this way resemble the traditional liminal groups described by Turner (1967), who operate as "a community of comrades and not a structure of hierarchically arrayed positions. This comradeship transcends distinctions of rank, age, kinship position, and in some kinds of cultic group, even of sex" (p. 100).

The final stage of reincorporation brings the therapy to its conclusion. It is through reincorporation that the alternative knowledges that have been resurrected and/or generated in therapy become authenticated in the presence of others. It is through reincorporation into the larger family and community system that the possibilities for a renewed identity can be realized.

OVERCOMING OBSTACLES TO REINCORPORATION

However, despite the possibilities that accompany the reincorporation metaphor, there are some obstacles to therapeutic practice that are suggested by it. For example, Kobak and Waters (1984), who also referred to the rite-of-passage metaphor, draw attention to the practical difficulties in linking the microworld of therapy to the world at large:

> In relation to his [*sic*] more "primitive" [*sic*] tribal counterpart, who manages a publicly recognized rite of passage, the family therapist is at a relative disadvantage in creating long-lasting, second-order change. The most apparent disadvantage is that the family therapist does not have the ties to the family's community and community norms that reinforce the changes that occur during the rite of passage once the participants return to ordinary life. . . . Such participation of the community in the change process serves to stabilize second-order changes that occur during the liminal rites. By operating without knowledge of community norms, the family therapist may create liminal change that is not sustained in the reaggregation phase. (p. 99)[3]

A developmental view of family problems may assist the therapist, yet the relative isolation of the therapist from the family's community remains a problem. Potential solutions to this dilemma have emerged in the form of involving the family "network" or, less extensively, by activating the family kin system. The rite-of-passage analogy suggests that such efforts should be further explored.

For a number of years, we have been experimenting, in various ways,

[3]In the translation of van Gennep's (1960) text, we prefer the term "reincorporation" over the term "reaggregation."

to overcome the sort of obstacles referred to above. The feedback that we have received in response to this experimentation has convinced us of (1) the pertinence of the rite-of-passage metaphor and the appropriateness of considering the concluding stage of therapy as reincorporation and (2) the inappropriateness of a strong emphasis on the termination-as-loss metaphor for this stage of therapy.

Because it has been our preference to construe the concluding stage of therapy as reincorporation, this has given us cause for celebration with the persons who have sought therapy rather than commiseration. We have been able to challenge the conception of therapy as an exclusive and esoteric social space or individual stage, necessarily bound by rigid rules of privacy and exclusion.

We have assisted persons to explore various ways and means by which to counter the practices informed by this conception—to protest the limitations of this privacy. We have participated with them in the publicizing and circulation of the alternative and preferred knowledges that have been resurrected and/or generated in therapy. We have joined with them in their attempts to identify and recruit audiences to the performance of these alternative knowledges in their day-to-day lives. And we have worked with persons in their efforts to document these knowledges in popular discourses and forms.

On reviewing our exploration of practices of reincorporation, we have classified various approaches that persons have found helpful. All these approaches include the identification and recruitment of audiences for the authentication and the legitimation of alternative knowledges. The ritual approaches include (1) celebrations, prize givings, and awards, attended by significant persons, including those who may not have attended therapy (White, 1986); (2) purposeful "news releases" whereby pertinent information as to the person's arrival at a new status is made available to various significant persons and agencies; (3) personal declarations and letters of reference; and (4) consultation with persons, in a formal sense, in relation to the solution knowledges that have enabled them to free their lives and in relation to the alternative and preferred knowledges about their lives and relationships.

We addressed the first three approaches mentioned here in *Narrative Means to Therapeutic Ends* (White & Epston, 1990). In this chapter we restrict our discussion to the fourth of these approaches, presenting a protocol for what we refer to as consulting your consultants.

CONSULTING YOUR CONSULTANTS

When persons are established as consultants to themselves, to others, and to the therapist, they experience themselves as more of an authority on their own lives, their problems, and the solution to these problems. This authority takes the form of a kind of knowledge and expertise which is recorded in a popular medium so that it is accessible to the consultant, therapist, and potential others.

Throughout, the relative inequality of "therapist as helper" and "client as helped" is redressed. the gift of therapy is balanced by the gift of consultancy. We consider this reciprocity to be of vital importance in reducing the risk of indebtedness and replacing it by a sense of fair exchange. In *The Gift,* Mauss (1954) eloquently draws attention to the hazards inherent in such inequality, noting that "to accept without returning or repaying more is to face subordination, to become a client and subservient. To receive something is dangerous not only because it is illicit to do so, but also because it comes morally, physically, and spiritually from a person" (p. 22). Thus, we view the rite of passage at the point of "graduation" from therapy as a time of "giving something back" to the therapist, the therapeutic community, and perhaps to future persons seeking assistance with similar problems.

Protocol for the Documentation of Alternative Knowledges

We conclude therapy with an invitation to persons to attend a special meeting with the therapist so that the knowledges that have been resurrected and/or generated in therapy can be documented. These knowledges will include those alternative and preferred knowledges about self, others and relationships and those knowledges of problem solving that have enabled persons to liberate their lives. They consist of the person or family's own constructions of their strengths, resources, and helpful patterns of relating that permitted them to transcend or resist the destructive influence of their "problem" and begin to write a new and more hopeful chapter in their life narrative.

In anticipation of the termination interview or interviews, persons are told that special attention will be given to an exploration of how they arrived at these useful knowledges and of how they "made these knowledges work" for them. This forewarning gives persons notice that they will be invited to provide some historical account of the struggle with their problems and of the discoveries that made it possible for them to free their lives. Such notice emphasizes that these knowledges are significant and that preservation of them through documentation is warranted.

Various means can be used for the purpose of substantiating and documenting these knowledges. Persons can choose from a variety of formats, including videotaping, audiotaping, autobiographical accounts, diaries, interview transcripts, and so on. If persons are concerned that they might have difficulty recalling relevant details, a sample of orienting questions can be supplied for them to reflect on. This sample usually assists persons in preparing for the consulting-your-consultants interview.

Upon convening the meeting, the therapist runs through a prologue that further orients persons to its purpose. During this prologue, future audiences (e.g., other therapists and persons with similar histories or problems) are presupposed and explicitly referred to. The therapist then asks persons to give an account of their transition from a problematic status to a resolved one and asks questions that encourage them to locate the significant events and steps in time in a sequential fashion. Alternatively, the therapist can provide his/her account of this transition and invite persons to comment on it, elaborate on it, make alterations to it, and contribute their reflections in ways that dramatically bring this account to life.

In the following text, we present a small sample of the sort of questions that have been helpful in encouraging persons to articulate these knowledges. Readers will note that these questions are constructed in a "grammar of agency" rather than one of passivity and determinism. In responding to these questions, persons achieve a sense of personal agency. This is the experience of being able to play an active role in shaping one's own life, of possessing the capacity to influence developments in one's life to the extent of bringing about preferred outcomes.

Encouraging persons to respond to questions in a grammar of agency—or, as Douglas (1982) might put it, in the "active voice"—effectively counters their tendency of solely imputing the therapist's actions as critical to the emergence of solutions, and is essential to the constitution of self-knowledge. As Harré (1983) observes, "self-knowledge requires the identification of agentive and knowing selves as acting within hierarchies of reasons. It follows that this kind of self-knowledge is, or at least makes available the possibility of, autobiography" (p. 26).

OWNERSHIP AND USAGE OF DOCUMENTS

We acknowledge that therapeutic productions are cocreated but consider the persons who seek therapy to be the senior partners in the ownership of this property. Thus, such persons have power of veto in relation to the use of any documents (including videotape) produced by their consultancy.

Persons are informed that these documents, which we refer to as *archives,* are considered to be on loan to the therapist for specific purposes and for specific periods of time, and that this loan can be retracted at any time. Despite this, many persons wish to deed these archives to the therapist to use at his/her discretion.

The therapist may suggest that persons consult the knowledges expressed in their own documents at certain points in time or request that these documents be made available, with discretion, to others who are experiencing problems or for teaching purposes, with an understanding that the responses of others will be recorded and made available.

The recording of the responses of participants in teaching contexts (e.g., seminars, training programs, and workshops) with the explicit goal of providing feedback to those persons whose documents are being presented, encourages participants in these training settings to more fully appreciate and respect the nature of their privileged position. This is a position in which participants are privy to the lives and relationships of those persons who have been willing to contribute to the development of "therapeutic knowledge." This recording of responses engages participants more fully in an understanding of the experiences of persons and mitigates against those responses that are the outcome of a position of detachment that is so easily arrived at by participants in teaching contexts.

Persons are almost invariably enthusiastic about receiving feedback from others in relation to their therapeutic productions. At times this feedback provokes ongoing and productive correspondences between these persons and others who are experiencing similar problems, or between these and workshop participants when these participants have appended an address to their comments.

DAVID CONSULTS BEN

The following is a typical consulting-your-consultants interview, although it is my (DE) second meeting with "Ben" and his parents, "Maggie" and "Jim." The first interview was an emergency consultation at a psychiatric hospital in the United States. The consultation was attended by Ben, his parents, the attending doctor, and all eight hospital staff who were involved with Ben while he was an inpatient. This meeting, scheduled at the request of Ben, occurred approximately two months later and took place at a family institute near his home. The reader should be aware that in the interval Ben remained in the care of the hospital staff.

This consulting your consultants is located (see Figure 13.1) in what is being referred to here as a genealogy of this "knowledge." It demonstrates the extent to which persons such as Ben, myself (DE), and his parents have recourse to this knowledge and contribute to it. For example, the videotape of this meeting was returned to both Tim and Al for their opinions as to Ben's candidacy for the award of the Diploma of "Impurfection" and then eight months later was forwarded to Ron and his family prior to our first meeting together. This "knowledge" is

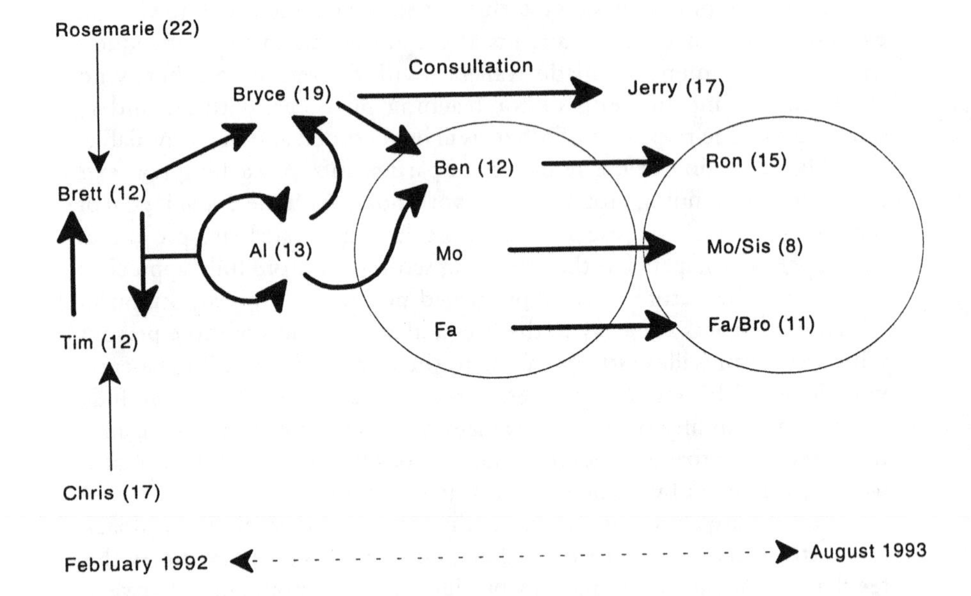

FIGURE 13.1. A community of connections. A heavy arrow indicates the exchangeof archival material; a fine arrow indicates that the therapist has read from letters or offered reminiscences from the therapy.

mediated through the therapist–archivist and passes backwards and forwards between members of the League. A league is what I refer to as a "community of concern," which may best be conceptualized as more virtual than real. Such communities form around shared concerns and the "knowledges" that emerge from them. The league discussed here has named itself the Anti-Habit League. The "problem" itself provides persons and their families with the right to membership in the League and the associated privileges. However, before availing ourselves of these privileges through the therapist–archivist, the conditions of consent and what Fran Morris (Epston, Morris, & Maisel, 1995) has referred to as respectful confidentiality is discussed at length. With the informed consent of the members, letters (Epston, 1994; White & Epston, 1990), videotapes, audiotapes, stories, and so on. become the shared property of the League itself. The therapist–archivist can be granted discretion to excerpt letters, exchange videos, and so forth, although each member may wish to have specific conditions attached to this use (e.g., to be known by their first name only or to be contacted ahead of time and to have their permission sought on each occasion of a "loan"). I have found people to be very generous indeed and much of what I have referred to as therapist discretion has to do with protecting members. My main concern would be the possibility of new members in distress putting undue demands on their sources. For this reason, all contacts are mediated through the therapist–archivist. At times of great risk or despair, I have arranged for face-to-face consultations. One example (see Figure 13.1) involved Bryce and Jerry. Bryce (age 19), a first-year university student, had tried to comply with the demand of the "curse of the idea of perfection" for his failure to achieve perfection in everything he did, especially combing his hair which could occupy up to four hours of his day. He "consulted" to Jerry (age 17), who had recently graduated from high school but failed to have a straight A+ average (thanks to one A–). Jerry had tried to take his life and his parents, justifiably, were desperately concerned about his welfare. We met prior to this consultation in order to cooperate around constructing appropriate questions for Bryce. We also agreed that I would intervene on Bryce's behalf should any further discussion seem to be intrusive. On this occasion, Bryce waived all my concerns in this regard. This was the only time Anti-Habit League members had ever met on purpose, although such meetings would certainly be worth considering. It is my practice in face-to-face consultations to split my fee 50/50 with my consultants. The consulting persons have to agree to this arrangement. If such "knowledges" are to be valued, they must be paid for.

In Figure 13.1, the "genealogy" of this league is charted through time (February 1992–August 1993) and from person to person and family to family. The heavy arrow indicates the exchange of archival material (e.g., letters, videotapes, audiotapes, stories, drawings, and slogans) whereas the fine lines indicate the therapist either excerpting and reading from letters or other reminiscences from the therapy (e.g., "The problem Bryce was experiencing was calling him names like. . . . Did your problem do anything similar or did it come up with some new insults?"). By detailed inquiry, cross-referencing of "knowledges," and so on, it does not take long to be knowledgeable yourself, nor does it take much contact with a problem through the people you meet before you get to know it reasonably well.

Ben's Thoughts and Recollections (December 1994)

"In October of 1992, I was diagnosed with OCD [obsessive–compulsive disorder]. I had been having symptoms for as long as I can remember but they were getting a lot worse. Depression also made things hard. Some of my symptoms were touching or doing things a certain number of times, counting, and repeating certain phrases. In general, I felt I needed to do things until it felt 'perfect.' I also had negative obsessions about my sister and felt compelled to behave aggressively toward her, which made it hard to live under the same roof. In February 1993 things got so bad that I had to be hospitalized at a psychiatric hospital. At the hospital things got worse. While doctors were experimenting with possible medicine combinations for me, I was suffering more, and spending a lot of time in the quiet room. Around mid-March two very important things happened. The first one was that the medicine was starting to help, and the second one was that I had a meeting with David Epston. At this meeting, David taught me a whole new way of dealing at my OCD. I didn't deserve to get pushed around by OCD. Although I had known it all along, I didn't know how to use it to my advantage. David really helped me turn my powerful OCD around, so that it barely affected me. Of course, there were still problems here and there, but they were a lot easier to handle. Thanks to the medicine, the great staff at the hospital, including the doctors, and the support of my family and friends, especially David, my life went from terrible to terrific. I am so thankful for David's help."

Interview with Ben, Maggie, and Jim

DAVID: We are making a tape to record this historic event, Ben, Maggie, and Jim. Also I think Al and Tim [veterans of the problem and now consultants in their capacities as president and vice-president of the Anti-Habit League of New Zealand] would be interested in hearing from you. They knew a little bit about you. But these people don't know very much about the fact that we met about . . . how long ago was it Ben? [*Note*: Dialogue continues on p. 290.]

I had met Tim, age 12, and his mother, Donna, over a 10-month period (December 1992 to October 1993) on eight occasions. When I first met Tim he had been involved with compulsive hand washing relating to concerns about dirt, animals, dust and "dirt" on TV. He would go berserk if anyone watched people kissing on TV and would not desist until they covered their faces with cushions like himself. He had had an eight-year-long headache and vomited most days on the way to school. He described himself as "suspicious." He felt himself to be forbidden to have friends because they were having fun, and he was not permitted to have more than "a minimum of friends." He was preoccupied with his schoolwork and, in the first session, described himself as "on the verge of a nervous breakdown."

This "story" was written after the second meeting and presented to me at the third:

> *Once my mind was plagued by guilt. I was forced by my mind to conduct a series of rituals, such as hand washing. My life was like a bowl of dust blowing away in the wind. I had hardly any activities or clubs to go to. My life usually centred around my schoolwork. I didn't have many friends and if I did, I would usually argue or get nasty to them as they were happy. My life was going down the drain. Then one day, a day in which freeness would finally invade the 'infected' areas of my mind, my mother decided, after seeing me go through a time of pain and guilt, to take me to see David Epston. After only one visit the shell of guilt that had covered me crumbled and light and freedom came to me again. I started making new friends and tying the old tethers back together that at one time had been left to rot and slowly decay. So after a long time of horror, I live in peace again.*

I had met Al, age 13, along with his mother and his father over a five-month period (July 1992 to December 1992) on four occasions. The problems commenced five years previously after the family moved from the capital city to a small rural town. Al was severely teased and had a series of overwhelming and distressing nightmares. This was followed by a succession and accumulation of what we referred to as "habits." He was currently obsessed by germs and the fear that he was suffering from a terminal illness such as AIDS. His schoolwork was deteriorating and he was refusing contact with others and when he was in contact with others was obliged to enter into touching back whenever touched so as to return the "germs."

This story was written after the third meeting and presented at the fourth:

> *It all started when I was eight. I moved from a large city and a happy life to a small town where I was plagued and terrorised by fears and habits. They first began with a dream and although I cannot and do not wish to remember it, it upset me a lot at the time, so much, in fact, that it opened the way for fears and the habits to enter my life. My main fear has always been disease and with it came many others. The first of my habits was a constant need to clear my throat and always needing to wash my hands. These habits have continued to terrorise me up until recently and although I have done my best against them, I still needed help to get rid of them. I believe if you know what habits are, you can get rid of*

> *them; otherwise they're invincible. Fear could have ruined my life, and it nearly did. I'm happy to be rid of it and I don't want it back!*
>
> *As a result of my nightmares, fears started to take over my life. After the move to the small town, I felt insecure and that opened the way for fear. My fears included fear of the dark, fear of disease and unnecessary worry. I seemed to catch worries off other people and accidentally used my imagination to scare myself. In the small town, I found it hard to make friends and was upset very easily. When I was nearly nine, my family moved back to Auckland. I was happier there but my habits still didn't leave. Once there, I felt more secure so I began trying to make my habits go away. It didn't work perfectly but it did help. As one habit went away, another came in its place. Some of the habits I've had were clearing my throat, blinking at things, washing my hands, not eating all my food, missing the top and bottom steps when I went upstairs and touching everything I walked past. My worst habit was that I felt other people were giving me germs so if they touched me I had to touch them back.*
>
> *The last habit is what made my mum look for help as she realized the habits weren't going to go away by themselves. After asking around, Mum found out about David Epston so she got an appointment with him. When I first went, I didn't know what to expect. We arrived early and were all nervous when we went in. But he told me there were other people with the same problems and best of all, it could be disposed of.*
>
> *Since then, I've visited him an three times. All my habits have gone and no new ones come. Well, to tell the truth, most have gone and the others are still disappearing into the background. With less to worry about, my schoolwork and attitude have improved. I'm glad I'm not afraid anymore.*

The therapist sets the scene by decreeing it to be an "historic event" rather than a mundane therapy event and specifying the potential audiences. In this instance, there are three potential audiences: Tim, Al, and the Anti-Habit League, those therapists attending this training at the Family institute of Cambridge, and what Lobovits, Maisel, and Freeman (Chapter 11, this volume) refer to as the introduced audience—those young persons, their family members, and possibly their therapists struggling with similar problems who may find a measure of relief and hope, ideas, or incitement to their own creativity in consulting such an "archive" of an "alternative knowledge." "These people" here are the audience of 35 professional therapists.

BEN: About two months ago.

MAGGIE: St Patrick's Day . . . March 17th.

DAVID: You wrote me a fax in Sweden. Is that okay if I read it out loud?

BEN: Go ahead.

DAVID: First of all, I was glad to hear about Mike. How is he doing?

[Mike was a young man suffering from severe cerebral palsy who required caretakers to support his efforts to walk and whose speech was quite aphasic. Until I met Ben on the first occasion, I had been informed that Ben had adopted the almost indecipherable speech of Mike. This made communicating with Ben extremely difficult. Almost within several interchanges on meeting Ben, Ben consented to my question: "Did Ben just say 'Hi!' or was that Mike speaking?" Ben replied: "Ben!" "I enjoy speaking to Ben. Do you mind continuing as Ben and I will be David?" And sure enough we did carry on for the next hour and a half as Ben and David. When I saw Ben on the second occasion, I inquired about Mike. I had heard from Ben's parents that Ben's relationship with Mike had changed after my first meeting with Ben. Although Ben had previously shown discomfort about his compulsive mimicking of Mike and had made some atoning gestures after our meeting, Ben began to reach out in a very heartfelt way to this boy who was the only child on the unit with physical disabilities and significant developmental delay.]

BEN: He is doing great! Well, when we both were in hospital in the same unit, some of the kids would make fun of him. And when I started feeling better I was very supportive of him. And I did stuff with him. I came to learn what a great person he was in that he expressed love to me as to how thankful he was.

DAVID: Was that a big surprise to you?

BEN: Yeah, it was . . . but that just proves more that he is a great person. I am glad he is doing well.

DAVID: Are you in touch with him?

BEN: No, but my doctor said he would try to get his address or phone number.

DAVID: Do you think if it wasn't for you, Mike wouldn't be living so happily with his new foster family?

BEN: I haven't thought about that.

DAVID: If you did think about it, what would you think?

BEN: I think I had some impact on him. I met his foster mum.

DAVID: Did you? Did you give her any advice?

BEN: I just told her he was a great kid. And she is very nice and caring. I think he would still be happy but not as happy.

DAVID: You know there are a lot of people in this world who for whatever reasons aren't able to show love. How did you bring that out in him?

BEN: By giving him love so that he would have the sense that he was loved. You know, set free the love that was trapped inside his heart!

DAVID: Was it touching for you to see his love get free of the trap that it had been in?

BEN: Very . . .

DAVID: Did it happen overnight or gradually?

BEN: It happened gradually over the course of time.

[This series of inquiries, aside from my interest in learning of Mike's well-being, also intends to implicate Ben in his own agency—that he could make an appreciable contribution to Mike's freeing his "trapped" love and his well-being, in spite of his physical disabilities and the humiliations associated with them. I wish I had been more explicit here and asked: "Did you learn this practice of 'giving love' so the other person could sense he or she was loved from your brother–sister relationship with [his sister] Julia? Or was it just a fresh hospital learning? Where did you learn this practice of giving love?"]

DAVID: Was that the highlight of your time in hospital?

[Undoubtedly there were "lowlights" and dark times during Ben's hospital admission but my preference here is to ask about the "highlights."]

BEN: That was one of them.

DAVID: What were your other highlights?

BEN: The meeting that I had with you.

DAVID: Why was that? Because you beat me in ping pong?

BEN: No, that wasn't it even though I liked that. It was sort of I felt someone really knew what I was going through, almost as if you were feeling the same pain I was feeling and could reach out and show me how to deal with it in the best way I could.

DAVID: Did you have some sense that I wasn't entirely happy with the way Mr. O had intruded upon your life?[4]

[For me, one of the most appealing advantages of an externalizing conversation is that it allows you out of the position of the "objective observer" or "fake neutrality." I have no problem whatsoever avowing my position against such a problem, given my experience-near "clinical knowledge." This was derived from relative influence questioning, that

[4] "Mr. O" was the name that Ben, his family, and the hospital staff arrived at to stand for "the problem," so that they could engage in an externalizing conversation about it.

is those questions that ask in an ethnographic rather than merely a psychological manner, "What effect is this problem having on your life and the life of those in your life?" I might add that that is an exceedingly complicated question and can best be broached by any number of questions. By allying all the concerned parties against the problem, my distaste for the problem does not have to be concealed by any such requirement of "being on everyone's side at the same time." I am on everyone's side against the influence of the problem. And you know, a problem such as so-called obsessive–compulsive disorder can be very compelling of professionals to find the perfect answer. Here the intention of this question is to review Ben's recollection of my avowed position against the problem. In the first meeting, I might have asked, if he was in doubt: "What do you think I think about the way this problem has intruded into your mind, heart, and soul? How do you think I feel about witnessing this happening to a nice, ordinary kid like you?"]

BEN: Well, you can't really help the problem because it sort of creeps up behind your back. But I think what you thought was "there's a problem so let's do all we can about it."

[For me, this comment is of profound interest and one that I have been researching ever since and that is, the spatialization of the problem. Once again, this is an experience-near "knowledge" and is hard won by ethnographically precise questioning "unpacking" such metaphors over Ben's experience of this problem. And in my research so far, some of it retrospective, this problem seems to be located behind the person and the solution seems to arise when the person relocates the problem in front of them. This would suggest to me such processual questions: "Where is the problem now? Behind you, beside you, above you, below you, or in front of you, or somewhere else?" If a person replied: "Beside me," I would further my investigation with: "Look last time we met, you indicated to me that it was behind you. Did you put the problem beside you in some way or other? Or did you command it to get out from behind you and stand alongside you? Or what? Can it pull you down from behind if it is beside you? Can you keep your eye on it better? etc."]

DAVID: I'm not asking you to be critical or anything but how were the other people helping you with the problem that was different? Did they have a different idea about problems?

[Such questions assist us as professionals to reflect on our practices regularly by having the people we see evaluate our helping efforts as we all know the way to hell is paved with good intentions but unexpected consequences.]

BEN: It wasn't so much what they were doing wrong but the amount of stuff they did right. Like my parents were very supportive but they didn't know as much about these things as you did. They did all they could but people like you who understand and can help you know. . . .

DAVID: But don't you think you are giving me overmuch credit here because I only met you for an hour or so and until I got your fax, I didn't know which way it was going for you? Are you sure you are not giving away too much here?

[It is important here to contest Ben's willingness to give me all the credit, for fear that by doing so he would be very likely to discount and disqualify all his efforts, "knowledges," and genius and that of his family, therapists, friends, and so on. This work concerns itself with generating "communities of concern" rather than therapist veneration. On the other hand, I am not arguing for false modesty or the assumption that therapists can't play an important role, but I construe that role as akin to opening a door, a door Ben had to walk through and then find his way from there.]

BEN: No. (*shaking head and grinning*)

DAVID: Well, that is very nice of you, especially saying that in front of all these people.

BEN: But just remember you owe me ten bucks afterwards. (*laughter all around*)

DAVID: We were talking amongst ourselves Ben about this young boy. What he said was that he thought he had a small problem but then found out it was a giant problem and that was what got his determination going. You know when I met you, your Mum said in the fax that you thought that you were the size of a crumb and your problem was the size of the Empire State Building.

[In the fax, Ben had metaphorically described his relationship with the problem (crumb vs. Empire State Building) at a point in time, "when I was going into hospital." This admits of the possibility of his revision of that relationship in the following series of questions.]

BEN: Yeah, I felt like when I was going into the hospital I was just a teeny little breadcrumb. This guy, Mr. O, was as big as the Empire State Building but as I grew over time, he shrunk. And now I am proud to say that I am taller than him.

DAVID: How tall are you? About 5′?

BEN: About 4′11″ and he is about . . . the size of my parakeet's brain. (*loud laughter all around*)

DAVID: Well, you have turned the tables! Just to give it some respect, how did it sneak up on you and how would you warn others. . . ?

BEN: I didn't expect it.

DAVID: Looking back now from where you are, what were its ways and means of sneaking up on a young person and taking over their lives like it did you? Do you have any warnings to other young people?

[These "warning" questions can only be asked of "veterans" of the problem and are asked on behalf of "others."]

BEN: Well, I guess the only thing I could say is that if something bad happens,just think about it. And make sure this problem doesn't get overblown because you can go through a lot.

DAVID: How would you warn another person that this problem was sneaking up on them and getting bigger than they were? Are there any signs or clues to forewarn another person?

BEN: A lot of stress was building up. . .

DAVID: What do you mean by that?

[It is important to have some consensual meaning for such a popular psychological term, for it is vital for me to understand what Ben understands by this rather than what I might mean.]

BEN: The normal stuff to do with school . . . I almost felt it was bigger because I didn't know about it.

DAVID: Hold on . . . are you suggesting that its knowing about the problem that made you see through it? Did you not know about it?

["Because I didn't know about it" catches my attention here and I will enthusiastically interrupt him in order to pursue the putative significance of his comment. At times, you have to be quick.]

BEN: Well, I knew I was compelled to do things but didn't know why. My parents said: "Well, you have a mild case of obsessive–compulsive disorder" but it got a lot worse and as I shrunk, Mr. O got a lot bigger.

DAVID: I guess the question that all of us are wondering is: "How did you shrink it?" "Did you shrink it, blow yourself up or do both at the same time?"

[Instead of asking, "How did it shrink you?" I go back to the above (4′11″ vs. the size of a parakeet's brain) and convert Ben's metaphor into a question implicating yet again his agency in relationship to the problem. This is a much richer question than say a straightforward solution-oriented question such as, "How did you do that?"]

BEN: Well,there a couple of things. One is that the medicine kicked in. Two is the support of everybody and *that* makes me feel stronger.

DAVID: What kind of support makes you feel stronger and what kind of support could weaken you? Is there a difference?

[Once again, I invite Ben to unpack the meaning of a rather taken-for-granted word in both professional and lay discourses—"support"—by asking about the potential effects on him of different kinds of support.]

BEN: Well, the support that makes me feel stronger is people letting me know I am a good person even though it seems like I'm not and let me know they are on my side. And in a way, this isn't you doing it, there is something inside of you that at that time you had no control over.

DAVID: Did you think for awhile that Mr. O was you? He owned your mind?

BEN: Yeah, because he did own my thoughts.

[My guess is that Ben at times must have felt unsupported by others and himself for attempting to physically harm his sister. The externalizing conversation has offered him the linguistic resources to think this anew and he certainly has asked us to "condemn the sin" rather than him. However this must not be understood to be an abrogation of any responsibility but rather the encouragement of responsible action on his part, supported by his "community of concern."]

DAVID: When you were a crumb, what percent ownership did he have of your thoughts?

BEN: Basically everything. I had a little basic common sense. I still knew how to walk. (*laughter all around*)

DAVID: Well, look this is quite a shock to me because when I met you, I thought there was a fair bit of you there? Do you remember on that day—March 17th? You were certainly ahead of Mr. O on that day?

[This is an attempt to resurrect an historical "unique outcome." My recollection of the hospital meeting with Ben convinced me at the time that he was a young man of considerable wit, charm, and grit. On that occasion his mind was certainly his own if I was to be asked to judge.]

BEN: Cuz of all the support. I was sitting in a room. Twelve people and I knew all of them were on my side and all of them cared about me. That gave me a lot of growing power. And in turn at that meeting I was a little taller than Mr. O.

DAVID: I thought so. Do you think Mr. O has any ways and means of separating people off from support? Turning you against people or turning people against you?

[This is an ethnographic question seeking for information as to the "practices" of the problem.]

BEN: Well, I think that to the normal person, if someone does something bad when really it is Mr. O . . . okay they think this guy has done something bad. The best way to look at it is to think of getting *him* help and wiping Mr. O out of the picture.

[Ben's account is an apt description of his "positioning" in this externalizing conversation—support for the person and opposition to the problem.]

DAVID: Okay, in your fax you offered some thanks to Tim and Al. These people won't know that Tim and Al are people who freed themselves from Mr. O in New Zealand. They sent you some letters, didn't they?

[I cannot recall what archives from the Anti-Habit League I sent Ben and his family, but the two "stories" on page 289 written by Tim and Al are regularly circulated and for me "speak" to this work far better than anything I know.]

BEN: You included some stuff about them in your letters.

DAVID: And you said: "Thank you, Tim and Al. Mr. O is a bad loser. Your strategy worked!"

BEN: It *did* work.

DAVID: What strategy of theirs did you put into use here in America?

[Can you imagine my curiosity here? I had no idea whatsoever what it was from the archival material that Ben selected out, put into his practice, labeled a strategy, and, more important, found effective, but I certainly wished to pursue this in some detail. I immediately discerned that "giving him one" was of vital importance. I wish I had reviewed this in reference to the externalization of the "curse of the idea of perfection" with such inquiries as: "Is this your means of sabotaging perfection? Would you consider this as getting back at it, a small dose of revenge? How did perfection react when you refused to do its bidding? Were you making fun of perfection? Does perfection expect to be taken seriously? etc."]

BEN: Because if I am getting really strong and I keep on beating Mr. O and then he is down for the count. And I am just standing there in the ring saying, "I am number one!" he will come up from behind and grab my leg or something because he is a very poor loser so I learned to get lots of stuff on him but give him one so he doesn't feel like he has to start creeping up on me again. That's even worse when you know the problem is there because he takes you by surprise.

DAVID: Did you become more vigilant, more watchful of Mr. O? You didn't turn your back on him?

BEN: Yeah I did. In the beginning, when I started to recover . . .

DAVID: Did you have to stand face to face?

[Here I am using the practice I have come to associate with the co-construction of "local knowledges" cross-referencing one person's experience with another and inviting the latter to comment on it (see Madigan & Epston, Chapter 12, this volume). This requires therapists to keep an available inventory of this at the forefront of their thinking/practice. If you expect a person, young or otherwise, to articulate a "local knowledge" without considerable "scaffolding," you will be waiting for a very rare bird. The therapist's contribution at this stage is considerable. This is certainly not a time to rest.]

BEN: (*after considerable reflection*) Yeah.

DAVID: That's funny because what Tim said was that he had to put him in front of him and keep him there for quite a while. He said: "Then Mr. O threw in the towel in the first round . . ."

BEN: That's very, very, very true.

[Ben's response is typical and is often associated with vigorous head nodding, grins of recognition, and so on. These are to be watched out for.]

DAVID: It didn't take very long. And then what he said was: "He would come back after a while but it wasn't much of a fight. It was more like a spat. And one flick of my finger and I could make it go away." Do you feel you are in Tim's shoes in terms of a return engagement?

[This is the "matching up" question, in an attempt to augment and thicken Tim's "knowledge." I very much like Kenneth and Mary Gergen's (1991) metaphor of "lamination" to describe this process rather than "reduction." This knowledge clearly builds in a very different manner than theory-generated positivist knowledge.]

BEN: Yeah, Yeah, I do but I also know not to get too overconfident because he will just take me from behind.

DAVID: So how do you keep yourself alert and attentive?

BEN: I don't know because I guess it has almost become an instinct. . .

DAVID: Second nature.

BEN: Because I feel like as long as this is inside of my head that Mr. O *is* a bad loser, I know that I can throw him one every so often. If I just keep on thinking I can beat Mr. O, "I'm the best," he's just going to grab your leg and take you down.

["Give him one" gets further elaborated into "throw him one." This is a very unique way Ben has of actively resisting the "curse of the idea of perfection." It is a very commendable conceit, one I intend to explore and elaborate in my future work opposing such a problem. I might have asked, "If Mr. O is a bad loser, as you say, does that mean you have to be a good loser to go against him? Would you describe your policy here as one of 'winning by losing on purpose'? How is this different from Mr. O's policy?"]

DAVID: You tell me that you have been working hard to to earn your degree in Impurfection. . .

BEN: Imperfection spelled with a U. . . . (*laughter all around*)

DAVID: Do you think you are ready to make your application for the New Zealand Diploma in Impurfection? Is it time yet or do you think you need more training in Impurfection?

[The steps of (1) preparation for application, (2) the application process itself, and (3) the award/nonaward of the application in this ritual process are taken very seriously, although I suspect some people reading this transcript may consider this a joke. This practice is clearly an application of the rite-of-passage analogy.]

BEN: There is only one more thing I have to do. I have to say this. I am "reedy"! (*mimicking my New Zealand accent; laugher all around*)

DAVID: You're reedy! Can I just check? I know it could be overconfidence talking here. (*to parents*) Do you think he is ready to submit his application for the New Zealand Diploma in Impurfection?

JIM: Yes

DAVID: What about you, Maggie?

MAGGIE: Mm hmm!

DAVID: This will have to go to Al and Tim because they are the president and vice president at the moment. Shall we write an application to them? And your Mum and Dad could be your references?

BEN: Sure. Tim and Al were in a way my teachers and they had been through it and they knew what to do and what not to do and they passed that knowledge on to me. And I am grateful to them for that.

DAVID: Can I write that to them?

BEN: Sure.

DAVID: (*writing*) "Tim and Al, I feel like you have been my teachers." What else did you say? I thought it was interesting what you said.

BEN: I said that because they had gone through what I was going through that they could tell me what to do and what not to do and pass that knowledge on to me. David, did you misspell a word in there?

DAVID: Yeah, look at that . . . see the d and the j. Well, I put them together. (*laughter all around*) These people don't know that one of the tests of impurfection is to make spelling mistakes on purpose. Now, I think Tim and Al might be interested to hear what it was you found useful from them. Was there anything you would like to say thanks to them for? Any ideas or practices. . .

[This tape is also being made for Al and Tim and I expected to forward copies to them. I can only guess what it was like for Al and Tim to review this tape. At this stage, I have a great fondness for "saying thanks" questions. Furman and Ahola (1992) have developed a parallel practice.]

BEN: They didn't have to tell me all this. They didn't have to give up some of their time to help *me*. But the fact that they did, I almost feel like they are really on my side and up in the front lines with me.

DAVID: They will be pretty pleased to hear that, I think. What evidence do you have to support your application for the Diploma in Impurfection?

BEN: Because I know and am aware of the *curse* of perfection.

DAVID: These people here might not know exactly what that is though they might guess. Can you fill people in on that?

BEN: (*shaking his head ruefully*) The curse of perfection. It's almost as if you try to be too perfect, something is bound to go wrong.

[In Ben providing his "evidence" and my assisting him to elaborate on it as to its significance qua problem, Ben's parents and I had many surprises in store for us, as is usually the case.]

DAVID: What else would you like to tell Tim and Al so they can be reassured that you are ready? Are there any good examples that you would like to say to them?

BEN: Well, a little story. Before I went into the hospital, I had a compulsion to make my last basketball shot. I needed to end on a perfect note. And about a week ago, I was at a doctor's appointment. And we were shooting around and I missed a shot. He asked: "Can you leave without making the last shot?" And I said: "Yes, I can!"

DAVID: And you did it? Was that hard?

BEN: (*smiling proudly*) No.

DAVID: Now in the old days when you were unaware of perfection and the effect it was having on your life, would you have been compelled to do that?

[These are important "bifurcative questions" (Karl Tomm, personal communication, 1991) that invite a person to compare his/her relationship with the problem at two points in time in order to draw distinctions (e.g., "a week ago" vs. "in the old days"). Note also the careful use of verb tenses to add considerable "pastness" to the past.]

BEN: I would have had to make my last shot. If I missed a layup, I would have to hit a layup.

JIM: What would happen if someone stopped you from doing that?

BEN: *At* that time, it was sort of inconceivable. I felt I couldn't stop this urge I had. And if someone did, I almost felt shattered.

DAVID: Was Mr. O lying to you about some things like it did to Tim and Al?

[This is an example of the personifications typical of work with "extreme" or "deadly" problems such as obsessive–compulsive disorder, anorexia/bulimia, life-threatening asthma, or psychotic experience (see White, 1995). Here the "problem" is enriched by personifying it, permitting it to have a "voice," tactics, strategies, personal characteristics, and indeed pathologies of its own (e.g., "What kind of problem do you think your problem has got? What would your diagnosis be for a problem with such 'a nature'?"[5])]

BEN: What do you mean by that?

DAVID: It told him that if he didn't do this, he wouldn't have any happiness for the rest of his life. Or he was trash. Or he would fall apart.

BEN: Yeah . . . Yeah.

DAVID: Did the New Zealand Mr. O speak in any way similar to the American one?

BEN: Very much so.

DAVID: Not any cultural differences?

[5]These questions were suggested to me by Rick Maisel at a Santa Rosa workshop in 1992.

[This is more than a jest. Such a question deprivatizes the problem and globalizes it as "worldwide . . . multinational." Still it is only a step down to "culture" (e.g., "Do you ever wonder if Mr. O is as prevalent in Polynesia or the Third World as it is in western capitalist countries?").]

BEN: Nope . . . no accents . . . It was like a feeling if I didn't do this, that I was nothing.

DAVID: Did it call you names if you didn't?

BEN: No, more like the thoughts I had. Then I realized that if I was going to be controlled by a bad force then I was a nothing.

DAVID: Well, I am glad you became your own person rather than a person for Mr. O. Tim and Al are insiders so they will know what you are taking about . . . what else would convince them that you are ready for this Diploma because you could help other people now?

[At this stage in the process, considerable reference is made to the "introduced audience," which also assists in marking Ben's new standing as "veteran" (e.g., "You could help other people now.").]

BEN: That I have strategies and one of these strategies is to think, say I have an urge to make my last shot, I try to reverse it and say: "I should have an urge to miss the last shot."

DAVID: Oh, really! Is this countercompulsions or something? An urge to oppose the urge.

[I think I would be hard put to find a better idea/strategy than this one in any professional text I have read over the years. This, to my way of thinking, is an act of genius and clearly Ben has a fine mind. But I want to reassure you that such ideas/practices "pop up" on a regular basis talking to young persons in this manner and with this expectation. As is the case here, the young person rarely considers informing his/her parents, even though I suspect Maggie and Jim would have been delighted to know about it.]

BEN: That was the most successful one. It doesn't work every time.

DAVID: Oh that's good, You don't want to be perfect.

BEN: (*crossing his hands in front of his face*) No, I wouldn't want that. (*laughter all around*)

DAVID: Where did that idea come from . . . was that your idea, your Mum's or Dad's or a hospital idea . . . where did it come from?

BEN: It just came from myself.

DAVID: Do you consider that a good idea? Would you recommend that to other young people?

[These are questions to discern the "genealogy" of this practice and the ideas that resourced it. Other questions are asked to have him evaluate it, both for his own use and for export to others. This kind of inquiry is at the heart of this work.]

BEN: I think that if it works for me it's not necessarily going to work for someone else.

DAVID: Give me an example . . . let me think of Al. Al was driven when he was coming down the stairs to miss the last step. . .

[Cross-referencing his "knowledge" back in time allows him to stand back from it and describe its deployment. By doing so, this practice will be more available for his use, should he require it.]

BEN: (*postulates*) *I had that!* I didn't have that very long. I had it some times.

DAVID: What else . . . oh, he felt he had to touch people.

BEN: I sometimes felt I had to do that.

DAVID: These are international. This is a multinational, Mr. O.

[Once again, many therapists might have been tempted to follow a pathology track here. Rather, once again, I return to the frame of reference of "culture."]

BEN: Worldwide.

DAVID: So say Al had that. Mr. O was compelling him to miss the last step, what would you recommend he do if he followed that particular strategy?

[This question invites Ben to refine and elaborate this strategy and at the same time to publicize it.]

BEN: He would miss the last two steps.

DAVID: Is that right! Is that like doing mischief? Being a bit noncompliant to Mr. O?

BEN: In that case, Yeah I guess.

[These questions invite Ben once again to refer this strategy back into a revised relationship with Mr. O—one in which he is certainly no longer Mr. O's puppet. Instead, "mischief" and "noncompliance" might appeal to a young man of Ben's age and feistiness.]

DAVID: Have you got any other ideas like that? (*to parents*) Did you know about these ones?

MAGGIE: No.

DAVID: That's a good idea, don't you think? Why do you keep those secret? Did you not think they were worthy of mention?

BEN: No, not that . . . they have just never really been brung up.

DAVID: Are you glad I brought it up because I think that is worth knowing about?

BEN: Everyone should know about it.

DAVID: Look I met Chris. He was about 17 and he felt compelled to shower and wash himself for hours on end. And the first way he opposed it was to go and have his usual shower but he would leave a little bit behind his knee undone to get back at the compulsion.

BEN: And work your way from there.

DAVID: Funny . . . the fact that he could do that it just vanished overnight. Did you find that by any chance that once you stood up to it, it pretty well backed down?

BEN: I was really afraid to. I mean. . . .

DAVID: How did it convince you to be afraid?

BEN: Well, it's almost like a big bully coming up to you, who is just really big. He is really afraid. . . .

[Here is another opportunity to "unpack" a metaphor and, in addition, to add it to my stock of counselor knowledge around such a problem (e.g., "Do you find that this problem is a bit like a bully?"). It increases the interviewed persons' responsiveness by adding "a bit like" rather than forcing the answer into a yes–no. This is critical when inviting persons to review their relationships according to metaphorical relationships (e.g., a bully in relationship to his/her "target" person). For example, "Why do you say that? Have you had some experiences of being bullied yourself? Or have you read about bullies? Or seen them on TV or in movies? etc."]

DAVID: You were afraid?

BEN: He's afraid . . . you are both afraid of each other. But I think he won't be afraid because he is this big guy. So I give him my lunch *but* if I say one day: "No, I am not going to give you my lunch," he'll say: "Okay, I'm sorry." (*laughter all around*)

[Once again, this is a revelation to me and something I intend to pursue in my coresearching efforts around such problems (e.g., "I know this is going to sound weird and I wouldn't have even thought to ask you about it if it wasn't for what Ben told me: He said, 'We are afraid of each other.' What do you guess he was getting at there?").]

DAVID: This is uncanny. Tim said the problem was like a big bully too. He said: "I realized it was hard on the outside but had a soft center".

[Here is another example of cross-referencing and "laminating" accounts/vocabularies/metaphors.]

BEN: Exactly!

DAVID: It's wearing a mask. There is a scared thing behind the mask.

[I regret I didn't pursue this line of inquiry: "Ben, where do you think you would be today—crumblike or a young man with growing power—if you hadn't come to think of it that way?" "Did that way of thinking pave the way, in a manner of speaking, for the road to recovery you have been walking the last month or so?"]

BEN: You just don't think of it that way at all.

DAVID: Can you be frank? For a while there did Mr. O terrorize you?

BEN: Yeah . . . for awhile there he was asking me to do his home-work, carry his back-pack. . . .

DAVID: Did you feel enslaved?

BEN: Yeah.

DAVID: When did you feel you got your freedom?

[The "enslavement" metaphor "naturally" allows for the next question: "When did you feel you got your freedom?" Again, such an agentic question is far preferable to less agentic questions such as: "When did you go free? Who let you go free? Was your time up?" Such metaphors have much more room in them than psychiatric/psychological metaphors such as diagnoses. I have always found that diagnostic descriptions limit a person's capability of expressing their experience, both the suffering and the freedom.]

BEN: It wasn't overnight. It was very gradual. I'd say . . . when I was in the hospital, I was an inpatient for a little over a month and a half . . . I was an outpatient for another month. And think after the first four weeks of my inpatient time, that's when things started turning around.

DAVID: I know there was a struggle but when you went ahead of it was that a very clear experience for you? Did you know it when it happened or is it only on looking back that you experience it that way?

BEN: Yeah, I guess I say I knew it but. . . .

DAVID: Did you tell anyone? Your Mum or your Dad?

BEN: I let them know I was feeling better.

DAVID: (*to parents*) Would either of you guessed exactly when that was? Can you date it?

[This is an attempt to locate this event in time so it can be marked ceremonially and remembered in years to come. I think you will agree that there is cause for celebration here, even if the problem is still hanging around in the background.]

JIM: February first he became completely overwhelmed. He was in the hospital February 22nd.

MAGGIE: David saw him March 17th. And I would say we were seeing very slight signs then but the month of April was just incredible. Every day he was so much. . . .

BEN: And late March.

JIM: It was over about a six-week period.

DAVID: If you were to celebrate freedom day, could you assign it to a date?

BEN: No. . . .

DAVID: What about even arbitrarily? Even somewhere in the middle so you could acknowledge it. I could send you a card next year.

JIM: Ben's first day out of the hospital being able to be in a social situation with the family was Margaret's birthday—April 28th. It was the first time the four of us were able to be together since December.

DAVID: Was that a special day for you? What do you think Julia thought about it. . . . Was she pleased?

BEN: It was almost like my birthday as well. I don't know exactly how Julia felt but I think she would be *extremely happy* to have the sense that a family of four could go out to dinner and have a nice conversation and sleep under the same roof.

[This interview goes on for another half hour with me closely interviewing Maggie and Jim as to their reasons for supporting Ben's application for membership. They added an immense amount of information to support Ben's "knowledge" being such loving and concerned parents, as well as close observers. I regret that I do not have the space to include most, if not all, of their commentaries.]

After reviewing the videotape of Ben along with his family, Al and Tim independently provided me with their decisions:

Dear David:

Thanks for your letter and video about Ben. I watched the tape and could understand his problems, though they were far worse than mine.

He must have worked really hard to overcome them. I think he has earned the New Zealand Diploma of Impurfection with Distinction. And in my capacity as Vice President of the New Zealand Society, I would recommend the award go to Ben, though I was a little surprised at my selection to the Vice President position but still honoured.

My habits are now well under control but occasionally they try to come back. This is getting less and less though. Since we last saw you, I have been fairly busy. In the May holidays, I went on a week long bike tour and was able to ride much faster without my habits dragging me back. In the August holidays, I went to stay on my uncle's farm again and really enjoyed my time there. I wasn't been afraid of the MUD!!! I have also joined a church youth group, partly because of the church side of the bike tour and also because I wanted to make new friends. We have now finished the aviary and as well as having four adult budgies and two adult quail, we now have an addition in the form of a newly hatched baby quail.

Next time you write to Ben, could you congratulate him from me on having beaten Mr. O. By the way, my Mum has the same birthday as his Mum. Thanks for your help in sorting out my life. Please keep in touch.

Yours (without habits),
Al

Dear David:

I was greatly impressed by Ben's battle with Mr. O. When I read your letter how he was before he was hospitalised and then seeing him on the video, I noticed his great change. He has really changed. I do believe he has worked hard enough to receive the New Zealand Diploma in Impurfection. At the moment, life is going good for me. I'm in the top class in the 3rd Form and have recently turned 14. The only bad thing has been the death of my grandmother some time ago and I am just about over it. And as for perfection, my borders have been closed to him. Mr. "O" as you called it has not visited me ever since.

Best wishes,
Tim

The letters along with a diploma were forwarded to Ben.

Eight months later, I was meeting with the Smith family along with a "team" whose members were attending a weeklong intensive training. The Smith family was invited to join this training week by their therapist, who was attending it. We met them on three consecutive days for a period of two hours. On the second to last day, I met with Ron, age 15, while the men attending met with Ron's father, Jim, and his young brother, Barry, age 12, and the women met with Ron's mother, Denise, and his younger sister, Carrie, age 10. The following is the letter faxed to Ben, Maggie, and Jim, which first outlines the desperation of the Smith's situation and then directs questions to Ben, Maggie, and Jim.

Dear Maggie, Jim and Ben:

I and a Team have been meeting with Denise and Jim Smith and their children, Ron, aged 15, Barry, aged 12, and Carrie, aged 10. They have driven up from a small New Zealand town, 400 miles south of Auckland. It seems that for the past four years, Ron has become more and more a slave to what he refers to as IT (this is his unique version of what you have called Mr. O). And by the way, Ron is a very unique person. He is required by IT to be perfectly clean which means he is living quite a lot of his life in the bathroom. He is becoming concerned that IT is driving him mad. Denise and Jim worry pretty much that this is the case. In fact, I suspect up until recently they have been more aware of the ambush Ron was innocently walking into than he was. His brother and sister are upset that they are losing their older brother to IT. At the moment, the only way they can relate to him is by being part-time slaves to IT and doing such things as opening doors and turning the TV on for Ron because IT "tells" him crazy stuff like he will be contaminated if he opens his own doors or turns his own TV on. Would you believe that IT has even trained him into turning on the TV with his feet and toes?

Maggie, Jim, and Ben, I suspect none of the above will be at all new to you. As you said, Ben, Mr. O (IT) is "worldwide" and "doesn't even have an accent." They watched your videotape before they came up to Auckland and not surprisingly, everyone was quite impressed with your family's opposition to Mr. O (IT). And if you had the time and energy we would all be grateful for a consultation with you. I am sorry I didn't have the time to fax you and ask for your permission in the first instance but things have reached a crisis for the Smiths. If this is inconvenient, we all, naturally, will understand; however if you could assist us, we would be more than grateful.

Questions for Ben from Ron

1. Do you think it is best in the beginning to give the problem a bit of your life while you get most of it back? Is it a bit like taming a wild animal where you throw a bit of meat to it every so often and it gradually becomes tamer?

2. Right now, what percentage do you have of your mind and what percentage does Mr. O have of your mind? This problem has been bugging me for four years but really started to get bad at the end of 1992. I have been thinking of a 90% (me)–10% (it) split? Is that a good way to begin from your point of view?

3. *How did you get around your attitude to other people who weren't supposedly "perfect" as Mr. O instructed you to be?*

4. *I think it is like a perfection syndrome because it wants you to be perfect. It is like trying to make everything perfect. How did you start opposing it? Did you begin with little or big things? I am confused as how to make my start.*

Questions for Maggie from Denise and Carrie

1. *Maggie, how did you cope before Ben started winning his life back from Mr. O?*

2. *Did you cope better when you gave in to Ben's compulsions or stood against them?*

3. *Did it go better for your family if you gave in to keep the peace or stood firm despite Ben's distress or rage?*

Questions for Jim from Ron and Barry

1. *Did the problem with Mr. O only have a bad effect on Ben? Or other people in the family as well? If so, what were the effects on other people?*

2. *How was your family able to help Ben increase the amount of time he was in control of the problem rather than the problem being in control of him?*

3. *How was the family able to help Ben oppose the problem head on rather than retreating from its influence?*

4. *Did you find that the problem had a "logic of its own"? Did you have any success trying to talk Ben out of Mr. O's "logic"?*

5. *When Ben took control over Mr. O, did this lead to Ben engaging in activities that he used to engage in before Mr. O took him over?*

6. *What tricks did Mr. O use to try to convince Ben he had no control? Did he have any tricks to try to talk Ben out of your capacity to help him oppose Mr. O?*

Thanks very much in anticipation. Sorry for the brevity of this. It is a race against time.

Yours sincerely,
David, Ron, Denise,
Jim, Carrie, and Barry

This is an excerpt of the response. I have deleted Jim's and Maggies' responses because of the limitations of space.

Dear Smiths:

I am very sorry to hear of your situation. I am sure that this must be a tough time for everyone in the family. Denise and Jim, seeing your son pushed around by IT must be heartbreaking. As parents of a son being pushed around by IT, you must want to have your son completely take control of IT. From experience, I know that IT is like a tyrant with a goal to control people's lives.

With David Epston and others giving help to you, you are in very good hands. With David Epston's help, cognitive–behavioural therapy, and medicine, I have been able to smash what I call Mr. O and you call IT. It was not easy to defeat Mr. O and sometimes he tries to get revenge, but he is weak and I am strong.

Barry and Carrie, it's tough knowing that your brother is going through tough times. As his siblings, it is good to support him in any way you can and show total disregard for IT. It will make your brother stronger and it will make your lives easier. Under all the blackness lies your brother, a good human being. Try your best to brush away the blackness and find your brother, pure and natural.

Answers to the questions that Ron asked Ben:

1. Yes, it is in many ways good to give the problem a little bit while you get your life back. It is too hard to carry a big load in one trip. Many trips of small loads will get the job done.

2. Right now, I have about 82% control and Mr. O has 18%. Mr. O has the 18% of my life that I value least—spare time. But when something important has to be done, Mr. O runs and hides. It is a very good idea to think of yourself as higher than IT with any numbers. It is terrific that you have such great confidence in yourself, but do not go higher than 90% or you will get overconfident and you will then be vulnerable to IT; 80–90% are the best numbers to start with. It is a good sign that you have such an accurate idea about the situation. This shows that you have control over your basic thinking. You have a very good approach to such an obnoxious enemy.

3. When Mr. O had the control to instruct me to be perfect, it made perfection such a big thing on my mind that it made me notice other people's imperfections. Then I thought, at least they don't have the inconvenience of being pushed around by Mr. O. Once I went into battle with Mr. O, who was my big problem, it was easier for me to feel sympathetic with other people who were battling big problems.

4. A good way to get started is to believe that you can defeat IT. Once you have that idea inside you, you're ready to make your start. Little things are good to begin with, but as time goes by, it is good to slowly change those little things to big things. If you want to climb a ladder with 12 steps it will always be tough to jump 6 of them. Go one at a time and as you get higher, it is good to slowly but swiftly beat IT to the top.

Good luck and remember Mr. O is scum; I would be happy to hear from you and to hear how things are going.

Your teammate against Mr. O,
Ben

CONCLUSION

In this chapter, we have described a process that we refer to as an archaeology of therapy. In this process, the solution knowledges that have been resurrected and/or generated in the context of the therapy and the history of, or conditions, that made the production of these knowledges possible become known. By using the rite of passage signaled by therapy termination to attend to and document the hard-won know-how that helped free persons from bondage to their problems, they become knowledge makers, and knowledge makers become knowledgeable. Both their knowledge-making capabilities and their knowledgeableness are authenticated, not only in the presence of the therapist but also in the presence of other relevant present and future audiences.

The consulting-your-consultants interview with Ben and his parents is an extension of this practice in that such knowledgeableness comes to reside with and be further coproduced by league members. Here, this league has named itself the Anti-Habit League of New Zealand and is merely one of many such leagues (see Madigan & Epston, Chapter 12, this volume). We have come to consider such a knowledge akin to what Foucault (1973) referred to as a "local knowledge," often hidden from view or lacking sufficient credibility to be either voiced or heard. And this knowledge might not only serve the interests of its membership but become "an effective criticism of the dominant knowledges" (White & Epston, 1990, p. 26). Many means have been explored to archive such "knowledges" and circulate them around the leagues. The league acts not only to legitimate these "knowledges" but also to discern gaps. Such gaps become the stimuli to further coresearched projects on behalf of coresearching participants and the league in general.

The practices outlined in this chapter encourage persons to deploy their knowledges more knowingly, increase their own authority in matters of their concern, and decrease their dependency on expert knowledges. We believe that such personal solution knowledges can be more viable, enduring, and efficient than imported "expert" knowledges, which too often disable those we seek to help and induce in them a stupefying patienthood. Viewed in this perspective, the artful use of therapeutic questions can help transform the process of therapy termination from one marked only by loss and diminishment to one offering the prospect of genuine gain and fuller authorship of the story of one's life.

ACKOWLEDGMENTS

Portions of this chapter originally appeared in the *Dulwich Centre Newsletter* (1990), No. 4 and are reprinted with permission.

REFERENCES

Douglas M. (1982). *In the active voice.* London: Routledge & Kegan Paul.

Epston, D. (1985). An interview with David Epston. *Family Therapy Association of South Australia Newsletter,* pp. 11–14. [Reprinted in Epston, D. (1989). *Collected papers.* Adelaide, Australia: Dulwich Centre Publications.]

Epston, D. (1987, Summer). A reflexion. *Dulwich Centre Newsletter,* pp. 16–17. [Reprinted in Epston, D. (1989). *Collected papers.* Adelaide, Australia: Dulwich Centre Publications.]

Epston, D. (1994, November/December). Extending the conversation. *Family Therapy Networker,* pp. 31–37, 62–63.

Epston, D., Morris, F., & Maisel, R. (1995). A narrative approach to so-called anorexia/bulimia. *Journal of Feminist Family Therapy,* 7(1/2), 69–95.

Foucault, M. (1973). *The birth of the clinic: An archaeology of medical perception.* London: Tavistock.

Furman, b., & Ahola, T. (1992). *Solution talk: Hosting therapeutic conversations.* New York: Norton.

Geertz, C. (1976). From the native's point of view: On the nature of anthropological understanding. In K. Basso & H. Shelby (Eds.), *Meaning in anthropology.* Albuquerque: University of New Mexico Press.

Gergen, K. J., & Gergen, M. M. (1991). Toward reflexive methodologies. In F. Steir (Ed.), *Reflexivity and research* (pp. 77–95). London: Sage.

Harré, R. (1983). *Personal being: A theory for individual psychology.* Oxford: Blackwell.

Hewson, D. (1990). *From laboratory to therapy room.* Unpublished manuscript.

Kobak, R., & Waters, D. (1984). Family therapy as a rite of passage: The play's the thing. *Family Process, 23*(1), 89–100.

Mauss, M. (1954). *The gift: Forms and function in archaic societies.* London: Cohen & West.

Turner, B., & Hepworth, M. (1982). *Confession: Studies in deviance in religion.* London: Routledge.

Turner, V. (1967). *The forest of symbols: Aspects of Ndembu ritual.* Ithaca, NY: Cornell University Press.

Turner, V. (1986). Dewey, Dilthy, and drama. In V. Turner & E. Bruner (Eds.), *The anthropology of experience.* Chicago: University of Illinois Press.

van Gennep, A. (1960). *The rite of passage.* Chicago: Chicago University Press. (Originally published 1908)

White M. (1986, May). Awards and their contribution to change. *Dulwich Centre Newsletter,* pp. 15–16.

White, M. (1988a, Winter) The process of questioning: A therapy of literary merit. *Dulwich Centre Newsletter,* pp. 8–14. [Reprinted in White, M. (1989). *Selected papers.* Adelaide, Australia: Dulwich Centre Publications.]

White, M. (1988b, Spring) Saying hullo again: The incorporation of the lost relationship in the resolution of grief. *Dulwich Centre Newsletter,* pp. 7–11. [Reprinted in White, M. (1989). *Selected papers.* Adelaide, Australia: Dulwich Centre Publications.]

White, M. (1989, Summer) The externalizing of the problem and the re-authoring of lives and relationships. *Dulwich Centre Newsletter,* pp. 3–21. [Reprinted in White, M. (1989). *Selected papers.* Adelaide, Australia: Dulwich Centre Publications.]

White, M. (1995). *Re-authoring lives: Interviews and essays.* Adelaide, Australia: Dulwich Centre Publications.

White, M., & Epston, D. (1985). Consulting your consultant's consultants. In B. A. Chable, R. A. Fawns, & T. R. Paterson (Eds.), *Proceedings of the Sixth Australian Family Therapy Conference.* Melbourne, Australia.

White, M., & Epston, D. (1990). *Narrative means to therapeutic ends.* New York: Norton.

CHAPTER 14

Family Reunions

COMMUNITIES CELEBRATE NEW POSSIBILITIES

Timothy Nichols
Cheryl Jacques

> All Hasidic tales are full of friendship. And to retell them is to communicate their promise. Listen to our Jewish tales, and you will know what hurts your friend. To listen well is to acquire all knowledge and experience. But who will teach modern man how to listen? To listen means to deny solitude, and solitude is the problem of man today.
>
> —*Elie Wiesel (Abrahamson, 1985)*

KIMBERLY WAS 12 years old. Donna was 31. They found themselves to be homeless. Even if they had a roof over their heads, they would have been unable to live together for fear that one of them would be hurt—physically and emotionally. The violence between the two was foreshadowed by drug addiction and abusive relationships that allowed chaos to flourish in their lives. The first six years of Kimberly's life were dangerous and unpredictable due to the intravenous drug addiction afflicting her mother. A collection of abusive, controlling men had come and gone over the past 12 years. Kimberly's and Donna's lack of faith in themselves encouraged violence and drugs to lurk near their home waiting for the opportunity to reenter. Their hostile relationship left them vulnerable to becoming instruments of violence as they assaulted each other. Their struggle continued despite Kimberly's psychiatric hospitalizations, prescription of psychotropic medication, and use of professional language to define the difficulties (i.e., "oppositional defiant disorder" and "impulse control disorder").

Meanwhile, an underlying current of hope was being nourished by Donna's successful seven-year stand against drug abuse, which was supported by her peers in the Narcotics Anonymous community. Kimberly and Donna loved each other, and sought to counter the social and cultural practices that marked them as a family ruined by drug abuse. They desired assistance and support, rather than control and judgment, from community and government organizations. They wanted encouragement to review and renew relationships with their community, extended family, and each other. Finally, they hoped to restore their faith in their own goodness and ability to enjoy life. In this chapter, the voices of Kimberly and Donna help us describe a treatment program that they (and other distressed families) helped to create for themselves.

The Beal Street Program and families such as Kimberly and Donna have worked together to develop and apply new treatment ideas that respect the client's voice and include their community in the process. Our goal is to safely reunite estranged families and restore their respect in the community. The resulting collaborative effort is organized around, and culminates in, the celebration of a family reunion. This approach was developed as an alternative to traditional "residential treatment" of adolescents who were unable to live safely in the community. Basic principles of the program include utilizing the expertise of families, treatment providing realistic opportunities to practice new ways of addressing problems in the community, and a value being placed on treatment in the least restrictive community setting. The end result is an approach that addresses many issues of language and power as new family stories are introduced to a community audience.

A narrative metaphor in the form of a "rite of passage" (Durrant, 1993; Epston & White, 1992; van Gennep, 1908) was adopted for the transition families were undergoing during the treatment process. In this framework the treatment effort begins with an agreement that a family reunion is a desirable outcome and with a conversation regarding issues that must be addressed as part of the practical preparation for this reunion. The family reunion then becomes the focal point for conversation, consensus, and decision making. It serves as a ritual that anchors a preferred narrative in the community in which the family lives. This reunion is a way for the community to unite behind the acceptance of an alternative narrative that restores integrity to individuals, relationships, and communities.

In this context, procedures are developed that support the deconstruction of problem-saturated narratives and the building of preferred alternatives. Potentially oppressive "realities" are deconstructed in the language and culture of the treatment setting, in the relationships that define lives, and in narratives of self. This process makes room for people to nurture a new family story. A family reunion then provides an opportunity to anchor this story in community life by enabling more people to be involved in the preferred story as coauthors and characters. The completion of the rite of passage becomes part of the family history as documents, symbolic items, audiotapes, and videotapes of the process are produced to become a part of a family archive.

ORGANIZATIONAL SUPPORT FOR SOLUTIONS

The organizational context within which the Beal Street Program operates has been an intimate part of how the solution-oriented treatment process has emerged. Program development was influenced by newness (a lack of history), financial realities of the times, the collaborative structure and educational culture of the parent organization, and the large number of organizations in the community that have a stake in the facility. The program began in 1990 with only one expectation: that the function would be to safely and permanently reunite, in as short a time as possible, adolescents and the families from which they were estranged.

The program opened amidst the transformation of the health care system in the United States. The accompanying need to cut costs translated into the need to provide care in community rather than in a residential setting whenever it was safe to do so. Therefore, it became necessary to strive for shorter residential stays or to use residential care as an alternative to lengthy or repeated hospitalizations.[1]

In addition, the program had very little pressure to conform to the traditional expectations of residential treatment in the United States, because it exists within the unique management structure of an educational collaborative. As such, the board of directors is made up of educational administrators from eight surrounding towns. As a result,

[1]Although actual figures are unavailable, a rough estimate is that similar clients in other residential care settings remain in residence between 18 and 24 months on the average. The average length of stay at the Beal Street Program is 7.2 months. Therefore, there appears to be a significant savings in time and cost.

Further savings are realized by enabling many of our residents to attend school within their town school system rather than having the town shoulder the cost of a private education at a treatment program. Also, up to a few years ago many of our clients would likely have been treated in private psychiatric hospitals. Although our lengths of stay are longer than most hospitalizations, the daily cost is approximately 15% of the daily cost of an inpatient hospitalization. The niche that we are filling is a combination of hospital diversion work and a shorter version of residential treatment. We believe that the Beal Street Program is a fiscally and programatically sensible way to address the needs of adolescents who are at risk in the community.

expectations of how things "should be done"clinically rarely hamper creative clinical solutions, partially because the board is situated in an educational rather than a clinical culture. The board members are more interested in reaching the goal of safely returning adolescents to their homes than they are in any particular clinical approach.

Other community organizations also have a significant interest in the facility. The residence is owned by a local housing authority and leased to the program. A state agency financed the construction of the building. The local office of the state department of social services is committed to having the program serve as a major resource for families in need. Overburdened local courts look to the facility as an alternative to incarceration. Private insurers use the facility as a cost-effective alternative to more expensive psychiatric services. Finally, area families look to the facility as a resource when all else has failed. This combination of factors has given many people a stake in helping the program reach the goal of reuniting families.

TREATMENT PRACTICES REVIEWED

In order to develop treatment practices that would support the goal of reuniting families, a review of relevant literature was conducted. This research indicated that there was a need both to deconstruct standard residential treatment procedures that were counterproductive to our goal and to institute alternative approaches that were conducive to reunification.

Many residential treatment facilities had a historical commitment to the long-term custodial care of children. In addition, the influence of psychoanalytic thought, behavior modification theory, and protective concerns encouraged program policy that supported separating troubled adolescents from their parents to facilitate the completion of a developmental task, as a consequence for undesirable behaviors in the community, or as an assurance that the child would be safe. As agencies embraced a new goal of returning children to family settings, the historical biases of institutional policies and procedures were difficult to overcome. Some problematic remnants of past policies include programs' inaccessibility to parents and the community, an assumption that parents seeking treatment are "bad" or "crazy," and a lack of institutional support for workers to see families in their homes (Gutterman & Blythe, 1986).

Relevant literature indicated that practices that included parents as valued partners in the treatment process and broke down traditional boundaries of the treatment setting facilitated the safe reunification of families (Gilliland-Mallo & Judd, 1986; Lewis, 1984; Nichols, 1989; Taylor & Alpert, 1973). Therefore, a commitment was made to invite parents to be consultants to the clinical process within the residence and to have program staff play an active role in the family home and community.

A FOUNDATION FOR CHANGE

A treatment process was developed that accepts the stated intent of parents to find ways to keep their child safe, attempts to minimize power differentials that exist between families and the professionals treating them, and uses the goal of returning home to focus treatment. Program practices were designed that are consistent with family members being consulted regarding all aspects of a transparent treatment process. Family workers pursue behavioral goals with strategies that can be duplicated by parents at home, and they avoid professional vocabulary that may exclude a family from comfortable participation in a conversation. A sampling of how these ideas actually translate into practice follows:

- As a part of an admission meeting, parents are congratulated for the commitment and care that led them to participate in the treatment process. They are accepted as valued consultants, countering an expectation they often have that they may be viewed as incompetent parents incapable of caring for a "bad" child.
- The family is informed that the program does not spend a great deal of time diagnosing or evaluating people. Rather, it serves as a place where families can safely practice making room for new stories in their lives. It becomes clear that the program intends neither to judge nor to set the agenda for treatment.
- Parents are told that the residence has no "visiting hours" because families are not considered visitors. They are always welcome.
- Parents are expected to be part of the team that runs the facility. They are recognized as program consultants with special expertise in the care of their own child. They are asked to commit to helping to operate the program and are consulted on a daily basis. This places parents in the position of being valued helpers rather than clients waiting to be told what to do.
- The physical space in which treatment occurs is stated to be flexible and without walls, only defined by the places members of the families live and work. The family home and various community venues are considered the ideal places for the family to practice the new stories that they are coauthoring. The building where residents may stay overnight is held in reserve for situations in which it is unsafe for an adolescent to be in the community.
- Recreational and vocational interests are nurtured in the com-

munity to contextualize the changes in the family's life. The location of the work anchors the newly respected narratives in the environment that will have to support them.

- The significance of behavioral change in the treatment milieu under the care of professionals is minimized, while new stories of safe life in the community are highlighted.
- Daily schedules and behavioral management structures of the program are designed to be easily duplicated in the community. This encourages solutions that are relevant to a home rather than an institution.
- Material and personnel resources (i.e., money, incentives for good behavior, or staff to monitor particular behaviors) used by the program reflect those available to particular parents. This is not the most effective approach to control behavior, but it does commit the program to living with the same risks and difficulties that the parents live with in their home. This parity of resources has the effect of building strong and tangible empathy between family workers and families as they face the same challenges with the same tools at their disposal.

THE FAMILY REUNION

In order to provide hope and place treatment in a context of growth, a rite of passage was adopted as a metaphor for the process that assists adolescents to move from the dependence of childhood to the responsibility of adulthood. The rite of passage consists of three stages of treatment: the separation phase, the liminal phase, and the reincorporation phase. The completion of this journey is marked at a ritual family reunion celebrating people's new roles in community life.

The separation phase refers to the separation of the family from the problem. This enables the parents, children, and family workers to join as a team in an effort to counter the difficulty that has been targeted for treatment. The separation is facilitated by externalizing the problem (White & Epston, 1990) with the help of the community.

The phase that characterizes much of treatment is the liminal or transitional stage, which involves the deconstruction of the dominant narratives to make room for alternative knowledge. Preferred stories about individuals, families, and communities are actively identified and authored in individual therapy, family therapy, the residential milieu, the family home, and community settings. This phase is often characterized by uncertainty and anxiety regarding people's self-images, the future of relationships, and the potential for the community to accept the new narrative. When a preferred story has become a newly dominant narrative that can support safe family interactions in the community, the reincorporation phase begins and the resident is ready to move home.

The reincorporation phase is the time for a celebration of a family's new skill in living a preferred story with community members present to validate the preferred narrative. Our facility found a need to develop a new ritual to mark the transition in treatment because the dominant theory regarding the "termination" of the treatment process emphasized the loss of the therapeutic relationship, which is inconsistent with the rite-of-passage metaphor for the process of change. An approach was needed that highlighted the significance of the reunification of the family in order to be consistent with the order and spirit of the process. Through a conversation among program staff, David Epston, and various participants at a conference, a ritualistic family reunion was conceived as a way to recognize and celebrate this transition in treatment.[2] When this idea was made a part of our practice, we found that the planning of the family reunion helps to focus the treatment process. The celebration provides the opportunity for a preferred narrative to be articulated and the supporting structure to be reinforced.

A large cast of characters participate in the reunion. The therapists entered the family's life specifically to coauthor an alternative story, so it is natural that they withdraw as central figures in the family's life at this point. The therapists do have a role at the reunion as historians documenting the narratives that have passed and those that have emerged. People from the community and the treatment center team (both paid staff and family consultants) are present at the reunion as part of the new social support system that will participate in the alternative narrative as it is lived. As the audience grows larger, the new narrative gains context because each person joining the conversation offers new family, social, economic, cultural, and racial perspectives to the discourse. This allows and encourages a variety of people to recognize and accept their part in the historically dominant narrative as well as the newly emerging alternative.

Reintegration into the community is symbolically marked by the family reunion, including invitations, food, music, reminiscing about the past, ruminating about hopes for the future, reacquainting oneself with old friends, establishing new relationships, games, awards, photographs, and videotaping. This process is intended to take advantage of the power of the community to author a story that will be privileged over other versions of the same "reality." Just as each family story is unavoidably integrated into the story of the community that embraces it, community

[2]The conference, "Case Conversations with David Epston," took place on June 18, 1993, at the Family Institute of Cambridge in Watertown, MA.

members are an invaluable coauthoring audience to the continually developing narratives.

The dialogue of the reunion often contributes to the creation or dissemination of a new use of vocabulary that enables all participants to express and thus authenticate previously unnoticed or unproclaimed narratives. The language of the community becomes privileged over professional language. Problems are separated from people and a commitment is made to a team effort to counter the problems.

The preferred story becomes embedded in the collective memory of the family and community by an appeal to all the senses of those present. Important clinical messages become associated with the sound of music familiar to the community, the taste and smell of food prepared by significant people, the feeling of the known furniture, and the decor of the home. Just as particular music may remind a person of a wedding or food of a christening, certain sensory experiences become associated with a child's successful return home. The planned touching moments and the unexpected surprises form memories that make the celebrated change a part of the family's daily consciousness.

As a part of the reunion, presentations are made and a citation is presented that offer an account of the developments that occurred in treatment. The language used is often from verbatim transcriptions of conversations that occurred in therapy. These ceremonies serve the purpose of renaming previously problematic stories and acknowledging the significance and prominence of newly noticed narratives.

The most prominent event at each reunion is the opportunity for each guest to make a statement to the family and community. These statements place the preferred narrative in a landscape of action and a landscape of consciousness (Bruner, 1986; White, 1991). The landscape of action establishes a sense of how stories have developed over time. The landscape of consciousness addresses the interpretations of the characters in the story and the interpretations of the readers as they try to enter the consciousness of these characters. The landscape of consciousness includes perceptions, speculations, realizations, and conclusions regarding desires, qualities, motives, and beliefs. The many characters participating in a family reunion engage in public conversation that serves to establish these landscapes for the preferred narrative, and this translates into a commitment to a lifestyle consistent with the narrative.

KIMBERLY AND DONNA'S FAMILY REUNION

As a part of the admission process to the Beal Street Program, Kimberly and Donna, together with program staff, agreed to work toward reuniting the family in a process that would culminate in a family reunion to be held in the home in which they would live together. Obstacles to the reunion were identified and family strengths elicited. The strengths included Kimberly and Donna's commitment to each other and the goal of reunion, the desire to talk about the situation, a determined spirit, and the support of both Narcotics Anonymous and friends and relatives. Obstacles included the fact that they were homeless at this point, a violent man was still an active part of their lives, drug abuse was still a temptation, and physical violence had become a way to settle differences in their lives. In the course of the family's six-month involvement with the program, Kimberly and Donna gradually developed a way to use their strengths to overcome these obstacles. Meanwhile, Donna was living with a formerly homeless family as arranged through a community program, and Kimberly resided at the residence. At the same time, they began planning a family reunion including details such as a guest list, invitations, food, and music.

Six months after beginning the Beal Street Program, Kimberly and Donna moved into a two-bedroom apartment together and the final preparations for the celebration took place. Family, friends, and family workers helped them move, unpack, and clean the apartment. People volunteered to bring food and drink. The invitations were sent out and an enthusiastic response was received.

The reunion took place late one afternoon in their crowded apartment. About 30 people were present. The participants included present and past residents of the Beal Street Program; family workers; therapists who had supported the family in the past and intended to support them in the future; relatives, including Donna's mother, whom they had not seen in two years; a guidance counselor from Kimberly's school; the woman and her children who had provided Donna with a home during the previous six months; the state social service worker assigned to the case; and family friends. A buffet of sweets and beverages was laid out on the dining room table in their basement apartment. Adults were continuously looking for more coffee and kids were looking for more cookies. The "rap" music that was playing was alternately being turned up by the teenagers and down by the adults. A few people were taking pictures and a video camera was capturing the event for the family. The celebration was engaging all the senses and becoming a part of the collective memory of what life in this new home is going to be like.

After people had socialized for a while, a brief introduction was given explaining that everyone would have an opportunity to make a statement or presentation. Another girl from the Beal Street Program, Beth, offered to begin. Early in the partnership between the family and the Beal Street Program, Kimberly kicked a hole through a wall when she was angry about a limit that had been set. As a part of the effort to repair the damage, the hole was cut from the wall when it was repaired. Beth presented the cut out hole as a humorous symbol of a past behavior that now seemed beyond what Kimberly would consider doing. The young woman who presented the hole stated, "This is a hole that Kimberly kicked in the wall at Beal Street. You can't see it at the residence anymore because it's been fixed, but we wanted Kimberly to have it to remember how things used to be."

Following this, a proclamation written by the family therapist, using Kimberly and Donna's words, was read by another young woman:

> *This document is to certify that Kimberly and Donna have successfully met the demands of their family reunion. Over the last seven months, both have worked to have "Big Ears." By that they mean to say that they have engaged in practices of listening to one another more patiently and working together toward more productive and satisfying ways of relating to one another. They stand before you, their community, and proclaim on this day that united they stand as a thirteen-year-old female who engages in typical thirteen-year-old practices and the Mom who tolerantly and patiently practices the art of mothering a teenage daughter. We, here at Beal Street, wish them continued success and hope to hear from them, and the community that welcomes them home, more about their future abilities to negotiate and master healthy family practices. Best of luck and congratulations. You both deserve it!!!!!*

The family's new, humorous, and memorable use of the words "big ears" and other language to describe their new skills becomes a part of the language familiar to the community. The family intention to commit to each other and against past difficulties is clearly stated. The idea that this new story will be carried into the future is presented.

At this point everyone was offered the opportunity to speak. A number of teenagers made brief statements wishing the family good luck, and joking about Kimberly's good looks and big ears. A family worker named Ed then commented: "It's been a pleasure to get to know you. I'm glad to see you've stopped beating up boys and are starting to date them instead. I'll miss you. I hope you come and visit, and *Ya Hoo*!" These comments marked Kimberly's passage from being a child of the community to being a young adult. The cheer occurs at each reunion that the teenagers attend and they anticipate Ed's doing it. It is one symbol of Kimberly's joining the ranks of program veterans.

Another family worker named John commented: "Today's a happy day for Kimberly and Donna. Donna, you're one of the parents I've seen helping out, giving us a hand. I think you deserve a lot of credit for that. You've been through a lot of stuff and you've hung in there. I think that's a pretty good accomplishment . I hope things go well and keep in touch."

A third worker named Maureen added: "I want to congratulate both Donna and Kimberly, and I hope things continue to go well for both of you. One of the best qualities of Kimberly is the strong respect she has for herself and her ability to give advice to others to respect themselves. I hope you keep in touch and come by and visit."

A woman who is part of a parent support group Donna attends offered: "Good luck, congratulations, and keep in mind that you have to have a lot of patience and listen to each other and things will work out fine."

Donna's mother said: "I'm shocked because I only thought there were going to be a couple of people here. I said 'who are all these people.' This is wonderful. I haven't seen her for what, two years? I think she looks marvelous."

The woman who took Donna into her home in recent months was holding one of her twin toddlers while Donna held the other. This woman stated: "When Donna called me and told me about this, I was thrilled to be here. Donna and I spent a lot of time together during the time that Kimberly was there and I'm real glad your home. I saw the work. I saw that it's a day at a time, and they've both worked real, real hard to make this happen."

Donna's sister Anne began crying, while saying: "Well, I've been with them for a long time and it's been a hard road, a very hard road, but I'm glad its here. Good luck, Kim. Good luck, Don. We're with you."

A guidance counselor from Kimberly's public school stated: "I want to say congratulations to Kimberly and Donna for all the hard work that you've done to rebuild your family, and also to the staff at Beal Street and the kids for all the hard work you've done because I don't think this would be happening so early otherwise. I don't think you know this, Kimberly, but in September when you left the hospital the principal had a lot of concerns about you returning to our school. You've just done a really marvelous job, and you should feel really proud of yourself."

These comments are typical of many that acknowledge the family strengths, state the desire for things to go well in the future, and make commitments to support the family in their new life together. This new narrative is contextualized by an audience that contains a varied cast of characters bringing diverse perspectives to the conversation.

At various times as the reunion progressed there were interruptions as more guests arrived, a stereo in another apartment was turned up loud, the cat scratched a guest, a neighborhood child looked in the windows, a toddler became restless, and a teenager was reprimanded for having a mouth full of food while talking. Instead of detracting from the ritual, these common occurrences seem to place the success being celebrated in the everyday life of the family.

After a variety of other people spoke, Cheryl, the therapist who had worked with the family throughout the process, commented:

> "It's been a very exciting fun-filled seven months. It's been quick, and I think that has a lot to do with how hard you've worked, Kimberly, and how hard your mom has worked. I feel proud to see you sitting here in this house and all these people here celebrating with and for you. I remember in the beginning how things were. You had a hard time just sitting in the same room together. You've come so far and I think that had a lot to do with you being honest with one another. And like most people here have already said, Donna, you being there five, six, or seven days a week offering us help, giving us advice on your daughter, cooking, and being the mother of Kimberly. Kimberly, you've survived so many difficult issues in your life, and I see you sitting there and you're so typically thirteen! I think a lot of that credit goes to your Aunt Anne, who when we asked early on in family therapy to consult to us, was there for our meeting without hesitation. And as Mrs. Gonsalves from school said, you've used the support of the kids and staff very well . For this occasion, I have an audiotape of a meeting that Kimberly, her mother, and I had. We taped this four months ago summing up the first big session where we talked about Kimberly getting ready to leave, and how well Kimberly and her mom started talking to and listening to one another. So, we thought we'd play it today."

The tape, which the therapist Cheryl narrated, was then played for the crowd:

> "Today I asked Donna and Kimberly what they've noticed about themselves that might lead them to get along better lately. I've asked them to notice what they've been doing differently that would lead them to this 'getting along.' Kimberly started by saying she's controlling herself better, she's taking space in her room, and she's not 'flipping out' on people. Her mother noticed that Kimberly has been listening better, she's more patient, and that she doesn't have to tell Kimberly to do things twice. Donna noticed that she is listening to Kimberly better. She's paying more attention when Kimberly is angry and more attention when she's successful as well. And Donna said she's sticking to her guns for the first time, being real consistent, and having more respect for herself and her efforts with Kimberly. Kimberly and Donna named these listening successes 'getting huge

> ears,' just like those of a little boy they know. We then talked about what other developments were going on in their lives at this time that might support them in listening to one another more effectively. Donna said there seems to be a lot less negative influence from the community. She noted several more positive influences developing for them since becoming homeless. Mary, the woman who offered her a temporary home and support, is one of these. Narcotics Anonymous is another. Donna noticed that being around Mary and watching her parent her three-year-old twins, helped her view firsthand the benefits of patience and positive attention with children. Donna, in dealing with these twins, began to experience herself as relating to children differently, with a better attitude, more patience, and in turn she received a better response from the kids. This ongoing experience, she felt, helped her efforts with Kimberly. Donna also noticed that Kimberly, by being at Beal Street and going to feedback meetings, groups, and Alateen was also developing skills. All these things have been put in place to help them to be patient and experience the benefits of positive attention. In finishing the summary of this session, Kimberly agreed to act as a consultant to kids coming to this program in the future, possibly with the use of this tape. She also said she would join us for Alateen and other groups following her family reunion. Donna agreed as well to act as a consultant and to return for parents group." [Then Kimberly pushed the button to stop the tape.]

Cheryl continued: "That was four months ago, early on in our planning for this family reunion. We were talking about who would be here and what food we would have. That just proves that if you really start planning and talking about these issues, a family reunion can occur and families do reach their goals."

Kimberly then said something brief to everyone in the room. She thanked people, told them she loved them, and offered liberal doses of advice on how they should live their lives. She then addressed her mother: "She's going to start crying. Mom, I love you. I'm glad that we've been working on things together. You are one of the most embarrassing persons that I have known. Congratulations on your six years sobriety. I know that if you haven't used by now, you won't. You did stick with it. I love you and everything." Everyone in the room applauded.

Donna then addressed the group:

> "I don't want to say something to people individually, but I just want to thank the staff that's always been there and was there to encourage me. That's what you guys did, encouraged me. And every time I

made another decision, or I did something else, or I didn't know what the hell to do, or I came running looking for some help, you guys were like 'all right Donna, good to see you're doing it, and good to see you here, and thanks for coming.' I wondered, are you guys told to say this (*everyone laughs*), you're all saying the same thing. (*Donna then imitates a staff person in high-pitched voice*) 'no, no, we're *really* glad you did it' (*more laughter*). That was what gave me the confidence to be able to keep going because I didn't have a lot of confidence in what I was doing. I was clueless as far as what to do. I just want to thank you all because all my insanity and all my insecurities and all my stuff are part of what Kimberly's going through. I just appreciate all your support. To my family, and my sister, and *my* therapist, thanks to everybody that came. Kimberly, *I love you.*"

That was the final formal part of the reunion, although people stayed around and socialized, ate, drank, and generally enjoyed themselves.

KIMBERLY'S AND DONNA'S COMMENTS ON THE PROCESS

Kimberly and Donna continued to consult with the program after their family reunion. They offered the following comments in response to questions posed by their family therapist, Cheryl, one month after the reunion.

CHERYL: Which abilities that helped you have a successful reunion do you think will be most helpful when you face future challenges?

DONNA: A lot of my vigilance, a lot of my "keep going." I've been where I've said I would be when I said I would be there. I've been making an effort to spend time with her, making an effort to find out what she's doing, why she's doing it, and if she ends up grounded, she stays that way.

CHERYL: How about you, Kimberly?

KIMBERLY: Work . . . togetherness . . . working together. You know what, my favorite thing is chaos (*smiling sarcastically*).

DONNA: I think you worked against creating chaos. You worked to the opposite. Chaos is something that we were used to being in and we get comfortable in it sometimes to the point we create it all the time. I think that Kimberly worked as hard as she could to find different ways. She also got real verbal.

CHERYL: Could you notice along the way when you were preparing to live back at home what you were doing to make that work out?

KIMBERLY: We work together, not against each other. Work together! Every question you ask that's going to be my answer, work together. I wasn't yelling, I was listening.

DONNA: We changed a lot of the influences in our lives and tried to create new ones.

CHERYL: Was there anyone else that noticed these things along the way and pointed them out to you?

KIMBERLY: My aunt.

DONNA: Everybody knew, everybody noticed how different I was with her, how different she was with me, how different she was with people, period. They noticed that she listens, that she's not as loud as she used to be. Some friends think it's remarkable, the change in her. They've known her since she was three years old. They say she's a lot calmer, she's a lot more focused on paying attention.

KIMBERLY: They would say . . . "oh, your mother's trying."

CHERYL: Was that something different they were telling you about your mother or was that something they told you all your life?

KIMBERLY: That was different.

CHERYL: When you first came into the program your family story included fighting and not getting along. Over time it seems that you have created a different family story for yourselves, this story of working together and controlling tempers. What discoveries or steps are you making now that will continue to invite this new story in the future?

DONNA: On a daily basis I'm surprised how well we treat each other. I love the leaps and bounds of growth that we've made. The relationship we have today is better than I could ever have imagined it would be.

KIMBERLY: That's normal.

DONNA: I think that's awesome. We're not fighting about things. She does nice little things for me lately, like the lilacs she picked me.

CHERYL: I want you to try to remember the comments that people celebrating your family reunion made to you about your family.

KIMBERLY: "I'm proud of you and your mother."

CHERYL: Right. Would it have been important for any people who weren't there to have heard all those people say, "I'm proud of you and your mother"?

DONNA: Her dad. To see these accomplishments we've made.

KIMBERLY: Yeah, my dad. Well, he missed out!!!

DONNA: Yeah! That we've accomplished something, that it took a long time, that it took six and a half years of a little bit of craziness, but were coming out on the other end (*tears*). People that were in our lives, people that saw us at our worst, people that saw me not be nice to her, that saw her not be nice to me, people that I haven't seen in a long time, part of what I say to them is that Kimberly and I have been through a lot of stuff but we're on the other side. Which before, I didn't see any other side. I saw complete insanity, and it was never, ever going to get any better.

CHERYL: How might you be able to let all these people know?

KIMBERLY: I've already let a lot of people know.

DONNA: I've been thinking about giving her dad a call or writing a letter to let him know that she has become responsible.

KIMBERLY: Who has? We have. Don't put it all on me.

DONNA: Sorry, Kim, that *we* have become a loving, caring family unit that works together and umm . . . (*tears*).

CHERYL: What is the single most important thing that you would say to another family entering the Beal Street Program.

DONNA: Don't stop.

KIMBERLY: Don't stop trying.

Six months later, during a conversation with Cheryl and Tim, who is the director of the program, Donna made the following comments regarding the significance of marking the end of treatment with a reunion held in her home.

DONNA: It was important to us that the reunion be at our apartment because you need to bring it home. This is where it's going to start again. It's a new beginning. When you first talked about a family reunion, I couldn't picture it. As it got closer I could see it, and we got really excited. It was more personal having it here. It was nice having it here because it was part of our new beginning in our new house. My mother was blown away by how many people there were here and the support we have. I was glad for her to hear who I am, who Kimberly is, and how far we've come. Having Mary [the woman who provided housing] here was important because she walked me through all the insanity. She was there at the beginning of it and at the and of it. It was important that her kids were here because they reminded me how important it is to be patient and tolerant with kids. It was important to have all the people who made up our support system here, without them we wouldn't be here. And it was important to have them here to help us celebrate. The reunion affirms that we have changed and that this is a whole new beginning. . . .

REFERENCES

Abrahamson, I. (Ed.). (1985). *Against silence: The voice and vision of Elie Wiesel* (Vol. 3). New York: The Holocaust Library.

Bruner, J. (1986). *Actual minds, possible worlds.* Cambridge, MA: Harvard University Press.

Durrant, M. (1993). *Residential treatment: A cooperative competency-based approach to therapy and program design.* New York: Norton.

Epston, D., & White M. (1992). *Experience, contradiction, narrative, and imagination.* Adelaide, South Australia: Dulwich Centre Publications.

Gilliland-Mallo, D., & Judd, P. (1986). The effectiveness of residential treatment for boys. *Adolescence, 21*(82), 311–321.

Gutterman, N., & Blythe, B. (1986, December). Toward ecologically based intervention in residential treatment for children. *Social Service Review,* pp. 633–643.

Lewis, W. (1984). Ecological change: A necessary condition for residential treatment. *Child Care Quarterly, 13*(1), 21–29.

Nichols, T. (1989). *The evaluation of specially supported aftercare programs for latency-age children: A comprehensive single subject design in conjunction with staff interviews.* Unpublished master's thesis, Smith College School of Social Work.

Taylor, D., & Alpert, S. (1973). *Continuity and support following residential treatment.* New York: Child Welfare League of America.

van Gennep, A. (1908). *The rites of passage.* London: Routledge & Kegan Paul.

White, M. (1991). Deconstruction and therapy. In D. Epston & M. White (Eds.), *Experience, contradiction, narrative, and imagination* (pp. 109–151). Adelaide, South Australia: Dulwich Centre Publications.

White, M., & Epston, D. (1990). *Narrative means to therapeutic ends.* New York: Norton.

CHAPTER 15

A Journey of Change through Connection

Janet Adams-Westcott
Deanna Isenbart

THE SECRECY AND SHAME experienced by adults molested as children often creates a sense of isolation. People we have worked with report that they have difficulty trusting or feeling connected to others. This chapter describes a therapeutic process that creates a rite of passage to help people overcome isolation and escape stories of victimization.[1] Based on a narrative approach to psychotherapy, a series of four groups were developed to help people (1) separate from stories about self that are defined by victimization; (2) recognize their own competence and expertise; (3) develop interpersonal patterns that invite mutuality and connection with others; and (4) experiment with stories about self that reflect the richness of their own lived experience.[2] Group members provide an audience for the emergence of preferred and more empowering narratives about self and relationships.

IDEAS THAT GUIDE OUR WORK

Personal Narratives

Our work is influenced by social constructionist ideas about "self" (Anderson & Goolishian, 1990; Gergen, 1991). As such, we assume that

[1]This is a revision of presentations given by the authors at the Texas Association for Marriage and Family Therapy, San Antonio, Texas, January 1993, and at Narrative Ideas and Therapeutic Practice, Vancouver, British Columbia, April 1994.

[2]These groups are funded, in part, by a Victims of Crime Assistance Grant and are offered at minimal or no cost to participants.

the self is an interpersonal rather than an intrapsychic phenomenon. A person's sense of self emerges when interpersonal conversations are internalized as inner conversations (Tomm, 1989b). These conversations are then organized into stories or personal narratives that we use to make sense out of our experiences.

Stories about self evolve from a variety of sources: Our lived experiences make the most important contributions to our stories about self and relationships (White & Epston, 1990). Our narratives about self are also shaped by cultural stories about who we should be as individuals, women or men, friends, or partners (Hare-Mustin, 1991; Weingarten, 1991; White & Epston, 1990). Narratives outside our experience also contribute to the stories we perform. We can be influenced by stories about who we are that were developed by family members prior to our birth (Parry, 1991). We can be invited by others to participate in interpersonal patterns that support particular narratives (Tomm, 1989b).

The dominant stories we perform about self create a "perceptual lens" through which subsequent life events are interpreted (White & Epston, 1990). We notice information that fits with the dominant story about our lives and relationships. As we look back through time, we interpret our experiences within the framework offered by the story. We interact with others in the present in a manner consistent with this interpretation. Figure 15.1 illustrates how these interactions can be added to lived experience in a way that reinforces the dominant narrative.

The stories we develop about ourselves can be empowering and generative or disempowering and oppressive. People experience personal agency when they internalize conversations about themselves that reflect the richness of their lived experiences (Adams-Westcott, Dafforn, & Sterne, 1993; Tomm, 1989a). Such stories allow people to consider a variety of possible explanations for events and choose viable solutions to the challenges of living.

Problems develop when people internalize conversations that don't allow them to access the full range of their lived experiences. These stories are experienced as oppressive because they limit the person's ability to consider alternative views and perceive available choices. Over time, people may develop a view of self that is problem-saturated (White & Epston, 1990). Experiences that don't fit the problem story are either not perceived as meaningful or interpreted in a way that supports a disqualified view of self.

The Process of Change

Anthropologists have examined how rites of passage help people in different cultures negotiate developmental transitions (Roberts, 1988).

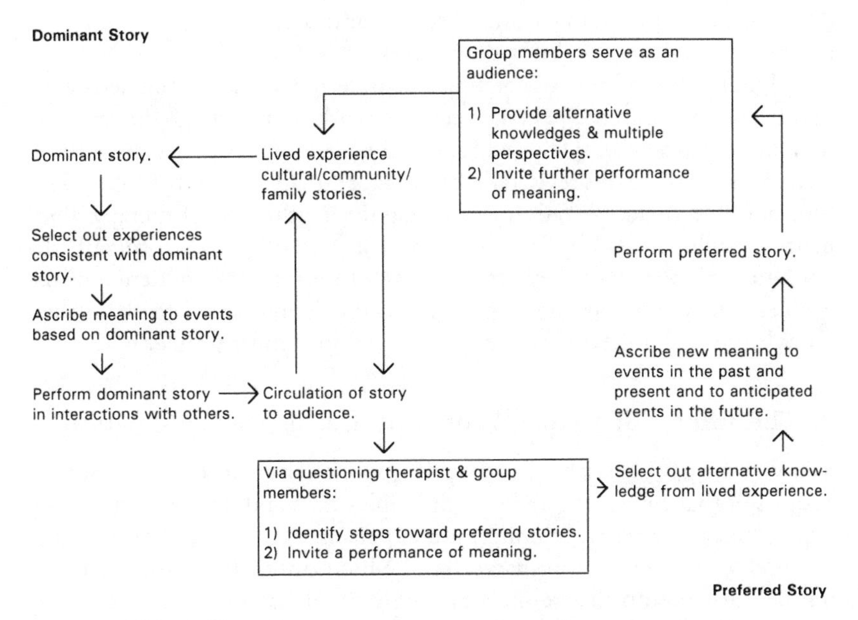

FIGURE 15.1. Group therapy as an audience for preferred stories.

Rites of passage begin when people start to separate from an old status or identity that no longer fits for them. They then experience a transitional period characterized by disorganization and experimentation with new ideas and behaviors. When the transition is successfully negotiated, the ideas and behaviors are incorporated into the person's evolved description of self. The community recognizes that change has occurred and acknowledges the person's new status.

The rites-of-passage analogy has been used to conceptualize change within the context of the narrative approach developed by Michael White and David Epston (Adams-Westcott & Isenbart, 1990; Epston & White 1990; White, 1986; White & Epston, 1990). This approach assumes that people present for therapy when significant aspects of their lived experience contradict the dominant story about themselves and their relationships. Symptoms and crises are considered evidence of progress and indicate that the person has already begun separating from a story that is no longer viable.

The separation process is facilitated by externalizing conversations (Epston, 1993; White & Epston, 1990). These conversations locate the problem or problematic beliefs, behaviors, or stories outside the person. Questions are asked that invite people to assume the perspective of an observer and reflect on their experiences. They gain access to experiences that contradict problem-saturated stories and begin to experiment with more preferred stories about themselves.

The process of reincorporating the preferred story is facilitated when significant people in the person's social network acknowledge the transformation. Significant people provide an audience to help the person authenticate and celebrate this revised description of self. Epston and White (1990) have adopted reincorporation as a metaphor for the end of therapy. They invite people to move from the role of "client" to "consultant" by documenting the steps they went through to escape the influence of the problem story. They create opportunities for "consultants" to share their knowledge with others who are struggling with similar problems.

The Effects of Sexual Abuse: Stories of Disqualification

Many of the people with whom we have worked have internalized stories about self that reflect the feelings of helplessness and powerlessness they experienced as a result of childhood experiences of abuse. These stories can create an "abuse-dominated lens" which only allows the person to notice information that reinforces a view of self as powerless. They may fail to notice or ascribe meaning to those lived experiences when they behaved in a competent manner or when others treated them as a person of worth (Durrant & Kowalski, 1990; Kamsler, 1990).

Access to alternative explanations from the person's own experience is limited by inner conversations that disqualify self-knowledge (Adams-Westcott et al., 1993; Gilligan, 1991). As a result, the person or others may doubt the validity of experiences that contradict the dominant narrative. The inner dialogue may invite the person to interpret these exceptions as evidence of their own psychopathology and to engage in self-pathologizing behaviors. They may participate in interpersonal patterns that have the effect of isolating them from the experiences of other people and, as a result, the experiences that other people have of them.

Often, persons in "authority" are viewed as the only legitimate source of knowledge, including knowledge about one's own experiences. As a result, many people turn to the media and self-help literature to try to make sense out of their experiences. Too often, these popular discourses reinforce disqualifying descriptions of self by focusing on deficits and dysfunction.

A Narrative Approach to Group Therapy

A series of therapy groups was developed to create a rite of passage to help people who have experienced child sexual abuse escape stories of victimization.[3] We have adopted a journey metaphor to describe the group series. We invite group members to develop connections and create a community that supports each participant's personal journey of change. This "community" provides an audience for members to (1) develop their own self-knowledge, (2) practice more validating stories about self, and (3) incorporate preferred narratives into their lived experience.

As therapists, we are interested in helping people develop their own self-knowledge. To accomplish this, we assume a collaborative role and ask questions or design activities that focus on the lived experience of participants. Whenever possible we are joined by consultants who have been members of previous groups. The consultant shares her experiences and provides hope to those people who are just beginning to challenge the effects of abuse.[4]

Over time, group members become consultants to themselves and to each other. They assume a reflecting position as they listen to each other discuss their struggles and successes (Andersen, 1991). When they compare their experiences to others, they begin to notice steps they have taken to overcome the effects of abuse. Multiple perspectives and possibilities are introduced when members share their experiences with each other.

The group becomes a place to experiment with new ways of thinking and interacting. Group members can offer each other perspectives that are not colored by the "abuse-dominated lens." They can turn down invitations to participate in "victim stories." They can interact in ways that validate each person's self-knowledge and worth. Group members provide an audience that witnesses the performance of preferred stories. They can help each other recognize and celebrate small steps in the direction of change. Figure 15.1 illustrates how group members invite each other to extend the preferred story and, in doing so, provide opportunities to cocreate lived experiences that support their evolving narratives.

During the last four years, more than 300 women and men have participated in the groups. The groups were developed in the context of a family service agency that serves a metropolitan area. Professionals from private practice and public agencies have referred people to these services. Some participants choose group as their primary involvement

[3]This chapter focuses on three groups developed for the person who experienced child sexual abuse. A fourth group was developed for couples where one partner was molested as a child. This group is titled Enhancing Connections and was designed to help partners escape the effects of abuse and develop healing interpersonal patterns.

[4]To date, all of consultants have been women.

with therapy. Other people choose to participate in group therapy as an adjunct to individual therapy. A minority of referring professionals consider themselves narrative or solution-oriented therapists.

Though the groups were designed as a series, people are invited to participate in particular group experiences that enhance their personal journey of change. Some people choose to complete the entire series, whereas others choose to participate in one or two of the groups.

The majority of participants have been women, although some groups have included both women and men. Participants have told us that they were initially uncomfortable with this arrangement but found the experience to be extremely valuable in challenging their beliefs about gender roles in general as well as the particular beliefs they developed about men and women as a result of their history of victimization.

We prefer that people struggling with suicidal behavior, self-mutilating behavior or delusional thinking develop skills to begin to challenge these problems prior to joining a group. We are sensitive to issues raised by the debate on the false memory syndrome and give careful consideration to requests for group services made by people who have no specific memories of sexual abuse.

Taking the First Step: Separating from Disqualifying Stories

"Taking the First Step" is a six-week psychoeducational group developed to help participants begin the process of separating from abuse-dominated stories and victim lifestyles. A classroom format is used to minimize the discomfort experienced by people who are beginning the process of escaping secrecy and isolation. The therapist attempts to avoid the expert stance this format invites by sharing the experiences, discoveries, and successes of people we have met in the course of our work. Discussion is invited, although some people attend the six sessions without participating in the conversation. People who chose not to participate in the discussion have told us later that the inner conversations they were having with themselves began to change as a result of their exposure to the ideas and experiences of others.

Over the course of the six sessions, a framework is developed to help participants begin to externalize the effects of abuse. The majority of participants begin the First Step group with the idea that whatever difficulties they are experiencing result from some personal defect. Those participants who have attended lectures or read the popular literature may believe that they have been permanently damaged by the experience of abuse.

A variety of interventions are used to externalize the effects of abuse. Many of the people we work with continue to be influenced by the story they developed to help make sense out of the experience of abuse when they were a child. This influence is demonstrated by asking participants to consider the experience of sexual abuse from the point of view of children at different developmental levels. For example, the concrete way that children think is illustrated by describing the experience of a five-year-old girl who was had been abused by her father and was living in a foster home. This child suddenly became terrified of going to a popular fast-food restaurant. Her therapist discovered that the child had heard a television advertisement saying that a visit to this restaurant could make all your dreams come true. The girl believed her nightmares would come true if the foster family ate at this restaurant.

Participants are asked to consider how that child might make sense out of the experience of abuse given her cognitive development:

- What story might she develop about herself?
- How might the fact that no one protected her influence the conclusions she makes about herself?
- What might she think about herself if her body responded with pleasure?
- How might the experience of abuse affect a child who thought she was the only person who had ever been molested?

Considering the perspective of a child invites participants to experience compassion for themselves. The conversation helps participants begin to entertain the idea that their descriptions of self might be stories rather than some essential reality about who they are as people.

Stories are shared with participants that demonstrate how people get recruited into stories of victimization. The events of one young person's life are described and participants are invited to speculate about the dominant story she develops about herself. Group members are asked to predict how the disqualifying story will influence the young person's development during adolescence and adulthood. A number of exceptions to the problem story are identified and participants are asked to consider how the person might interpret these experiences within the framework of her dominant story.

Participants are also asked to speculate about how that person might begin to escape from an abuse-dominated story. They are invited to offer a different description of the person that takes into account the exceptions to the disqualifying story. Participants are asked for their ideas about how this person might be invited to see herself the way they see her.

They are asked to consider how the person might interact with others in more healing ways.

Aspects of dominant and alternative stories identified in the conversation are juxtaposed using Venn diagrams that elementary school teachers employ to demonstrate the concept of sets and subsets. Different colors are used to depict events that fit with dominant or alternative stories. Participants are asked for their ideas about how to help the person highlight events in the alternative story and move these events into the foreground of the person's experience so that the events that make up the dominant story recede into the background. Within the context of the alternative story, participants begin to suggest new meanings for events the person experienced in the past.

Participants are invited to speculate about how this person might respond to stressful events in the future. Given that the disqualifying story remains in the background of the person's experience, participants begin to see setbacks as potential responses to stressors or crises. This discussion opens space for participants to be less harsh on themselves when circumstances invite them into old ways of thinking and behaving.

This conversation helps people begin to escape from a view of the problem as caused by some personal defect. They begin to view the problem as the consequence of their experiences of oppression and disqualification. This dialogue has the effect of introducing a view of change that is evolutionary and optimistic.

The stories of previous participants are shared to validate and normalize experiences that invite participants to "feel crazy." For example, participants are asked to compare the reactions of people who "survive" tornadoes and people who "survive" child sexual abuse. They are also asked to compare how observers might interpret these reactions. They often conclude that both categories of survivors might experience difficulty sleeping, flashbacks, and other similar reactions. They believe that observers are likely to empathize with the behavior of a tornado survivor and interpret the behavior of the abuse survivor as pathological.

People who experience intrusive flashbacks seldom understand the connection between sensory cues related to the abuse and the onset of these disturbing perceptual experiences. Participants are invited to recognize the sensory cues that have the potential to evoke these responses. Practical solutions developed by previous group members are offered as strategies to minimize the influence of flashbacks on participants' daily lives. These strategies often combine symbols of safety with visual images that include the experience of mastery. One group member interrupted flashbacks of abuse by touching a piece of jewelry she had been given by a group of friends. This reminded her that she was in the present rather than the past and surrounded by supportive friends.

Another person carried the remote from her videocassette recorder as a reminder that she would "pause" or "stop" the images. Another participant pictured herself growing from a vulnerable child into a strong adult as the person who molested her became smaller and eventually disappeared.

Stories are also shared to help participants normalize struggles they might have with intimacy and sexuality. A distinction is introduced between sex and violence by summarizing Sanders (1988), "When an assailant assaults a victim with the intent of robbery and uses a hockey stick, we don't call it 'hockey,' we call it assault" (p. 26). A description of sexual intimacy that focuses on each person's experience is introduced for discussion. For an interaction to be sexually intimate, Sanders argues that both partners must experience choice, mutuality, arousal, vulnerability, and trust. Interactions that do not include these elements are not sex. Depending on the context, penetration of a woman by a man without sexual intimacy may be described as business, duty, reproduction, or violence. Participants are asked to consider how they might interpret their experiences differently if they adopted this definition of sexual intimacy.

Stories are shared that describe resourceful young people who developed habits such as dissociation, alcohol abuse, reading, or overeating to experience a sense of safety and to cope with the experience of abuse. Participants are encouraged to identify any habits they might have developed and to consider how those habits were helpful. They are asked to evaluate whether these habits continue to work for them now that they are adults.

Group members are invited to identify other resources they have available to them through a variety of solution-focused techniques. Participants have found the interventions described by Dolan (1991) to be especially helpful. A series of questions is asked to help participants identify possible solutions and recognize what they are already doing that is helpful.

- What will be the first sign that you are beginning to escape the effects of sexual abuse?
- What will you be doing differently?
- What will you be thinking about instead of thinking about the abuse?
- Are there times when this is already happening to some extent?
- What is different during those times when it is already happening?
- What do you think the people who are important to you will notice when the abuse is less influential in your life?
- What differences will these changes make in your relationships?

Participants are invited to imagine a time in the future when they are old and wise (Dolan, 1991). They are asked to consider what advice their older, wiser self might offer to help them make it through this difficult time in their present life. The older, wiser self is invited to reflect on what personal resources and new ways of thinking and interacting she discovered that helped her escape the effects of abuse.

Consideration of these questions helps shift the focus of participants from the past to the present. Answers to these questions also help participants begin to develop concrete treatment goals. Identifying small changes provides participants with the experience of hope as they begin to understand how they can make a difference in their own lives.

Escaping the Past: Internalizing Personal Agency

"Escaping the Past" is a 16-week psychotherapy group developed to help people negotiate the transitional phase of this rite of passage. New groups are scheduled to begin two weeks after the last session of the Taking the First Step group. Most often, Escaping the Past combines participants who have completed the six-week group and people who have had previous group experiences or who have been in individual therapy for an extended period of time.

The psychotherapy group is less structured than the psychoeducational group. The content of the conversation is developed from the recommendations of group members. The therapist organizes conversations and activities to help participants (1) continue the process of externalizing disqualifying self-stories, (2) access self-knowledge and ascribe meaning to lived experiences that contradict the disqualifying story, and (3) begin to describe a story about self that recognizes the person's own agency.

The development of personal agency is an important aspect of our work with people who have experienced child sexual abuse (Adams-Westcott et al., 1993). The process of separating the person from the problem begun during the Taking the First Step group creates space for participants to begin to recognize their own knowledge and give voice to their experiences. The process of separating the person from the problem is continued in the Escaping the Past group. Participants are invited to examine their inadvertent participation in disqualifying self-stories. Questions are asked that map the relationship between their inner conversations and interpersonal interactions. This examination of experience promotes the experience of choice: Participants discover that they can choose to continue to embrace ideas and behaviors that maintain the experience of disqualification and victimization or to interact in more self-validating ways.

Depending on the preferences of group members, this examination can be accomplished by asking questions about specific situations experienced by individual group members or by designing activities that deconstruct disqualifying self-stories in general. One activity asks group members to consider what beliefs and behaviors a person would embrace who describes herself as a victim, a survivor, or a person whose life is no longer defined by the experience of abuse (one group labeled this latter category "transcenders"). These descriptions are then juxtaposed in a chart developed through group discussion or depicted in collages created by individual participants.

This activity deconstructs beliefs and behaviors that maintain stories of victimization. Entertaining the survivor and transcender descriptions invites people to consider alternative beliefs and behaviors and discover how they might already be thinking and interacting in these ways. They begin to recognize these exceptions as examples of competence that had been disqualified in the past.

An exercise has evolved that externalizes the disqualifying inner conversations. The exercise begins with one group member describing a situation or relationship that he/she finds particularly difficult. A second group member agrees to give voice to the disqualifying conversation, while a third group member articulates an alternative and more healing conversation. Remaining group members assume a reflecting position and observe the dialogue between the group members participating in the exercise. When the difficulty is with a particular relationship, a fourth member might join the exercise to role-play the person in question. The group member who has identified the difficulty interrupts the role-play from time to time to consult with group members offering the disqualifying or healing dialogue. At the conclusion of the interchange, the team members ask questions and offer their observations.

Group members serving as participants and team members have described this exercise as particularly liberating because they are able to use the ideas offered by the healing conversation in their daily lives. The exercise has been modified in a number of ways in response to the particular needs of group members. For example, someone might serve as a "coach" to the person providing the validating conversation, or several group members might operate as a "healing chorus" when the disqualifying dialogue exerts a strong influence on the person presenting the difficulty.

Questions modeled by the therapist and consultant encourage a growing recognition of the competence. The therapist is eternally curious about how group members were able to take steps in the direction of the preferred story:

- How did you get ready to take this step?
- What does it mean about you as a person that you were able to take this step?
- What personal qualities helped you prepare to take this step?
- Does taking this step open up possibilities for the future?

Questions that collapse time backward are asked to highlight progress. For example, group members might be asked to compare their reaction to a current challenge with how they might have handled a similar challenge at the time when they began attending the groups. These questions invite the person to notice and account for positive changes they have made.

Group members challenge the process of disqualification by sharing their personal experiences of the changes the person has made over time. Progress is highlighted and hope for the future is provided when group members comment about the changes they have witnessed.

By the end of the 16-week group, participants have begun to recognize their competencies and experiment with more preferred stories about themselves and their relationships. We often observe a shift away from a critical self-observation to a position of curiosity. Group members begin to notice and celebrate small steps in the direction of their preferred story.

Building New Futures: Incorporating Preferred Stories

An open-ended ongoing therapy group is available to help participants incorporate a preferred story into their description of self. Circulation of the preferred story to a community is an important aspect of the reincorporation stage of a rite of passage. Members in the ongoing group assume a collaborative role. Most often, the conversation focuses on performing the preferred story in relationships outside of the group context. Conversations also focus on continuing to help the person revise his/her relationship with self.

- What does it mean about you as a person that you were able to share your experiences with your partner?
- How will sharing your experience with your partner affect how you see yourself?
- How will it affect how you treat yourself?

Group members have worked together to cocreate rituals that punctuate progress and celebrate change. A catching-up ritual has developed where participants introduce themselves to new members by sharing the most important thing they have learned about themselves or the most important step they have taken since beginning group. Participants appreciated this reminder of their progress and asked to begin each group by considering small steps they have taken since the previous meeting. Several members reported that this ritual reminds them to "make things happen" during the week.

One group of participants spent several weeks cocreating a ritual to circulate the changes they had made to significant people outside of the group. They began by identifying the beliefs they no longer held and patterns of interaction in which they did not want to continue to participate. These beliefs and behaviors were written on individual cards and burned in a ceremony conducted during a group session. A "wake" was held to celebrate the "passing" of the disempowering stories. More healing beliefs and interpersonal patterns were written on birth announcements to be shared with family members and friends.

Group members are encouraged to develop daily rituals that maintain their transformed story about self. One member made an audiotape of healing conversations suggested by participants so she could listen to the tape everyday on her way to work. Another member sent daily affirmations to herself via electronic mail.

A number of different graduation rituals have been created by group members to recognize members who are ready to leave the group. One participant referred to the group as her "home base" and discussed her apprehension about maintaining changes after leaving the group. At her last session, group members wrote their observations of the changes she had made on an actual base and that was given to her as a symbol of her progress.

CLINICAL EXAMPLE

An excerpt from a session of an Escaping the Past group is used here to illustrate the way in which the group members provide an audience for emerging narratives. Early sessions of the group focused on helping members to challenge difficulties such as flashbacks, angry outbursts, depression, and self-criticism. Several members made decisions to escape secrecy and began to share their experiences with important people in their lives. One member chose to directly challenge the person who molested her and insisted he assume financial responsibility for her therapy. Several members began to challenge shame. Others began to stand up for themselves at work or with members of their extended families.

During the ninth session, group members began discussing trust, vulnerability and emotional closeness. They decided to invite their partners to the eleventh session and developed a list of questions that guided the conversation with their partners. They were particularly interested in creating interactions in which they and their partners experienced mutual support. They invited their partners to consider questions such as:

- What is it about your partner as a person that has allowed her to begin to take her life back from the abuse?
- What have you learned that you wouldn't have learned if it weren't for your partner's courage to escape the effects of abuse?
- What is it about you as a person that has allowed you to help your partner escape the effects of abuse? What do you think you are doing that appears to be the most helpful in assisting your partner to escape the effects of abuse? What would she say you do that helps her escape the effects of abuse?
- What will be different about your relationship as each of you continues to escape the effects of abuse? What will be different about how the two you interact? What new ways will you discover to support each other? What difference will this make in the future of your relationship?

The next session focused on changes group members had made since beginning the group. One member discussed the "new chapter" he was writing about his life. Members were invited to collapse time backwards by comparing titles of the chapter of their present life with the chapter they were living when they began the group. This conversation helped participants punctuate their progress and revise their description of themselves. By considering the title to the "next chapter," the conversation also helped them collapse time forward and consider how they could help create a preferred future. For each participant, the current chapter included enhancing sexual intimacy in their relationship with their partners. The following excerpt is taken from the beginning of this conversation.

STACEE: If someone asked me what intimacy is, I'm not sure if I could tell them what it is.

LAURA: I feel as if my experience of intimacy is so complicated I don't know if I could cover it in a half an hour [the time remaining for the session].

STACEE: Intimacy is so hard for me not to automatically think of as sex.

LAURA: That's exactly what I think.

ANGIE: That's exactly what I think, too.

THERAPIST: Maybe that conversation would be interesting for a start.

ANGIE: Talk about a struggle—a struggle for me is letting myself enjoy it.

SUSAN: Enjoy "it," meaning?

ANGIE: Sex! Making love. I can't be free. I'm still in this confined little space where I'm so terrified. Finding ways to break out of this is what I need to do.

LAURA: That's my problem.

SALLY: Yeah, I think [it is] for me, too. I think being in touch with my body enough to let go and enjoy it is important. I have to constantly remind myself to relax and not think about how the abuse reminds me of this. I'm so busy thinking about it all the time that I am not relaxing, which defeats the purpose of the whole thing.

ANGIE: I'm still this terrified person that can't breathe [when trying to be sexual].

SALLY: Something you [Angie] said last week, something as simple as needing to keep your eyes closed. Whether it is your eyes or needing to keep the lights out or the position that you are in, it has to be controlled or else we are reminded of the abuse.

THERAPIST: What if I asked the two of you [Angie and Sally] more questions about intimacy and we asked the three of you [Susan, Stacee, and Laura] to listen from the perspective of a person who isn't pushed around by abuse? We could then have our listening team respond to the conversation they heard. What do you think?

GROUP: Yeah, okay . . .

THERAPIST: So tell me a little more about how this struggle influences your life.

ANGIE: Even though I have the desire, it's very hard for me to act on it. To even be verbal about it. I'm trying to get myself to say one thing.

THERAPIST: So is this one of those small goals you were talking about earlier?

ANGIE: Yes. That's right, that's a goal. And just opening my eyes [while being sexual] is another goal.

THERAPIST: Are there ideas or beliefs that seem to get in your way of you meeting this goal?

ANGIE: I think for me it is still a feeling of being dirty. That this was bad. That type of thing. It's got a hold over me.

THERAPIST: That being sexual is bad?

ANGIE: Right, that feeling pleasure. Of course when the incest was going on if you felt yourself feeling pleasure it was like, "How can this be happening? I can't feel that way or else I'm bad."

THERAPIST: I see.

ANGIE: I think that's what it is for me and also the trust. I don't know if I totally trust my husband or maybe I don't trust myself.

THERAPIST: Can I back up just a minute? You talked about still struggling with this idea that when you were little and you responded, there was something bad about you.

ANGIE: When I had sex I feel bad. I'm just like you said you were Sally, so tense and trying to overcome all these things. It defeats your whole purpose of having sex. It's work, keeping your mind on what you're doing.

SALLY: It takes all your energy just staying focused on what's going on.

ANGIE: That's right.

SALLY: Mine is not related to pleasure as much as just that sex is just something that men do to women.

THERAPIST: And by sex, do you mean intercourse?

SALLY: Yeah. Those old messages. "It's not suppose to be pleasurable. It's just a duty that you are performing." So, I never initiate it. It is just suppose to be pleasure for the man. And that's the problem I have with it, in thinking of it that way. I know it's wrong thinking, but I can't get my mind set away from that thinking when it is occurring.

THERAPIST: How did this idea get so much power over you that it robbed you of your judgment and your experience of pleasure?

SALLY: My abuse occurred in a very cold situation like on the bathroom floor. There was no love or even any pleasure in it. [She tells a story of several experiences that lead her to believe she has current physical problems created from the abuse.] It was so cold. It wasn't loving in any way.

THERAPIST: It sounds as if you experienced it as violence.

SALLY: It was violence. It was physically violent. It was the holding you down, "do what I tell you" kind of thing. It was very violent. I remember the floor was so cold and it was very violent. And it was so many times. I think of it as, "this was something you do for men and this is a woman's role."

ANGIE: As if you are here for their taking.

SALLY: Right. You are on earth for their pleasure and not for your own.

THERAPIST: I see. And those ideas still . . .

SALLY: Very much so.

THERAPIST: Are these ideas you want to give up sometime in the future or are they ideas that you need to hang on to?

SALLY: I would like to give them up. Yeah! I would. I would like to be the one to initiate for a change. [Sally discusses the desire to determine whether she has physical scarring from the abuse that might make intercourse painful. This will allow her to be free to explore the emotional aspect of her abuse. She relates that she would like to be able to discuss sexual experiences with close women friends. Sally refers to her abuse as "sex."]

THERAPIST: It seems for you sex means violence. That for you they are very much connected. There is this psychiatrist that takes offense with sexual abuse being called "sexual abuse." He thinks it should be called "genital assault." It is his idea that if you hit someone with a frying pan, you don't call it cooking. If you hit someone with a hockey stick, you don't call it hockey. He argues that what happened to you wasn't sex at all. It was violence. I'm curious, it you were to think about what happened to you not as sex but as violence, what does that bring to mind?

ANGIE: Anger!

SALLY: I've always related the word sex to a meeting of the bodies and not with love. If I could try to think of sex as intimacy and love and all those things we talk about and not violence, then I might be more open to think about it [being more sexual].

THERAPIST: So what possibilities might that open up for you?

SALLY: I feel strongly about the way my husband talks about it. He has to say "make love" or he has to say something that sounds like he cares and not just say, "Come on, Baby, let's go do it." That turns me off right away. Any little bit of desire I might have had is gone.

THERAPIST: What possibilities would it open if you began to think of your abuse as assault?

SALLY: Anger and hate, like she [Angie] said. It is hard to believe that someone so close to you assaulted you like that.

ANGIE: Maybe it [thinking of abuse as assault] would help you direct it [feelings of anger and hate] toward the person that did it [the abuse], not the person you are with.

THERAPIST: How might that happen?

ANGIE: I just know that sometimes it is real easy to take my dad into the bedroom with me. I have to remind myself that this [my husband] is someone that loves me and would never hurt me. It would make it easier to separate the two.

THERAPIST: Have there been times when you have been able to do that?

ANGIE: Maybe a little bit more lately.

THERAPIST: What's that like when you are able to do that, to separate?

SALLY: It's a lot nicer. You can enjoy it . . .

ANGIE: . . . [When I] don't let that part of it play such an important role and just try to enjoy the togetherness, maybe it [sexual pleasure] will come.

THERAPIST: Is that what you tried to do?

ANGIE: Yes.

THERAPIST: And has that been helpful?

ANGIE: Yes, it has.

THERAPIST: Has it helped you achieve the kind of closeness you want?

ANGIE: Yes.

THERAPIST: I've argued that what has happened to you is violence and not sex and I keep asking, "by sex, do you mean intercourse?" What difference would it make if you started thinking about sex as including experiences other than intercourse?

ANGIE: It's hard to do that. Just being intimate—that is what I would like to do.

THERAPIST: And what attracts you to being intimate?

ANGIE: Relaxation. A sense of being able to enjoy everything. Just easing into it instead of just the act of sex.

SALLY: The first few years [of a relationship] you do a lot of intimate stuff—a lot of cuddling. I think in my case you start to learn that that leads ultimately to intercourse and so you do less and less and less of it until you get to the point that in my case I back off when he reaches out for a hug or a kiss.

THERAPIST: I know we haven't finished this conversation, but why don't we invite the folks who were listening to react to our conversation from the perspective of somebody whose life is not overtaken by the abuse.

SUSAN: For me it was easy to take the perspective of the person because it sounded like any conversation between women.

STACEE: That is what I was thinking. That conversation wasn't really just about women who are abused. They grew up to learn that that is their role—to be the "receptors," I guess I could say.

LAURA: It sounded like women's communication.

THERAPIST: Does that surprise the two of you to know that they heard the conversation as similar to a discussion between women friends?

[Stacee shares that she knows of a friend who is just as oppressed by the belief that it is a woman's duty to please her husband sexually with no consideration of her own feelings. Stacee states that she finds this idea "gross."]

THERAPIST: What is it about that perspective that you find "gross"?

STACEE: Because she is like a doormat . . .

THERAPIST: What was it like for the two of you [Laura and Stacee], listening to the conversation? What was it like from the perspective of what has happened to you—the sexual abuse—as being violence?

LAURA: It was really enlightening. I seem to feel more compassion for the child that was violated. By thinking violence, it is easier to feel sadness for that child.

[Stacee referred to the sympathy and outrage of people in response to five rapes reported on the news that week. She contrasted this reaction with the lack of empathy she believes most persons who have experienced incest receive. She stated that instead of thinking of incest as a "dirty secret," it needs to be viewed as violence.]

LAURA: I think it [this conversation] will help me separate what happened to me from intimacy. What happened to me was a violent crime. I just don't stop and think about it like that and I should and I shall.

The conversation between Angie, Sally, and the therapist introduced distinctions between violence and sex and intercourse and sex. Beliefs that maintained the experience of victimization, such as "being sexual is bad" and "sex is women's duty to men," were externalized.

The remaining group members assumed a reflecting position. By listening "as if" their lives were no longer influenced by abuse, members of the audience imagined themselves in a preferred future that provided an alternative understanding. Rather than viewing Angie's and Sally's concerns as resulting from some personal defect, they considered the larger social context. From this larger perspective, group members were invited to experience compassion for themselves.

CONCLUSION

This group approach has proven to be a cost-effective intervention for helping people overcome the effects of abuse.[5] Reports of outcome data indicate that this approach has made a positive difference for the women and men who have participated in the groups.[6]

In January 1993, 12 participants (11 women and 1 man) agreed to consult with us about their experiences in the group.[7] They told us that they found the group experience to be more helpful than individual therapy for a number of reasons. They experienced the group as extremely validating. The experience of getting to know and respect other people who were molested as children helped them challenge secrecy, overcome shame, and develop compassion for themselves. Several members discussed the effect of listening to others talk about their experiences. While listening, they discovered what they thought and felt, often for the first time. By comparing their experiences to others, they noticed their own progress and found hope for the future. The group experience provided them with the opportunity to practice new ways of relating to each other. One consultant explained her experience in this way:

> "Instead of saying, 'I am a victim,' I can set it out here (*holds out her hands at arm's length*) and instead say, 'I was victimized.' The discussions in group have helped me make that distinction: I no longer feel like a victim. In the past, I was victimized. I choose not to act like or think like a victim any more. Group gives me an opportunity to practice a different way of thinking for a long enough period of time that I can set aside thinking and acting like a victim."

[5]These services are provided at an average unit cost of $34 per person.

[6]Though we recognize the inherent contradiction in conducting an objectivist assessment of an approach derived from social constructionist ideas, we were intrigued by the results of pretest and posttest comparisons of measures of self-esteem, self-efficacy, and posttraumatic stress. Over the past four years, participants in the psychotherapy groups have demonstrated the largest increases in their sense of mastery. This is consistent with the focus on helping participants recognize their competence, develop self-knowledge, revise their relationship with themselves, and experiment with more preferred patterns of interaction.

[7]Videotapes of this consultation were presented at the Texas Association for Marriage and Family Therapy, San Antonio, Texas, January 1993.

Those of us who have worked with the men and women who have attended these groups have been privileged to be included in their journey from an identity dominated by abuse to a story about self described by possibilities.

REFERENCES

Adams-Westcott, J., Dafforn, T., & Sterne, P. (1993). Escaping victim life stories and co-constructing personal agency. In S. Gilligan & R. Price (Eds.), *Therapeutic conversations* (pp. 255–270). New York: Norton.

Adams–Westcott, J., & Isenbart, D. (1990). Using rituals to empower family members who have experienced child sexual abuse. In M. Durrant & C. White (Eds.), *Ideas for therapy with sexual abuse* (pp. 37–64). Adelaide, Australia: Dulwich Centre Publications.

Andersen, T. (Ed.). (1991). *The reflecting team: Dialogues and dialogues about the dialogues.* New York: Norton.

Anderson, H., & Goolishian, H. (1990, November). *Changing thoughts on self, agency, questions, narrative and therapy.* Paper presented at the Reflecting Process, Reflecting Teams Conference, Salzburg, Austria.

Dolan, Y. (1991). *Resolving sexual abuse: Solution-focused therapy and Ericksonian hypnosis for adult survivors.* New York: Norton.

Durrant, M., & Kowalski, K. (1990). Overcoming the effects of sexual abuse: Developing a self–perception of competence. In M. Durrant & C. White (Eds.), *Ideas for therapy with sexual abuse* (pp. 65–110). Adelaide, Australia: Dulwich Centre Publications.

Epston, D. (1993). Internalizing discourses versus externalizing discourses. In S. Gilligan & R. Price (Eds.), *Therapeutic conversations* (pp.161–177). New York: Norton.

Epston, D., & White, M. (1990). Consulting your consultants: The documentation of alternative knowledges. *Dulwich Centre Newsletter,* pp. 25–35.

Gergen, K. (1991). *The saturated self: Dilemmas of identity in contemporary life.* New York: Basic Books.

Gilligan, S. (1991, March). *Healing trauma survivors: An Ericksonian approach.* Paper presented at the Family Therapy Networker Conference, Washington, DC.

Hare-Mustin, R. (1991). Sex, lies and headaches: The problem is power. In T. Goodrich (Ed.), *Women and power: Perspectives for family therapy* (pp.63–85). New York: Norton.

Kamsler, A. (1990). Her–story in the making: Therapy with women who were sexually abused in childhood. In M. Durrant & C. White (Eds.), *Ideas for therapy with sexual abuse* (pp. 9–36). Adelaide, Australia: Dulwich Centre Publications.

Parry, A. (1991). A universe of stories. *Family Process, 30,* 37–54.

Roberts, J. (1988). Setting the frame: Definition, function, and typology of rituals. In E. Imber-Black, J. Roberts, & R. Whiting (Eds.), *Rituals in families and family therapy* (pp. 3–46). New York: Norton.

Sanders, G. (1988). An invitation to escape sexual tyranny. *Journal of Strategic and Systemic Therapies, 7*, 23–34.

Tomm, K. (1989a). Externalizing the problem and internalizing personal agency. *Journal of Strategic and Systemic Therapies, 8*, 54–59.

Tomm, K. (1989b, October). *Pips, tips, & slips: A heuristic alternative to the DSM–III*. Paper presented at the meeting of the American Association of Marriage and Family Therapy, San Francisco.

Weingarten, K. (1991). The discourse of intimacy: Adding a social constructionist and feminist view. *Family Process, 30*, 285–305.

White, M. (1986). Ritual of inclusion: An approach to extreme uncontrollable behavior of children and young adolescents. *Dulwich Centre Review*, pp. 20–27.

White, M., & Epston, D. (1990). *Narrative means to therapeutic ends*. New York: Norton.

✷

Closing Reflections

ON COMMUNITIES, CONNECTIONS, AND CONVERSATIONS

Steven Friedman

To become open to multiple layers of vision is to be both practical and empathic.

—*Mary Catherine Bateson*

IN THIS VOLUME the reader has been exposed to an emerging set of ideas and methods in the changing terrain of family therapy. Shifting away from theoretical certainties and objective truths, the approaches presented reflect a respect for differences, a tolerance for ambiguity, and an openness to multiple points of view. The techniques, structures, and absolutes of positivist thinking are replaced by a context of mutual discovery. The therapist and his/her team are coparticipants or partners in a meaning-generating process that is collaborative, respectful and hopeful. The therapy process becomes a more public one, with people recruited to construct, witness, and circulate new narratives. The therapeutic conversation serves as a medium for expanding the range of voices available to the client. The therapy process is like a tapestry or weaving in which therapist and client co-construct pattern out of their conversation, giving it coherence and meaning (Chenail, 1993).

The main threads of this therapeutic tapestry are outlined below.

1. Our dialogues with ourselves and with others come to define our views and determine our actions. We are "storied" animals. As we have seen, the stories we come to tell about ourselves become lenses that shape the ways we process new information. The reflecting process can be useful in expanding both the client's and therapist's lenses so that new

ways of "seeing" are possible and increased options made available. The therapist is included as part of the therapeutic system. Because meanings are inherently negotiable and ambiguous, the conversational process has the potential to "render [both the client and therapist's] world newly strange" (Bruner, 1986, p. 24).

2. As therapists we are not immune to dominant cultural discourses (Hare-Mustin, 1994; Law & Madigan, 1994) regarding gender, class, and race and we need to be vigilant so that we do not perpetuate oppressive ideologies in our practices. By making the practice of therapy more public, the therapist's values and prejudices are no longer hidden; and they are more open to scrutiny by the people we serve. In this way, the therapist becomes accountable. By making our ideas and actions "transparent," the client gains an understanding of the therapist's thinking. Rather than hiding behind formulaic interventions, the therapist is challenged to be authentic in presenting the thinking that underlies the idea. The reflecting process offers a forum for the client to question team members and requires the therapist/team to situate their thinking in their own life experiences. In so doing, the therapy process becomes a more human and normalizing event that establishes both client and therapist as equally susceptible to life's obstacles and predicaments.

3. The therapist leaves space in the interview for clients to tell their stories and to reflect on their inner and outer conversations.

> Conversation was never begun at once, nor in a hurried manner. No one was quick with a question, no matter how important, and no one was pressed for an answer. A pause giving time for thought was the truly courteous way of beginning and conducting a conversation. Silence was meaningful with the Lakota, and his granting a space of silence to the speech-maker and his own moment of silence before talking was done in the practice of true politeness and regard for the rule that, "thought comes before speech." (Luther Standing Bear, Oglala Sioux Chief, cited in *Native American Wisdom,* 1993)

4. The reflecting process allows the therapist (and his/her team) to spontaneously generate ideas that may or may not resonate with the client. In this way the client is free to use or "hear" what is valuable and relevant and discard what isn't. The therapist working in this manner must nurture his/her creativity, imagination, and spontaneity, playfully engaging the client around metaphor and meaning.

5. The professional is emerging from behind closed doors, to a position alongside the client. By so doing the pejorative jargon of pathology (and distance) is replaced with the language of the everyday.[1] Instead of the therapist gossiping with his/her colleagues, ideas, thoughts,

and speculations are shared in an open forum that requires team members to place their comments in a positive frame such that the client, rather than feeling judged or evaluated, feels listened to, respected, and understood.

6. The postmodern therapist co-constructs goals and negotiates direction in therapy, placing clients in the driver's seat as the expert on their own predicaments or dilemmas. It is the client's request that serves as the starting point for therapy and it is this request that must be respected and taken seriously. Instead of relying on invisible and illusory explanatory structures with their set of defined ideas about what represents "health" and "dysfunction," the therapist opens space for new ideas and preferred developments that stand outside "normative" realities. Therapy becomes more time-effective when the client's goals are given priority (Friedman & Fanger, 1991). When driven by the therapist's goals, therapy often goes on longer than is necessary. Ironically, by slowing the therapy process down (i.e., listening to the client's story and not prematurely imposing meaning or direction on the process), therapy actually becomes briefer. The goal is not one of imposition, of one idea over another, but of respect for the client's systems of meaning, introducing ideas into the dialogical field such that the client's lens or framework expands. Leaving space allows clients to generate their own solutions.

7. When lives are defined by fixed categories and those categories are ones of deficit and dysfunction, people come to view themselves in negative and pessimistic ways. The therapist, rather than becoming a detective for pathology and reifying rigid diagnostic distinctions, needs to search for and amplify client competencies, strengths, and resources. The postmodern therapist maintains a sense of optimism about change and an affiliative and affirmative stance (Hoffman, 1993). The therapist's curiosity is better focused on how people have been able to overcome adversity rather than on how they have succumbed to life's hardships.

8. The therapist and client invite others to join in the therapy process, to offer ideas and witness changes. This puts the client in touch with local knowledge via affiliations with others in the community. How do we build bridges of connection, networks of support, that afford opportunities for local knowledge (in contrast to expert knowledge) to be privileged? How do we open the doors to indigenous community knowledges?

---

[1]Johnella Bird (1994) suggests several ways to "protect" ourselves from engaging in "professional talk." Only a few of these will be mentioned here: "When talking at any time, imagine your client is also present. . . . Ask yourself, 'what would the client think if he/she heard what I thought?'. . . When writing notes from a . . . session, make these available to the client. . . . When writing letters to professionals either write these letters together with the client, or send the client's a copy of the letter" (p. 45). See also the ideas of Pilkington and Fraser (1992) on being accountable to clients.

> In a neighborhood in Brooklyn, New York, tensions had developed between Blacks and Jews leading to several violent incidents. Several members from each group began meeting to "achieve respect for one another." A proposal was made for young people from each community to join together to create a mural honoring two children who had died in the neighborhood. In addition, the women of each community came together to make a memorial quilt. This led to people inviting their neighbors to visit their homes building links that created a new sense of community, harmony and connection. (Teltsch, 1991)

> In traditional Hawaiian culture members of the extended family would come together for a "Ho'oponopono" to resolve problems and set things right. The focus of this ritual was on restitution and forgiveness. A transgression ["hala"] was visualized as a "cord," binding the offender to his or her deed and to the victim. The ritual of Kala encompasses the idea of loosening or releasing another person from some trespass or misbehavior. "As you loosen your brother from his trespass you loosen yourself, too. As you forgive, you are forgiven." (Pukui, Haertig, & Lee, 1972)

9. We need to be sensitive to the methods and processes we use in our professional endeavors. How can we avoid become a "colonial presence" (Hoffman, 1991; Kearney, Byrne, & McCarthy, 1989) in the lives of our clients? As Foucault (1965) emphasized, our explanations and objectified truths can place powerful constraints on our freedoms. Ideas can imprison.

In the late 19th and early 20th centuries a lieutenant in the United States Army, Richard Henry Pratt, initiated a project to "civilize the American Indian." He recruited Native American children into group homes where their hair was cut and styled to look like the hair of "other" Americans, their traditional clothes were taken away and their customs were viewed as primitive vestiges requiring resocialization. Pratt's goal was to make Native Americans into "intelligent, industrious citizens." The dominant societal discourse reflected a view of the Native American as a primitive savage who needed to be civilized "in the white man's image." During his time Lt. Pratt was perceived as an innovative and benevolent public servant. In fact, on his tombstone are the words "A friend and counselor to the Indians." Was Lt. Pratt a benevolent and loving friend of the Indian or a ruthless oppressor with the goal of destroying Native American culture? Depending on one's historical perspective, the events of that era can be viewed in very different ways (Lesiak, 1992).

How often do we as therapists think of ourselves as helping or liberating when we may be acting in the role of oppressor? Is labeling people using psychiatric terminology a benevolent act that opens options for change or does it oppress people by imposing "totalizing descriptions" on them? Is imposing a professionally driven treatment plan on a client a therapeutic act or a process of subjugation? Is keeping a set of client records containing negative and pejorative commentary a professional responsibility "in the best interests of the client" or a way of distancing the therapist from the client's humanity and struggle? Is the psychiatric hospitalization of a child an act of medical necessity or a way to disqualify the family as the child's most knowledgeable resource? Is labeling a set of behaviors as a psychiatric disorder (e.g., attention-deficit/hyperactivity disorder or posttraumatic stress disorder) a simple way to classify and categorize information to improve treatment planning or a process that reifies diagnoses in ways that increase their visibility, and by so doing, their prevalence?

Postmodern approaches offer a lens from which therapists can critically consider the impact of their actions as social agents. Therapists can begin to transform social structures by collaboratively negotiating with people in sharing power for codetermining the process and goals of therapy. The reflecting process is one medium that allows the therapist to relinquish power in providing a more level and balanced playing field. The reflecting process functions to break down barriers that professionalism has created about who can be helpful. By advocating for involvement of consumers in institutional policy development, and by supporting policies that are people-oriented rather than technology-driven, we can have a positive impact on social institutions.

In summary, several significant threads connect to form a pattern in the postmodern tapestry: (1) a commitment to *privilege the individual's knowledge of self* over expert knowledge; to listen to and honor people's stories without imposing our own normative views on the process; (2) a sensitivity to the *power of the sociopolitical and cultural context* and the ways dominant discourses serve to oppress people; (3) a belief in the *community as an indigenous resource,* providing archives of preferred knowledges that open the door to alternative narratives; (4) *therapist transparency*—a willingness to situate our thoughts and ideas in a personal frame, to spontaneously present our comments rather than hide behind rehearsed formulas; and (5) a *rebalancing or recalibrating of the power dynamics inherent in the therapy* situation by providing the space for clients to both ask questions about the process and determine the goals and direction of the therapy.

Are we in danger, as some authors point out (e.g., Amundson, Stewart, & Parry, 1994) of falling prey ourselves to the modernist agenda believing the "narrative frame" to be the "final story," the "one truth"? These authors suggest that the way to avoid this possibility is by continually reinventing ourselves, by seeing our work as an evolving story that will change continuously over time. The ideas and practices represented in this book reflect this evolutionary process. The contributors are all endeavoring to articulate their own voices in the unique contexts in which they work. I feel honored to have been a part of this project and am grateful to the authors for providing, in such transparent form, a momentary glimpse into their current thinking and practice.

ACKNOWLEDGMENTS

Special thanks for Donna Haig Friedman, PhD for her constructive suggestions on this chapter.

REFERENCES

Amundson, J. K., Stewart, K., & Parry, A. (1994). Whither narrative? The danger of getting it right. *Journal of Marital and Family Therapy, 20,* 83–89.

Bird, J. (1994). Talking amongst ourselves. *Dulwich Centre Newsletter,* pp. 44–46.

Bruner, J. (1986). *Actual minds, possible worlds.* Cambridge, MA: Harvard University Press.

Chenail, R. (1993). Making maps. In A. H. Rambo, A. Heath, & R. J. Chenail (Eds.), *Practicing therapy: Exercises for growing therapists.* New York: Norton.

Foucault, M. (1965). *Madness and civilization.* New York: Random House.

Friedman, S., & Fanger, M. T. (1991). *Expanding therapeutic possibilities: Getting results in brief psychotherapy.* New York: Lexington Books/Macmillan.

Hare-Mustin, R. (1994). Discourses in the mirrored room: A postmodern analysis of therapy. *Family Process, 33,* 19–35.

Hoffman, L. (1991). A reflexive stance for family therapy. *Journal of Strategic and Systemic Therapies, 10,* 4–17.

Hoffman, L. (1993). *Exchanging voices: A collaborative approach to family therapy.* London: Karnac Books.

Kearney, P. A., Byrne, N. O'R., & McCarthy, I. C. (1989). Just metaphors: Marginal illuminations in a colonial retreat. *Family Therapy Case Studies, 4,*. 17–31.

Law, I., & Madigan, S. (1994). Introduction to power and politics in practice. *Dulwich Centre Newsletter, pp. 3–6.*

Lesiak, C. (Producer). (1992, February 13). *In the white man's image.* Lincoln, NE: Nebraska Educational Television Network.

Native American Wisdom. (1993). Philadelphia: Running Press.

Pilkington, S., & Fraser, N. (1992). Exposing secret biographies. *Dulwich Centre Newsletter, pp. 12–17.*

Pukui, M. K., Haertig, E. W., & Lee, C. A. (1972). *Nana I ke kumu [Look to the source].* Honolulu, HA: Hui Hanai.

Teltsch, K. (1991, September 1). Youth groups edge closer in Brooklyn. *The New York Times,* p. 35.

*

Index